T0155530

Certified Ophthalmic Assistant

Assistant

Exam Review Manual

Third Edition

Certified Ophthalmic Assistant
Assistant
Exam Review Manual
Third Edition

Janice K. Ledford, COMT

EyeWrite Productions

Franklin, North Carolina

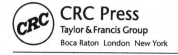
CRC Press
Taylor & Francis Group
Boca Raton London New York

CRC Press is an imprint of the
Taylor & Francis Group, an **informa** business

Janice K. Ledford, COMT has no financial or proprietary interest in the materials presented herein.

First published 2012 by SLACK Incorporated

Published 2024 by CRC Press
2385 NW Executive Center Drive, Suite 320, Boca Raton FL 33431

and by CRC Press
4 Park Square, Milton Park, Abingdon, Oxon, OX14 4RN

CRC Press is an imprint of Taylor & Francis Group, LLC

Ledford, Janice K..
  Certified ophthalmic assistant exam review manual / Janice K. Ledford. -- 3rd ed.
    p. ; cm.
Includes bibliographical references.
  ISBN 978-1-61711-058-0 (alk. paper)
I. Title.
  [DNLM: 1. Diagnostic Techniques, Ophthalmological--Examination Questions. 2. Ophthalmic Assistants--Examination Questions. 3. Vision, Ocular--Examination Questions. WW 18.2]

  617.7'0232076--dc23

                        2012006995

ISBN: 9781617110580 (hbk)
ISBN: 9781003522942 (ebk)

DOI: 10.1201/9781003522942

Dedication, First Edition

This book is dedicated to TJ and Collin.
With two such fine, inquisitive sons, I should be used to answering questions by now!

Dedication, Second Edition

For Kelly and Katie—my girls.

Dedication, Third Edition

For you, Mom. I like you best.

Contents

Acknowledgments

It seems like the more I write, the more help I need! I have been blessed with many wonderful folks willing to assist, and here is where I get the pleasure of thanking them.

I tried something new with this book and got a personal coach. Not a writing coach (although she is an author herself and very capable of doing that), but a motivational coach. Pam Keyser met with me and helped monitor my progress through the first difficult 6 months or so of this project. Pam, I can't begin to thank you enough.

At Pam's suggestion, early on, I recruited a set of Voices of Wisdom (VOWs). First and foremost of these has been Susan Larson of the Joint Commission on Allied Health Personnel in Ophthalmology (JCAHPO®). Without her help, this book would not have been possible. In the ophthalmic field, my VOWs were Al Lens, COMT; Barbara Harris, COMT; Lindy DuBois, COMT; and Bob Campbell, MD. Each is a busy professional in the field who faithfully answered my questions and gave me input…for months!

I want to thank Jennifer Briggs who worked with me from start to almost finish. I'll miss you, Jennifer, and thank you for your patience! April Billick has also assisted, particularly with photographs. And to my publisher, John Bond, thanks again for the opportunities you continually afford me. I couldn't ask for better.

Thanks are also due to Todd Hostetter, COMT; John D. Gross, MD; Ken Woodworth, COMT; Faith Race, COT; Donna Leef, COMT; Sheila Nemeth, COMT; Aaron Shukla, COMT; Ken Daniels, OD; Brian Duvall, OD; Sandra Gay, COT; Robert Kalapp, Director of Professional Relations at Marco; and Susan Manier, Marketing Coordinator at Marco.

Finally, there are two individuals who have stuck by me, encouraged me, and generally put up with me during the long months of this project: Cheryl Pelham and Cheera Roadarmel (Mom). You are both so dear, and I love you to pieces.

About the Author

1. **The author's preferred appellation is:**
    a) Janice
    b) Jan
    c) Your Majesty
    d) Hey You

2. **The author studied on her own for which of the following certification exams?**
    a) Assistant
    b) Technician
    c) Medical Technologist
    d) all of the above

3. **The author has been in the field of ophthalmology for _____ years.**
    a) 10
    b) 20
    c) 25
    d) more than she cares to count

4. **The author lives where and with whom/what?**
    a) Western North Carolina mountains with two cats
    b) Middle Georgia with three guinea pigs
    c) Western North Carolina mountains with her mom and a Labrador retriever
    d) North Georgia mountains with Sean Connery

Explanatory Answers

1. b) While c may sound correct (and may actually be correct on certain days), the best answer is b.
2. d) Because Jan took all three of the exams via self-study (versus a formal program), she has a special place in her heart for others doing the same.
3. d) Jan started in the field in 1982, but says she's still going strong and hopes to continue for another 17.5 years.
4. a) Jan lives in Franklin, North Carolina, with her two kitties, Angel and Nadia…but would trade them both for Sean Connery. (Not really!) Mom lives right across the road. Her older son is in the Air Force National Guard in North Carolina, and her younger son is a computer program tester in Franklin. Her grandkids live in Middle Georgia.

Introduction

Writing this third edition of the *Certified Ophthalmic Assistant Exam Review Manual* has been one of the most challenging jobs of my career.

The exam criteria have changed, in some areas rather drastically. This is necessary, of course, in order to reflect new technology (exciting advances in imaging come to mind immediately). Research offers much as well, and the certifying exams must call upon candidates to stay current.

The new criteria are definitely more task-based than ever before. The Joint Commission on Allied Health Personnel in Ophthalmology (JCAHPO®) Task Analysis Survey asked ophthalmologists to rank approximately 80 tasks performed by technicians, in order of their importance to the practice. Ranking number 1 in the survey was history taking, and its inclusion in the exam criteria is appropriate and undisputed.

Problems arose, however, as I faced writing questions and answers in other areas. With the criteria now being task-based, what does one study? Regarding tonometry, for example, the criteria look much like a checklist for performing the skill without mentioning the academic knowledge one needs for understanding aqueous dynamics (which used to be listed, itself). Is the knowledge implied? If so, how will someone new to the profession know that this will be "on the test" if it is not listed in the criteria? One might learn how to perform applanation tonometry without understanding the basics of intraocular pressure (although I should hope not). Along the same lines, the Schiøtz tonometer is no longer listed. Yet, when I questioned this, I was told that the candidate would be expected to know about it. In yet other circumstances, I was unwilling to omit material just because it does not appear on the criteria list. These are identified by footnotes throughout the book.

I appreciate the fact that my queries have often put my JCAHPO® Voice of Wisdom (VOW) in a very awkward position. Please know that over all my years of writing the exam review books, no one at JCAHPO® has ever told me "what will be on the test." They have, however, helped define what is meant by specific criteria items. (For example, what's the difference between cleaning the applanation tonometer and disinfecting it that makes it necessary to list both?) I have dealt with these details using footnotes in the text itself, as well.

One change that I hope you will find helpful is that the explanatory answers are at the end of each chapter, instead of grouped together in a chapter at the end of the book. This should make it easier for you to find the information and should be the instant reinforcement you need as you study.

In the end, I must say that I have done my best and that I had a lot of help (see the Acknowledgments)! Always feel free to contact me through the SLACK Incorporated Books division by sending an email to bookspublishing@slackinc.com. It is especially helpful to know if anything has been left out that would have been helpful to you as you studied or if any material is extraneous. It has been my distinct pleasure over the years to help aspiring ophthalmic medical personnel attain certification and offer the best patient care possible.

Chapter 1

History Taking

Ledford JK.
*Certified Ophthalmic Assistant: Exam
Review Manual, Third Edition* (pp. 1-14).
© 2012 Taylor & Francis Group.

General[1]

1.   **A history is obtained by:**
      a) asking a series of organized and specific questions
      b) observing the patient's actions in the exam room
      c) allowing the patient to discuss anything he or she wishes
      d) asking the same questions of each patient during every exam

2.   **The history should be recorded:**
      a) by writing down the patient's entire story, word-for-word
      b) by condensing the patient's story, including pertinent facts
      c) by interpreting the patient's story and suggesting a diagnosis
      d) by copying patient information from a questionnaire

3.   **When taking a history on a school-aged child, it is important to:**
      a) listen only to the parent's account of the illness
      b) listen only to the child's account of the illness
      c) talk to the parent outside of the child's hearing
      d) get an account of the illness from both the parent and child

4.   **Which of the following statements is *false*?**
      a) A thorough history can direct a physician toward a final diagnosis.
      b) All information given by the patient can be shared with insurance companies without patient permission.
      c) Statements made by the patient should lead the assistant into additional questions that can be asked.
      d) All patient information is private unless a consent release form is signed.

5.   **Which of the following is *not* a part of a history?**
      a) presenting complaint
      b) medications currently used
      c) family eye disease
      d) visual acuity

Presenting Complaint[2]

6.   **The "presenting complaint" is:**
      a) the main reason that the patient has come to the office
      b) always the most serious of the patient's many complaints
      c) the only item with which the history is really concerned
      d) the main reason the patient should be dilated

---

[1]While the JCAHPO® criteria do not specifically list the parts of a history, I have included them here.

[2]The current JCAHPO® criteria list only "Ocular History"; I have chosen to separate them into *Presenting Complaint* (which is generally ocular) and *Past Ocular History* (referring to ocular history both related and unrelated to the presenting complaint).

7. **An example of a question relating to onset would be:**
    a) "Can you still function at work?"
    b) "When did you first notice the problem?"
    c) "What treatment have you tried?"
    d) "Has the problem worsened?"

8. **The question "Does your head hurt so badly that you have to leave school early?" relates to:**
    a) onset
    b) duration
    c) progression
    d) severity

9. **To obtain the most important information about the presenting complaint, you should ask questions relating to:**
    a) location, timing, aggravating and alleviating factors, and family history
    b) location, quality, severity, timing, and aggravating and alleviating factors
    c) location, severity, timing, drug allergies, and past surgical procedures
    d) present illness, past ocular history, family history, and description of pain

10. **A symptom is:**
    a) something you notice when you look at the patient
    b) something that can always be tested and proven
    c) a change noticed by the patient
    d) any change that results from injury

11. **An example of a sign is:**
    a) the patient tells you what part of the eye hurts
    b) an elevated intraocular pressure reading
    c) the patient complains of blurred vision
    d) the patient complains of a pressure sensation behind the eyes

12. **A 56-year-old patient complains of a sudden onset of double vision. It is most important to ask:**
    a) "Does the doubling go away if you cover one eye?"
    b) "Are the eyes also red?"
    c) "Do the eyes ache?"
    d) "Does anyone in your family have a lazy eye?"

13. **An old photograph of the patient will be most useful to the physician if the patient complains of or exhibits:**
    a) eye protrusion, double vision, or floaters
    b) lid droop, pupil abnormality, or head tilt
    c) redness, pain, halos around lights at night, and decreased vision
    d) headache, rash, or lid droop

14.   **Your patient has a cut eyelid. It is important to know what caused the injury because:**
a) this will determine how the doctor will repair the lid
b) if the object was organic (plant or animal matter), there is a greater risk of infection
c) if the object was metal, there is a greater risk of infection
d) the injury needs to be reported to the National Ocular Injury Registry (NOIR)

15.   **A patient presents with a corneal foreign body, and your supervisor asks how the foreign body got into the eye. This is an important question because:**
a) if the patient was not wearing safety glasses, Workers' Compensation will not pay
b) if the particle was under high speed, there might be internal ocular damage
c) this determines whether or not you should check the patient's vision
d) this determines whether or not you should irrigate the eye

16.   **The patient is not wearing contacts, but would like to be fit for them. The most relevant question is:**
a) "Have you tried contact lenses before?"
b) "Are you interested in disposable lenses?"
c) "Do you have trouble seeing to read?"
d) "Are you allergic to thimerosal?"

Past Ocular History[2]

17.   **A 52-year-old patient hands you his single-vision glasses, the only glasses he has. Which of the following is the most important question in determining the patient's refractive status?**
a) "How long have you had these?"
b) "Do these help you see better?"
c) "Do you wear these for driving or for reading?"
d) "Do the frames hurt your ears?"

18.   **A patient reports that he sleeps in his contact lenses. An important question would be:**
a) "What type of lenses are they?"
b) "Do you have astigmatism?"
c) "Why haven't you had LASIK?"
d) "Are you legally blind without the contacts?"

19.   **The patient gives a history of having a cataract removed with a laser. You should:**
a) record the cataract surgery without mentioning the laser, because the patient does not know what he or she is talking about
b) use this as a "teachable moment" and inform the patient that cataracts cannot be removed with a laser
c) ask the patient if the surgery was done in a hospital while lying down or sitting up in a chair (to an instrument like a slit lamp)
d) not record this, because the patient is obviously confused

20.   The patient gives a history of having a laser treatment, but is not sure what it was for. You might discover more by asking:
      a) "Have you had cataract surgery?"
      b) "Do you have diabetes?"
      c) "Do you have glaucoma?"
      d) all of the above

21.   The patient states she used to wear contact lenses, but went back to her glasses. A pertinent question would be:
      a) "Do you have astigmatism?"
      b) "Do you think the lenses were improperly fit?"
      c) "Why did you stop wearing them?"
      d) "Do you have dry eyes?"

22.   A 76-year-old new patient tells you that he caught astigmatism from his brother when they were both children. You should:
      a) tell him he is wrong because astigmatism is not a disease
      b) agree with him because astigmatism can run in families
      c) ask him what he means by "astigmatism"
      d) explain that astigmatism is a refractive error

23.   Knowledge of a past ocular injury is needed because:
      a) it might help explain current complaints and findings
      b) it might indicate a reason why the patient's vision should not be checked
      c) it might indicate the reason for an allergy to eye drops
      d) a careless, accident-prone patient is likely to be noncompliant

24.   The patient states she has prism in her glasses. Which of the following is the *most* important question to ask?
      a) "Have you ever had surgery to straighten your eyes?"
      b) "Does anyone in your family have a lazy eye?"
      c) "Have you recently tried glasses without prism?"
      d) "Were you dilated during your last eye exam?"

25.   A mother brings in her 4-year-old son. The mother says he has a lazy eye. What do you need to find out?
      a) Was the birth premature?
      b) Who else in the family has a lazy eye?
      c) Does the child rub one eye frequently?
      d) What does she mean by "lazy eye?"

Medical

26.   An example of a systemic illness is:
      a) Down syndrome
      b) senility
      c) past surgical procedures
      d) cardiac problems

27. **Questions asked of a hypertensive patient should include:**
    a) method of blood pressure control, sensation of pressure in the eyes, last blood pressure reading
    b) weight loss, last blood gases reading, visual stability
    c) method of blood pressure control, decrease in vision, last blood pressure reading
    d) method of blood pressure control, onset of double vision, last blood sugar reading

28. **Questions asked of a diabetic patient should include:**
    a) loss of depth perception, visual stability, type of insulin used
    b) method of sugar control, visual stability, last blood sugar reading
    c) weight loss, last blood gases reading, type of insulin used
    d) injection sites used, increased floaters, frequent urination

29. **A patient with heart problems:**
    a) may need to eat something during an eye exam
    b) cannot be dilated
    c) may have hardening of the arteries in the eye
    d) always has high cholesterol

30. **Knowledge of a patient's breathing or lung problems would be important if the patient also has:**
    a) dry eye
    b) glaucoma
    c) macular degeneration
    d) oxygen deficiency color blindness

31. **Your patient states that he has rheumatoid arthritis. You should now ask symptom-related questions to find out if he has:**
    a) dry eye
    b) angle-closure glaucoma
    c) decreased central vision
    d) a visual field loss

32. **Sickle cell disease:**
    a) is hereditary and occurs primarily in the black population
    b) is hereditary and occurs primarily in the white population
    c) is hereditary and occurs equally in all populations
    d) is hereditary and occurs primarily in the Latino population

33. **Sickle cell disease may affect the eye:**
    a) by causing a paralysis of the extraocular muscles
    b) by causing posterior subcapsular cataracts
    c) because the abnormally shaped cells can block the optic nerve
    d) because the abnormally shaped cells can block the eye's blood vessels

34. **Knowing a patient's past history of surgical procedures is important because:**
    a) it may reveal precautions needed before eye surgery is undertaken
    b) it reveals whether or not the patient is likely to be compliant
    c) it may reveal whether or not the patient is a hypochondriac
    d) it reveals whether or not the patient may be reluctant to have future surgery

35. **Major infections that can affect the eye include:**
     a) Human immunodeficiency virus (HIV), gonorrhea, tuberculosis, and herpes simplex
     b) gonorrhea, tuberculosis, Down syndrome, and leukemia
     c) sickle cell disease, HIV, tuberculosis, and toxemia
     d) herpes simplex, herpes zoster, anemia, and gonorrhea

36. **Your patient is a 4-month-old who was born prematurely. Which question will be** *most* **important in predicting the occurrence of eye disorders related to prematurity?**
     a) How much did the baby weigh?
     b) Was the mother exposed to measles during pregnancy?
     c) Did the baby receive oxygen after birth?
     d) Has the baby steadily gained weight since birth?

Medication[3]

37. **In which of the following ocular disorders would it be** *most* **important to know what eye drops a new patient is using?**
     a) cataract
     b) glaucoma
     c) macular degeneration
     d) retinitis pigmentosa

38. **Which situation poses a potential problem in a patient taking aspirin-containing medications?**
     a) the patient with a cataract who will be having surgery
     b) the patient with migraine headaches
     c) the patient with headaches from convergence insufficiency
     d) the patient with diplopia

39. **While taking the ocular history of a new patient, she mentions that her last ophthalmologist told her she has macular degeneration. This should trigger you to specifically ask about which of the following?**
     a) aspirin use
     b) steroid use
     c) vitamin use
     d) artificial tear use

40. **Patients taking a diuretic might have which special need during the exam?**
     a) frequent trips to the restroom
     b) an increase in the amount of oxygen they are receiving
     c) frequent stops to use an inhaler for breathing
     d) an early appointment because they tire easily

---

[3]See also Chapter 9, section *Drug Reactions*.

41. **A patient taking a diuretic probably has which health problem?**
    a) asthma
    b) heart trouble
    c) emphysema
    d) diabetes

42. **High blood pressure is frequently treated by:**
    a) nonsteroidal anti-inflammatory drugs (NSAIDs)
    b) oral steroids
    c) beta-blockers
    d) analgesics

43. **If a patient with glaucoma is to be treated using beta-blockers, it would be *most* important to know if the patient is currently being treated for:**
    a) diabetes
    b) gout
    c) sinus
    d) high blood pressure

44. **It is important to know if a patient is taking birth control pills because:**
    a) an overdose can cause blindness
    b) these hormones can cause loss of depth perception
    c) these hormones can cause changes in the retina
    d) forgetting to take them can cause loss of depth perception

45. **A patient who has been taking oral steroids for long periods should be evaluated for possible development of:**
    a) dry eye
    b) cataracts
    c) iris cysts
    d) macular degeneration

46. **Conditions for which a person might take oral steroids include:**
    a) rheumatoid arthritis
    b) diabetes
    c) hypertension
    d) hypoglycemia

47. **Patients often fail to report the use of over-the-counter medications because:**
    a) they consider them to be unimportant and unrelated to eye care
    b) over-the-counter medications have no ocular side effects
    c) only prescription medications are important because they are stronger
    d) patients do not want to admit they use them

48. **The patient has said he has no heart problems, but you notice that he is taking two heart medications. For the most complete history, you should:**
    a) simply record the medications
    b) not record the medications because the patient must be mistaken
    c) ask the patient what he takes the medication for
    d) confront the patient with his misinformation

49. **Diabetes medication includes:**
    a) diuretics and beta-blockers
    b) insulin injections and "sugar pills"
    c) steroids and analgesics
    d) antibiotics and NSAIDs

50. **An example of an analgesic is:**
    a) insulin
    b) aspirin
    c) sulfa
    d) nitroglycerin

51. **Which patient is most likely to be using hormone replacement therapy?**
    a) a woman who has not yet reached menopause
    b) a woman who has had a hysterectomy/oophorectomy
    c) a pregnant woman
    d) a woman who has had a mastectomy

52. **A male patient is going to be scheduled for cataract surgery. Which of the following medications is of *most* concern?**
    a) sildenafil citrate
    b) hydroxychloroquine
    c) amiodarone
    d) testosterone patch

53. **Your patient says she is allergic to something common, but cannot remember the name. You suggest:**
    a) penicillin, sulfa, or codeine
    b) niacin, sulfa, or codeine
    c) penicillin, sulfa, or caffeine
    d) penicillin, sulfur, or codeine

54. **Your patient says that beta-blockers make him nauseated. This is:**
    a) an allergy
    b) a side effect
    c) an unrelated occurrence
    d) unimportant

55. **Your patient says that erythromycin makes her break out in a rash. This is:**
    a) an allergy
    b) a side effect
    c) an unrelated occurrence
    d) unimportant

56. **Your patient is scheduled to have a chalazion excision. It is most important to know his previous reactions to:**
    a) general anesthesia
    b) local anesthesia
    c) neomycin
    d) fluorescein

57. **Your patient is unsure if she has ever had any local anesthesia. You could ask if she:**
    a) has ever had a numbing injection for a dental procedure
    b) has ever been put to sleep for any surgery
    c) has ever had an applanation tension test
    d) has ever had drops to numb the eye

58. **Your patient reports an adverse reaction to dye injected for a kidney evaluation. This could affect:**
    a) performing applanation tonometry
    b) performing a fluorescein angiogram
    c) testing tear function
    d) dilating the pupils

Social

59. **Knowing a patient's occupation may be important in:**
    a) prescribing bifocals or trifocals
    b) deciding what type of medication to prescribe
    c) knowing the patient's risk of eye injury
    d) all of the above

60. **A patient's social history would include all of the following *except*:**
    a) tobacco use
    b) living arrangements
    c) hobbies
    d) therapeutic drug use

61. **Your patient has been referred to your practice for cataract surgery. You ask if there is anyone at home who can help the patient instill eye drops. This is part of the patient's:**
    a) family history
    b) ocular history
    c) social history
    d) medical history

Family

62. **The *most common* ocular disorders that run in families are:**
    a) cataracts, macular degeneration, and color blindness
    b) strabismus, myopia, and glaucoma
    c) glaucoma, color blindness, and albinism
    d) retinitis pigmentosa, strabismus, and albinism

63.   **A 25-year-old white woman comes in as a new patient because her mother has just been diagnosed with glaucoma. This information:**
a) is unimportant because the patient is under the age of 45
b) is unimportant because glaucoma is less prevalent among whites
c) is a good reason for a full eye exam
d) is insignificant because glaucoma is passed through the father, not the mother

64.   **A mother brings in a 2-year-old child with esotropia. Which of the following is significant for the history?**
a) Does anyone in the family have crossed eyes?
b) Is anyone in the family blind?
c) Does anyone in the family have Down syndrome?
d) Has anyone in the family been born prematurely?

65.   **Examples of hereditary systemic disease include:**
a) shingles, diabetes, hypertension, and gout
b) diabetes, hypertension, arthritis, and cancer
c) cancer, diabetes, arthritis, and meningitis
d) hypertension, acquired immune deficiency syndrome (AIDS), and shingles

66.   **Which of the following is *not* potentially a hereditary disorder?**
a) keratoconus
b) secondary glaucoma
c) migraine headaches
d) nystagmus

Explanatory Answers

1.   a) The questions should be organized and specific, directing the patient's narrative and tailored to the problems at hand.
2.   b) The assistant should avoid writing down the patient's every word or trying to interpret. Diagnosis is the physician's realm. Questionnaires have their place, but cannot be used for an entire history because each patient is different.
3.   d) A normal school-aged child is usually able to give a fairly good history, with the parent affirming the information.
4.   b) The patient must sign a consent to release information, even to insurance companies.
5.   d) Visual acuity is part of the examination, not the history.
6.   a) The presenting complaint is the patient's main reason for coming in. An accurate history might include other complaints as well, however.
7.   b) Onset relates to when the patient first noticed the problem.
8.   d) The severity of a problem relates to the amount of disability a patient suffers.
9.   b) Location, quality, severity, timing, and aggravating and alleviating factors are all pertinent questions regarding the presenting complaint. Family history, drug allergies, past surgical procedures, and past ocular history are all important parts of the history, but not the most important regarding the presenting complaint.
10.   c) A symptom is a change that the patient notices, whether from injury, illness, or other situation. It cannot always be proven (eg, pain) or seen by looking (eg, pressure sensations).

11.   b) A sign is something that you can observe in the patient, such as an intraocular pressure reading. The other answers are symptoms.

12.   a) Double vision in an adult is potentially serious. If vision is single with one eye covered, this indicates a muscle balance problem, which could indicate a possible brain tumor or nerve disorder. If vision is double in one eye only, the eye itself has a problem. The other answers are irrelevant to the situation.

13.   b) If any of the conditions listed in this answer are present in the photograph, this indicates that the problem is longstanding.

14.   b) Any laceration that was caused by or infused with organic matter has a much greater likelihood of becoming infected. The physician might choose to give an oral antibiotic. (There is no such thing as the NOIR!)

15.   b) A foreign body at high speed might cause serious internal damage. The patient's vision is checked regardless of how the injury occurred. While it is true that you should not irrigate an eye if you suspect the globe has been penetrated (nor is irrigation usually used for a corneal foreign body), b is still the best answer.

16.   a) It is most important to know a patient's past experience with contacts. Answers b and c are not wrong, but they are not the best. Thimerosal is a preservative that was formerly used in contact lens solutions, but was largely discontinued when many people developed a sensitivity to it.

17.   c) While all the questions are good ones, you can determine the patient's refractive status only if you know how he uses the glasses. At his age, he has been presbyopic for a number of years. If the glasses are for driving, he is myopic. If the glasses are for reading, he is probably emmetropic with presbyopia.

18.   a) You need to know about the lens material. It may be okay to sleep in a disposable extended-wear lens, for example, but some contacts should never be left in during sleep, and the patient is doing something potentially harmful.

19.   c) When a patient says something that does not make ophthalmic sense, ask more questions before writing it in the history. She may be referring to having a laser capsulotomy for a so-called "secondary cataract."

20.   d) Laser treatment might be used after cataract surgery (laser capsulotomy), in the case of diabetes (photocoagulation), or glaucoma (trabeculectomy or iridotomy).

21.   c) Answers a and d are not bad questions, but they are not the best. Answer b could imply a judgment on the patient's past care, which is not ethical as it calls into question the competency of another practitioner.

22.   c) The patient obviously has a misconception about the origin of astigmatism, or he may have misapplied the term to some type of infection. Ask him.

23.   a) A patient's current problems may stem from past injury (such as recurrent erosion syndrome).

24.   a) Prism is usually prescribed to overcome motility disorders; hence, asking about surgery to straighten the eyes is in order.

25.   d) What does the mother mean by "lazy eye"? She may mean an eye that "looks weak" or crosses. Or, she might mean amblyopia. Answers b and c are good, but are not key. Answer a is mostly irrelevant in this case.

26.   d) "Cardiac problems" is the only systemic illness listed. Down syndrome may have systemic effects, but it is a genetic condition, not an illness.

27. c) You need to know how a hypertensive patient controls the blood pressure (medications can affect the eyes), any decrease in vision (possible symptoms of hypertensive retinopathy), and the last blood pressure reading (to compare with the one obtained today).

28. b) A diabetic patient should tell you how he or she is controlling his or her blood sugar (diet, pills, or injections), whether or not vision seems stable (fluctuations indicate uncontrolled blood sugar and may affect the refractometric measurement), and his or her last blood sugar level (preferably the A1C, a single test that evaluates levels over a 90 day period).

29. c) Ocular disorders associated with heart problems include hardening of the arteries and/or blood vessel blockage. Patients can be safely dilated in most cases. Answer d is wrong because of the word "always."

30. b) Certain glaucoma medications are contraindicated in patients with lung disease.

31. a) Dry eye is strongly associated with rheumatoid arthritis.

32. a) Sickle cell disease occurs mainly in the black population and is hereditary.

33. d) The abnormally shaped cells in sickle cell disease can block blood vessels in any part of the body, including the eye.

34. a) A patient's reaction to prior surgery (eg, excessive bleeding or panic) can be a good indicator of how he or she will tolerate future procedures.

35. a) Each item in answer a is an infection. Down syndrome, leukemia, sickle cell disease, toxemia, and anemia are not infections; they are conditions or disorders.

36. c) Oxygen therapy after a premature birth has been linked to retinopathy of prematurity. Answers a and d are good, but not related to the question.

37. b) A new patient who states he or she has glaucoma should be asked what eye drops he or she is using to control the pressure. Conditions in answers a, c, and d do not require medication.

38. a) Aspirin and aspirin-containing medications thin the blood. Thus, the patient taking them runs a greater risk of hemorrhage during or after surgery.

39. c) Patients with diagnosed macular degeneration have probably been put on a vitamin regimen of some kind.

40. a) Diuretics act to reduce the body's fluids. Thus, the patient may need a break to go to the restroom during the exam.

41. b) Heart patients are placed on diuretics to reduce excess fluid in the body, thereby reducing heart strain. Asthma and emphysema are breathing problems. Diabetes is related to blood sugar.

42. c) Beta-blockers are frequently used to treat hypertension. NSAIDs and steroids are used to treat inflammation. Analgesics are for pain.

43. d) If the patient is already taking a beta-blocker for hypertension, the physician may not want to prescribe an additional beta-blocker for the glaucoma.

44. c) Birth control pills can cause changes in the retina, including retinal artery and vein occlusion.

45. b) Cataract formation has been associated with the long-term use of oral steroids.

46. a) Steroids are anti-inflammatory drugs and, thus, are used in the treatment of rheumatoid arthritis.

47. a) Patients tend to think that over-the-counter medications are not important (or they would be regulated), nor have an effect on the eye.

48.   c) When in doubt, ask. In some cases, a drug is prescribed for a condition other than its "usual" use. Recording the medicine without delving a little further, or not recording it at all, would be irresponsible. Confronting the patient is unnecessary.

49.   b) Diabetes is treated with oral medication ("sugar pills") and injectable insulin. (Of course, a diabetic does not take pills made out of sugar, but many patients call oral diabetic medicine a "sugar pill.") Do not feel bad if you missed this one!

50.   b) An analgesic is a pain reliever, such as aspirin.

51.   b) A woman who has had her ovaries removed is most likely on a hormone replacement therapy. Hormones are generally contraindicated in women who are pregnant or who have had a mastectomy for breast cancer. A woman who has not reached menopause presumably still has functioning ovaries.

52.   a) Medications for erectile dysfunction, such as Viagra (sildenafil citrate), have been implicated in intraoperative floppy iris syndrome, a complication of cataract surgery. Plaquenil (hydroxychloroquine) is an antimalarial drug sometimes used in the treatment of arthritis. Its side effects can include disturbance of the macula. Amiodarone is used for irregular heartbeat and can have ocular side effects (eg, corneal deposits). The testosterone patch is a male hormone replacement therapy.

53.   a) The most common drug allergies are to penicillin, sulfa, and codeine. An allergy to niacin or caffeine is possible, but not common. Sulfur is a mineral.

54.   b) Nausea is a side effect and should be recorded in the patient's chart. (Examples of an *allergy* are rash, itching, and shortness of breath.)

55.   a) Rash (urticaria) is a common allergic response.

56.   b) A chalazion excision is done under local anesthesia. An exception might be general anesthesia for a small child, but the question does not give you this kind of detail.

57.   a) A numbing injection prior to dental work is local anesthesia. Answer b refers to general anesthesia. Answers c and d refer to topical anesthesia.

58.   b) Dye is injected into a vein during a fluorescein angiogram. Fluorescein involved in procedures a and c would be topical.

59.   d) A patient's occupation may affect the prescription of a bifocal or trifocal (because of work distance), medications (eg, those causing blurred vision or drowsiness), and the types of ocular risks to which the patient is exposed (eg, the need for safety glasses).

60.   d) "Therapeutic" implies that the medication/drug is used as a treatment for an illness or condition. Use of "recreational" drugs *would* be part of the patient's social history.

61.   c) A patient's living situation is one component of the social history. (***Note***: Family history covers hereditary disorders.)

62.   b) While all the disorders listed may be hereditary, strabismus, myopia, and glaucoma are the most common.

63.   c) A family history of glaucoma is reason for a full exam, regardless of the patient's age or race. There is no evidence that glaucoma is linked to the X chromosome.

64.   a) Strabismus tends to be familial.

65.   b) The tendency to develop diabetes, hypertension, arthritis, and cancer can be linked to heredity. The other conditions (except gout) are infectious diseases.

66.   b) The term *secondary* was your clue that the glaucoma was caused by something (eg, steroid use, injury, etc) and not inherited. The others can be hereditary or not.

Chapter 2

Pupillary Assessment

Ledford JK.
*Certified Ophthalmic Assistant: Exam
Review Manual, Third Edition* (pp. 15-22).
© 2012 Taylor & Francis Group.

Measure

1. **Any pupil smaller than what size is considered miotic?**
   a) 1 mm
   b) 2 mm
   c) 3 mm
   d) 4 mm

2. **Any pupil larger than what size is considered mydriatic?**
   a) 3 mm
   b) 4 mm
   c) 5 mm
   d) 6 mm

3. **Which of the following groups tend to have smaller pupils?**
   a) children
   b) myopes
   c) people with light blue eyes
   d) older people

4. **Unequal pupil size is termed:**
   a) anisocoria
   b) anisometropia
   c) anisochromia
   d) aniseikonia

Compare[1]

5. **The pupil evaluation includes:**
   a) size, shape, and reaction to light
   b) iris color, roundness, and reaction to light
   c) angle depth, iris diameter, reaction to light
   d) reaction to cycloplegia, light, and accommodation

6. **An iris coloboma usually causes a pupillary shape defect:**
   a) at 12 o'clock
   b) at 3 o'clock
   c) at 6 o'clock
   d) at 9 o'clock

7. **Constriction of the pupil can be accomplished by any of the following *except*:**
   a) shining a bright light into the eye
   b) having the patient focus on a near object
   c) using miotics
   d) dimming the room lights

[1]My JCAHPO® VOW says that *compare* "refers to assessing and comparing the pupil reaction."

8. **Dilation of the pupil can be accomplished by any of the following *except*:**
   a) shining a bright light into the eye
   b) pinching the patient's neck
   c) having the patient focus on a distant object
   d) dimming the room lights

9. **Direct pupillary response refers to:**
   a) the reaction of both pupils to light
   b) the reaction of one pupil to light
   c) the reaction of both pupils to near
   d) the reaction of one pupil to near

10. **Testing of the consensual light response in healthy eyes is possible because:**
    a) each pupil reacts to light independently
    b) if one pupil reacts to light, the other reacts with it
    c) the pupils react to light in reverse order
    d) the pupils react to near stimuli independently

11. **When checking consensual pupil responses to light, all of the following should be done *except*:**
    a) dim the room lights
    b) have the patient look at a distant object
    c) shine the light source from the side
    d) cover the eye not being tested

12. **To test pupillary response to accommodation:**
    a) observe the pupils as the patient looks from a distant object to a close-up object
    b) observe the pupils as the patient looks from a close-up object to a light source
    c) observe the pupils as the patient reads the near card
    d) observe the pupils as the patient reads the distant chart

13. **To evaluate a patient for tonic pupil (or Adie's tonic pupil), one would use which method?**
    a) pupillometer
    b) slit-lamp evaluation
    c) cycloplegia
    d) accommodation response test

14. **Each pupil constricts to direct light. This indicates:**
    a) there is no relative afferent pupillary defect (RAPD) present
    b) the pupils react equally
    c) light is passing through each optic nerve
    d) equal reaction to accommodation

Evaluate[2]

15. **Testing that reveals normal-appearing pupils that react appropriately is documented by the acronym:**
    a) PERRLA
    b) RAPD
    c) CSM
    d) PEAR

16. **The most common cause of a false-positive pupillary defect is:**
    a) glaucoma
    b) papilledema
    c) RAPD
    d) weak flashlight batteries

17. **Each of the following could cause abnormal pupil shape *except*:**
    a) surgery
    b) trauma
    c) birth defect
    d) Marcus Gunn

18. **Each of the following disorders can cause a change in pupil size *except*:**
    a) iritis
    b) angle-closure glaucoma attack
    c) drug reactions
    d) open-angle glaucoma

19. **Argyll Robertson pupils are often:**
    a) unreactive to direct or consensual light
    b) unreactive to accommodation
    c) reactive to light
    d) sluggishly reactive to accommodation

20. **You discover that your patient has an Argyll Robertson pupil. This pupillary defect is associated with:**
    a) acquired immune deficiency syndrome (AIDS)
    b) syphilis
    c) gonorrhea
    d) rubella

21. **Which of the following is associated with ptosis, miosis, and lack of perspiration (anhydrosis) on the affected side?**
    a) Adie's tonic pupil
    b) Horner's syndrome
    c) Argyll Robertson pupil
    d) Marcus Gunn pupil

[2]My JCAHPO® VOW says that *evaluation* "refers to the information (regarding the pupils) that was gathered based on the assessment or comparison after testing."

22. **Horner's syndrome is caused by:**
 a) nerve damage
 b) keratoconjunctivitis
 c) syphilis
 d) Herpes zoster

23. **Adie's tonic pupil (or tonic pupil) is caused by:**
 a) systemic rubella
 b) sympathetic ophthalmia
 c) gonorrhea
 d) nerve damage

24. **You might first suspect that the patient has a tonic pupil when:**
 a) the response to direct light is slow
 b) the pupil enlarges in direct light
 c) that eye also has a ptotic lid
 d) the patient is photophobic

Relative Afferent Pupillary Defect

25. **A relative afferent pupillary defect (RAPD) is identified by using the:**
 a) cross cover test
 b) pupillometer
 c) swinging flashlight test
 d) direct flashlight test

26. **The presence of a RAPD:**
 a) demonstrates a totally blind eye
 b) indicates a problem in the optic nerve
 c) indicates a defect in the facial nerve
 d) indicates a problem in the cerebral cortex

27. **An eye with a RAPD usually has:**
 a) redness and pain
 b) subnormal visual acuity
 c) delayed extraocular muscle responses
 d) irregular astigmatism

28. **Another name for a RAPD is:**
 a) Argyll Robertson pupils
 b) Adie's syndrome
 c) Marcus Gunn pupil
 d) tonic pupil

29. **You are performing a swinging flashlight test. The right pupil does not react at all when you shine the light in it. When you swing over to the left eye, the left pupil constricts rapidly. When you swing back to the right eye, there is again no reaction. This indicates:**
    a) a normal reaction
    b) RAPD OD by reverse
    c) RAPD OS by reverse
    d) a tonic pupil

Explanatory Answers

1.   b) If a pupil is 2 mm or smaller, it is considered miotic.
2.   d) A pupil that is 6 mm or larger is considered mydriatic.
3.   d) Children, myopes, and those with light blue eyes tend to have larger pupils. Older people tend to have smaller pupils.
4.   a) Anisocoria is the term for unequal pupil size. (The other answers are all real terms that you might want to look up if you do not know them.)
5.   a) Evaluation of pupils includes checking each pupil for its size, shape, and reaction to light (and sometimes to accommodation). After that is done, one pupil is compared to the other. Are they the same size? Shape? Do they respond to light (or accommodation) to the same degree?
6.   c) Iris coloboma is a congenital defect where the iris fails to fuse, usually inferiorly (ie, at 6 o'clock).
7.   d) Dimming the room lights would make the pupils enlarge.
8.   a) Shining a bright light into the eye causes the pupil to constrict, not dilate.
9.   b) The reaction of a single pupil to light is a direct pupillary response.
10.   b) The consensual light response compares the response (to light) of one pupil to the response of the other pupil. This is possible because healthy pupils are innervated to do the same thing at the same time, regardless of which eye has the light shining into it.
11.   d) Consensual light response testing requires that you be able to see both pupils, so covering is not appropriate. Covering either eye during any type of pupil check is unnecessary.
12.   a) To see the pupillary change that occurs in accommodation, have the patient look into the distance (accommodation relaxed), then at something up close (accommodation stimulated), or vice versa.
13.   d) In Adie's tonic pupil, there is a rapid/normal reaction of pupillary constriction when looking at a near object, but dilation is markedly slow when the patient shifts to look at a distant object. The pupil is also slow in its reaction to light. A pupillometer is used to measure the pupil's diameter. (*Note:* Do not confuse a pupillometer with the instrument that measures pupillary distance, which should properly be called an interpupillometer.)
14.   c) The direct test evaluates each pupil on its own and is not meant to compare the reaction of one pupil to the other. All you can say at this point is that at least some light is traversing the optic nerve of each eye. In order to find a RAPD, you would need to additionally perform the swinging flashlight test. Testing pupillary reaction to accommodation would involve having the patient look at a near then distant object and back, watching the pupillary response as he or she does this; a light is not used.

15. a) PERRLA stands for "pupils equally round and reactive to light and accommodation."

16. d) You probably will not see this question on the test, but it does make an important point. Any time you detect a pupillary defect, double-check with another penlight.

17. d) The Marcus Gunn pupillary defect affects the pupil's reaction, not its shape. An example of a congenitally abnormal pupil shape is the coloboma.

18. d) Open-angle glaucoma has no effect on pupil size. Some medications for glaucoma do (the miotics), but that was not the way the question was worded. Iritis causes a smaller pupil, angle-closure causes a larger pupil, and drug reactions can go either way.

19. a) The hallmark of Argyll Robertson pupils is their lack of response to direct or consensual light.

20. b) The Argyll Robertson pupil is a sign of syphilis.

21. b) Horner's syndrome is identified by the triad of ptosis, miosis, and anhydrosis on the affected side.

22. a) Horner's syndrome is caused by nerve damage that specifically affects eyelid position, pupil size, and facial perspiration to varying degrees.

23. d) Damage to the short posterior ciliary nerves is the cause of Adie's tonic pupil.

24. a) A tonic pupil will have a slow reaction to direct light. A pupil that enlarges in direct light most likely has a Marcus Gunn, or RAPD defect. Horner's syndrome exhibits ptosis on that same side.

25. c) The swinging flashlight test is used to test the consensual light response, comparing the light reaction of one pupil to the other. This is how an RAPD is identified.

26. b) The Marcus Gunn pupil can be identified by shining the light in one eye, then the other, also known as the swinging flashlight test. An eye with a Marcus Gunn pupil usually has poorer vision than the normal eye, but is not necessarily blind. It generally indicates a problem with the optic nerve.

27. b) RAPD indicates optic nerve damage, so visual acuity is usually compromised to some degree.

28. c) Another name you may hear for RAPD is Marcus Gunn pupil.

29. b) Usually, a RAPD is identified when the unaffected eye constricts rapidly and the affected eye dilates when you swing back to it. But one can still identify an RAPD in a fixed pupil by the reaction of the other (reverse), reactive eye, as in this scenario.

Chapter 3

Contact Lenses

Ledford JK.
*Certified Ophthalmic Assistant: Exam
Review Manual, Third Edition* (pp. 23-38).
© 2012 Taylor & Francis Group.

Measure[1]

1.   **In order to determine the base curve for a patient's contact lens, one must perform:**
     a) keratometry
     b) lensometry
     c) refractometry
     d) slit-lamp exam

2.   **Soft contact lens diameter can be selected by measuring the patient's:**
     a) pupillary distance
     b) vertex distance
     c) visible iris diameter
     d) corneal curvature

3.   **For most contact lens fitting purposes, it is acceptable to measure corneal diameter:**
     a) using an ophthalmoscope set on +10.0 and a millimeter rule
     b) by measuring the visible iris with a millimeter rule
     c) by using a pachymeter
     d) by anesthetizing the eye and using calipers

4.   **Which of the following is *not* a factor in determining the appropriate power of a contact lens?**
     a) pupil diameter
     b) refractive error
     c) vertex distance
     d) astigmatism

5.   **Your patient, a 63-year-old woman, wants to try contact lenses. Which of the following should be done?**
     a) tear evaluation
     b) pachymetry
     c) glare test
     d) conjunctival biopsy

6.   **Your patient is going to be fit with rigid gas permeable (RGP) lenses. In addition to the usual parameters, you should also measure:**
     a) corneal thickness
     b) palpebral fissures
     c) axial length
     d) contrast sensitivity

[1]See also the section titled *Fitting* (later, this chapter); Chapter 6, Keratometry; and Chapter 14, Refractometry.

Patient Instruction[2]

7. **A good rule of thumb when instructing patients regarding contact lenses is to:**
    a) provide a training session offering oral and written instruction
    b) provide written instruction and tell the patient to call with questions
    c) provide a training session and oral instruction
    d) develop a support group where successful lens wearers teach others

8. **The first rule to teach patients about handling contact lenses is:**
    a) always use a mirror
    b) work over a clean surface
    c) always wash hands first
    d) never touch the lens itself

9. **Before inserting a soft lens, the patient should make sure it is not inverted. This can be done by:**
    a) visual inspection or the taco test
    b) visual inspection or the jelly roll test
    c) inserting the lens in an inversion tester
    d) viewing the lens' reverse image in the mirror

10. **To insert a soft lens:**
    a) the lens should be dry and the finger wet
    b) the lens and finger should be dry
    c) the lens should be wet and the finger dry
    d) the lens and finger should be wet

11. **The patient should be instructed to place a contact lens:**
    a) directly on the cornea
    b) on the inferior sclera, then slide it up
    c) on the margin of the lower lid
    d) on the nasal sclera, then slide it over

12. **Use of lotion or moisturizer before handling lenses or use of makeup, hair spray, or face cream after inserting contact lenses can cause:**
    a) lens film
    b) corneal edema
    c) degradation of the lens
    d) giant papillary conjunctivitis

13. **The patient asks what he or she should do if the contact lens drops into the sink while trying to insert the lens. You tell the patient:**
    a) rinse the lens with saline and insert
    b) rinse the lens with rewetting drops and insert
    c) clean and disinfect the lens as per solution instructions
    d) replace the lens

[2]Per my JCAHPO® VOW, *patient instruction* refers to the proper use of the lenses.

14. **Soft contact lenses are most easily removed by:**
    a) using a plunger cup
    b) blinking them out
    c) squeezing them out
    d) pinching them out

15. **Damage to soft contact lenses is frequently caused by:**
    a) enzymatic cleaners
    b) rolling them between the fingers
    c) long fingernails
    d) defective materials

16. **Rigid contact lenses are often removed by blinking them out. For this technique to work:**
    a) the lens should be moved onto the sclera first
    b) the lens must be centered on the eye
    c) the patient must flip the edge of the lens with the finger
    d) the patient must squint and look up

17. **All of the following are helpful/proper techniques for using a plunger to remove a rigid lens *except*:**
    a) locate the lens on the eye before applying the plunger
    b) wet the plunger with wetting solution first
    c) run the plunger over the cornea and sclera to locate a "lost" lens
    d) carry an extra plunger in your pocket or purse for emergency removal

18. **Soft lenses should be cleaned immediately after removal because:**
    a) grunge is easier to remove at body temperature
    b) the patient might forget to do it later
    c) grunge is harder to remove once the lens has dried out
    d) otherwise enzymes are needed

19. **The difference between cleaning and disinfecting is:**
    a) cleaning is mandatory; disinfecting is optional
    b) cleaning removes film and debris; disinfecting kills germs
    c) cleaning kills germs; disinfecting removes film and debris
    d) cleaning is optional; disinfecting is mandatory

20. **When using a one-step contact lens solution, what should one do upon removing a lens from the eye?**
    a) put the lens directly into the case with fresh solution
    b) place the lens in the palm, add solution, and gently rub with fingertip
    c) rinse lens with solution and rub vigorously between the thumb and index finger
    d) rinse the lens under the water faucet and gently rub with fingertip

21. **Enzymatic cleaners may be used weekly for daily-wear soft lenses and gas-permeable lenses in order to:**
    a) sterilize the lenses
    b) prolong the life of the lens material
    c) remove protein deposits
    d) reduce splitting and chipping

22. **When not being worn, even rigid lenses should be stored in soaking solution because:**
    a) this prevents warping
    b) this reduces the chances of chipping the lens
    c) this maintains the power of the lens
    d) this maintains the integrity of the plastic

23. **If a gas-permeable lens dries out:**
    a) it must be replaced
    b) it can still be worn immediately
    c) it should be soaked for at least 4 hours
    d) it should be soaked for a week before wearing

24. **If soft contact lenses are not going to be worn for a few days:**
    a) add more soaking solution periodically to keep the lenses covered
    b) screw the case lid on tight to prevent evaporation
    c) use only nonpreserved saline as a soak
    d) change the soaking solution every day to maintain disinfection

25. **Which of the following regarding "topping off" cleaning/disinfecting solutions is *false*? ("Topping off" refers to the practice of adding a little fresh solution to what was left in the case from the last cleaning.)**
    a) it weakens the lens material
    b) it contaminates the solution
    c) it dilutes the solution
    d) disinfection is compromised

26. **Wetting solutions are used to:**
    a) keep lenses sterile while stored in the case
    b) enable tears to spread evenly on the lens surface
    c) make the lens resistant to deposit build-up
    d) prevent scratches on the lens surface

27. **Rewetting solutions are used to:**
    a) disinfect the lenses while on the eye
    b) remove deposits
    c) rehydrate the lenses while on the eye
    d) treat ocular redness

28. **Which of the following is the *least* sterile of these unapproved, ill-advised, and dangerous rewetting fluids?**
    a) saliva
    b) tap water
    c) urine
    d) water from a swimming pool

29. **Every patient who wears extended-wear contact lenses should be told to:**
    a) remove the lenses and clean them daily
    b) allow the lenses to remain in the eye for up to 1 month
    c) use lubricating drops every morning and during the day
    d) endure occasional pain and redness as a matter of course

30. **All of the following are true regarding a contact lens case *except*:**
    a) it can be boiled in water
    b) it should be washed weekly with hot water and soap
    c) it should be rinsed daily with fresh lens solution
    d) the interior is disinfected along with the contacts

Patient Counsel[3]

31. **Patients who work around smoke, dust, and chemical fumes should be told:**
    a) they are not good candidates for contact lenses
    b) they should wear rigid lenses, which will not absorb fumes
    c) they should not wear contacts at work
    d) they should change jobs if they want to wear contacts

32. **The contact lens patient should be told that if the eye ever becomes red or painful:**
    a) try another lens
    b) irrigate the eye
    c) bear with it
    d) remove the lens

33. **Corneal vascularization can result from chronic:**
    a) hypoxia
    b) solution sensitivity
    c) conjunctival injection
    d) giant papillary conjunctivitis

34. **The area of the cornea that most commonly becomes vascularized is the:**
    a) inferior limbal area
    b) superior limbal area
    c) 9 o'clock limbal area
    d) 3 o'clock limbal area

35. **Corneal edema is caused by:**
    a) excess oxygen permeability
    b) insufficient oxygen
    c) excess carbon monoxide
    d) excess tear production

36. **Symptoms of corneal edema include:**
    a) blurred vision
    b) rainbows around lights
    c) injection and burning
    d) all of the above

---

[3]Per my JCAHPO® VOW, *patient counsel* refers to any suggestions regarding concerns the patient may have about use of the lenses.

37. **Which of the following has been associated with *Acanthamoeba* infections in contact lens wearers?**
    a) nonpreserved saline
    b) thimerosal-preserved solutions
    c) homemade saline
    d) sample bottles of solutions

38. **Patients who remove his or her extended-wear lenses only once a month experience a higher percentage of all of the following *except*:**
    a) decreased need for artificial lubrication
    b) redness
    c) corneal anesthesia
    d) exposure keratitis when lenses are removed

39. **Giant papillary conjunctivitis is suspected to be:**
    a) an allergic response
    b) an infection
    c) a response to mechanical irritation
    d) a sign of overwear

40. **In addition to mucus formation, itching, and lens intolerance, the hallmark of giant papillary conjunctivitis is:**
    a) corneal ulcers
    b) inflamed pinguecula
    c) papillae on the palpebral conjunctiva of the upper lid
    d) papillae on the bulbar conjunctiva under the upper lid

41. **The patient with excess tear secretion may experience:**
    a) "sucked on" lens syndrome
    b) increased risk of neovascularization
    c) excessive lens movement
    d) circumcorneal indentation

42. **Patients using the monovision technique might experience problems:**
    a) taking the driver's license vision test
    b) in very bright light
    c) looking from the desk to the board in classroom situations
    d) when peripheral vision is checked by confrontation

Fitting

43. **The advantages of soft lenses include all of the following *except*:**
    a) they are more comfortable than rigid lenses
    b) they provide crisper vision than rigid lenses
    c) there is less lens displacement
    d) there is less lens loss

44. **One of the main disadvantages of soft lenses is:**
    a) frequent lens loss
    b) poor durability
    c) low oxygen permeability
    d) corneal injury on insertion

45. **The characteristic of soft lens material that is responsible for most of the lens' advantages (and disadvantages) is its:**
    a) tear exchange under the lens
    b) ability to absorb water
    c) resistance to deposits
    d) larger diameter

46. **One of the main risks of wearing soft contact lenses is:**
    a) modifications are impossible
    b) residual astigmatism
    c) infection
    d) lens discoloration

47. **Which patient is a poor candidate for soft lenses?**
    a) a patient with dry eye
    b) a patient with a spherical refractive error
    c) an infant or child
    d) a recreational basketball player

48. **Fitting a dry eye with a soft lens can be difficult because:**
    a) tear supplements cannot be used with soft lenses
    b) the lens will move excessively
    c) the diameter of the lens will change as it dries
    d) the optical properties of the lens will change as it dries

49. **All of the following are poor candidates for extended-wear lenses *except*:**
    a) those who work in a dusty environment
    b) those with chronic blepharitis
    c) those taking blood thinners
    d) those with pre-existing giant papillary conjunctivitis

50. **Which of the following probably would be a poor candidate for the monovision technique?**
    a) a public speaker
    b) a teacher
    c) a bookkeeper
    d) an actor

51. **Monovision contact lens fitting for presbyopia involves:**
    a) fitting both eyes for distance and using reading glasses for near
    b) fitting one eye (usually the dominant eye) for distance and the other eye for near
    c) fitting one eye (usually the dominant eye) for near and the other eye for distance
    d) wearing a contact lens for near in one eye and leaving the other eye uncorrected

52. **The lower the water content of a soft lens:**
    a) the more durable the lens
    b) the greater oxygen permeability
    c) the less frequently it needs to be cleaned
    d) the smaller the diameter

53. **A soft contact lens with a high water content will:**
    a) be more stable if lens dehydration occurs
    b) allow for greater oxygen transmission
    c) need to be disinfected by thermal methods only
    d) be more durable if it is made of hydroxyethyl methacrylate (HEMA)

54. **The "Dk value" of a contact lens refers to its:**
    a) carbon dioxide permeability
    b) oxygen permeability
    c) carbon monoxide permeability
    d) deciliter per kilogram value

55. **The oxygen supply to the cornea can be increased by selecting a lens:**
    a) with a high Dk value or reduced thickness
    b) with a low Dk value or reduced thickness
    c) with a high Dk value or increased thickness
    d) with a low Dk value or increased thickness

56. **Selecting the power of a spherical soft contact lens is based on:**
    a) the spherical element found on refractometry
    b) the cylindrical element found on refractometry
    c) the spherical equivalent of the refractometric measurement
    d) the refractometric and keratometric measurements

57. **To obtain the spherical equivalent:**
    a) add half of the sphere to the cylinder algebraically, keeping the cylinder
    b) add half of the cylinder to the sphere algebraically, keeping the cylinder
    c) add half of the sphere to the cylinder algebraically, deleting the cylinder
    d) add half of the cylinder to the sphere algebraically, deleting the cylinder

58. **You want to fit a spherical soft contact. The refractometric measurement is −3.00 + 1.00 × 180. Your lens choice is:**
    a) −3.00 sphere
    b) −3.50 sphere
    c) −2.00 sphere
    d) −2.50 sphere

59. **With spherical soft lenses, a small amount of corneal astigmatism is:**
    a) increased
    b) eliminated
    c) tolerated
    d) a reason to fit toric lenses

60. **The amount of astigmatism that is present after the patient is fitted with lenses is referred to as:**
    a) residual astigmatism
    b) corneal astigmatism
    c) lenticular astigmatism
    d) irregular astigmatism

61. **The most common source of residual astigmatism in contact lens wearers is:**
    a) the tear lens
    b) the cornea
    c) the crystalline lens
    d) the retina

62. **The patient with astigmatism may tolerate spherical soft contact lenses up to the point that the astigmatism is:**
    a) less than one-third of the total refractive error
    b) less than half of the total refractive error
    c) lenticular
    d) with the rule

63. **You plan to fit a soft toric contact lens. Which of the following is *true* regarding the refractometric measurement?**
    a) it must be converted to plus cylinder
    b) you will use the spherical equivalent
    c) you want the patient to accept the most cylinder power possible
    d) you want the patient to accept the least cylinder power possible

64. **The major difficulty with fitting toric lenses is:**
    a) patient discomfort
    b) lens stability on the eye
    c) arriving at the correct prescription
    d) obtaining accurate over-refractions

65. **An aid in evaluating the stability of a soft toric lens is:**
    a) the movement gauge
    b) etch or laser marks on the lens
    c) a protractor in the slit-lamp ocular
    d) the contact lens gauge

66. **Most practitioners would prefer to fit a gas-permeable contact lens instead of a traditional hard polymethylmethacrylate (PMMA) lens because:**
    a) vision with a gas-permeable lens is better
    b) gas-permeable lenses are easier to handle
    c) gas-permeable lenses are available for astigmatism
    d) corneal warpage is less with gas-permeable lenses

67. **Which of the following makes a patient a poor candidate for gas-permeable contact lenses?**
    a) history of giant papillary conjunctivitis
    b) exophthalmos
    c) corneal irregularity
    d) neovascularization from soft lenses

68. **The fact that gas-permeable contact lens material allows more oxygen to the eye means that:**
    a) the lens can be larger than a PMMA lens
    b) the lens is more comfortable than a PMMA lens
    c) lens movement is not an important factor
    d) the lens can be allowed to rest on the lower lid margin

69. **The average life of a rigid gas-permeable lens is:**
    a) 6 to 9 months
    b) 12 months
    c) 18 to 24 months
    d) 36 months

70. **Over-refractometry of a contact lens is useful in fine tuning:**
    a) lens power
    b) lens diameter
    c) lens centration
    d) lens base curve

71. **When taking a refractometric measurement over a contact lens of a patient over 40 years old:**
    a) first find out how the patient is corrected for presbyopia
    b) measure each eye for distance only
    c) measure each eye for near only
    d) measure the right eye for distance and the left eye for near

72. **Bandage contact lenses are routinely used for all of the following *except*:**
    a) correction of a refractive error
    b) promoting healing and protection
    c) patient comfort
    d) drug reservoir

73. **The key in selecting a bandage contact lens is:**
    a) the patient's refractive error
    b) the patient's ability to handle the lens
    c) oxygen permeability
    d) the patient's corneal curvature

74. **Even if a patient has a hyperopic refractive error, it is best to try a plano bandage lens first because:**
    a) refractive correction may trigger ciliary spasms
    b) a plano lens is thinner
    c) a plano lens has a higher water content
    d) the patient should avoid using the eye anyway

75. **All of the following are suitable bandage contact lenses *except*:**
    a) a collagen disintegrating lens
    b) a disposable soft lens
    c) a low water content lens
    d) a thin soft lens

Explanatory Answers

1. a) The keratometer measures the curvature of the cornea. The base curve of the lens is then selected to complement this measurement.
2. c) A soft lens should extend beyond the limbus, so one needs to measure the visible iris diameter (limbus-to-limbus).
3. b) A millimeter rule is adequate for measuring the limbus-to-limbus value.
4. a) Pupil diameter could possibly figure in on the design of a *rigid* contact lens, but is not a factor in the *power* of a soft or rigid lens.
5. a) Tear production and quality is an important consideration when fitting a woman of menopausal age or anyone in whom dry eye might be a concern. A Schirmer's tear test, tear break-up time, and slit-lamp exam are the most common tear evaluations.
6. b) RGPs are more dependent on eyelid structure than soft lenses because it is critical that they move with each blink. The distance between the upper and lower lids (the palpebral fissure) should be measured with a simple millimeter rule.
7. a) Patients should be given a training session that includes verbal instruction plus written instructions to refer to at home. Providing only written instruction or no written material at all is an invitation to failure. Trusting patient instruction to other patients is ill-advised.
8. c) Patients should be taught to wash his or her hands before handling lenses. (This is one of the rare times where "always" does not signal a wrong answer!)
9. a) Patients can be taught to recognize an inverted lens by both visual inspection and the taco test. The taco test involves holding the lens on thumb and forefinger and gently squeezing. If the lens edges flip inward, like a taco shell, then it is *not* inverted. (There's no such thing as the jelly roll test or an inversion tester.)
10. c) Inserting a soft lens is easiest if the lens is wet (not dripping) and the finger is dry (to prevent sticking).
11. a) The lens should be placed directly on the cornea, bull's-eye style. Sliding is not a good idea with a rigid lens, as this can cause a corneal abrasion. A lens on the lid margin is almost sure to be blinked out.
12. a) To prevent a filmy build-up on the lens, only hand soap that is free of moisturizers and other additives should be used. Makeup, face cream, and hair spray should be used before inserting lenses. Hand lotion should be used after.
13. c) A dropped lens should be cleaned and disinfected before wearing. No exceptions.
14. d) Soft lenses are pinched out with thumb and forefinger at the 9 and 3 o'clock positions. A plunger could tear a soft lens. Blinking and squeezing do not work.
15. c) Long fingernails are the nemesis of soft contact lenses. A person who is unwilling to cut the nails can learn to adapt, however, by turning the fingers slightly to keep the nails away from the lens and eye.
16. b) Blinking out a rigid lens requires the patient to look down, open both eyes wide, and pull the temporal canthus with thumb or finger. The lens must be centered on the eye for this to work.
17. c) Teach your patients never to apply the plunger to the eye unless they know exactly where the contact lens is. "Fishing" for a lost lens with the plunger is disastrous and painful if the plunger adheres to cornea or sclera. A drop of wetting solution helps the lens stick to the plunger, and carrying an extra plunger is always a good idea.

18. a) Body temperature grunge is easier to remove. A soft lens should not be allowed to dry out.

19. b) Neither cleaning nor disinfecting is optional. Disinfectant cannot reach all the surfaces of a dirty lens. Cleaning removes dirt, film, and deposits; disinfectant kills germs.

20. b) It is recommended that the contact be cleaned with solution and gentle friction even when using a "no-rub" or all-in-one formula.

21. c) Enzyme cleaners are used to remove protein build-up on soft and gas-permeable lenses. They do not provide the advantages listed in answers a, b, or d.

22. a) A rigid lens that is stored dry for a period of time can warp.

23. c) If a gas-permeable lens dries out, the base curve may change. It should return to normal after soaking for 4 hours or overnight.

24. d) For disinfection to be maintained, the disinfecting solution should be changed daily. Adding a little active disinfectant to a chamber of old disinfectant dilutes the active solution, rendering it too weak for the purpose. Saline (preserved or otherwise) does not disinfect.

25. a) Topping off simply adds a *little* fresh solution to used solution that is "used up." But once you stick your finger in the solution to put the lenses in, it is contaminated. Top off a couple times in a row, and there is no disinfecting going on.

26. b) Wetting solutions, used with rigid lenses, cause the tear film to spread evenly over the lens. This increases comfort. Wetting solution does not sterilize, reduce deposits, or prevent scratches.

27. c) Rewetting drops are used to ease dryness and mild discomfort caused by dryness during lens wear. This increases lens movement and comfort.

28. a) Gross as it may be, urine is more sterile than saliva. (Telling your patients this may discourage the terrible habit of wetting a rigid lens in the mouth!) Saliva harbors all kinds of nasty, infection-causing bacteria. Tap water and pool water (although "cleaner" than saliva) are not the right solutions either and can cause the lens to adhere to the cornea, as well as cause corneal edema.

29. c) See answer 38. It is not necessary for every patient to remove and clean the lenses every day, although some do and should, nor is it advisable to blithely allow every patient to wear them for a month at a time. Most physicians recommend weekly removal. If the eye is red or painful, the lens must always be removed.

30. b) The contact lens case should *not* be washed with soap because residue could interfere with the disinfectant or cause a film on the lenses. The entire case should be replaced every couple of months.

31. c) A patient who works around smoke, dust, and fumes still can wear contacts, just not at work!

32. d) Before the new contact lens wearer walks out the door, the final, cardinal rule to be emphasized is to remove a lens if the eye becomes red and/or painful. No exceptions.

33. a) Vascularization, or the development of new, abnormal blood vessels in the cornea, results from a lack of oxygen (hypoxia).

34. b) The superior limbal area of the cornea (under the upper lid) is most often the spot where vascularization occurs.

35. b) Corneal edema is caused by a lack of oxygen to the cornea.

36. d) Symptoms of corneal edema include blurred vision, halos around lights, redness, and burning.

37.   c) *Acanthamoeba* has been linked with homemade saline using salt tablets and distilled water.

38.   a) Every patient who wears contact lenses on an extended basis needs to lubricate the lenses regularly, especially every morning. Corneal anesthesia is a loss of sensation.

39.   a) Giant papillary conjunctivitis is considered to be an allergic response of the body to the protein deposits on a contact lens (usually soft). As the deposits break down, an allergic response is triggered.

40.   c) The signs and symptoms of giant papillary conjunctivitis include itching, mucus, lens intolerance, and the formation of large papillae on the inner surface of the upper eyelid. (The palpebral conjunctiva lines the lids, and the bulbar conjunctiva covers the sclera.)

41.   c) Excessive tears equal excessive movement as the lens floats around on the surplus fluid. Answers a, b, and d are seen in a tight/dry lens situation.

42.   a) The test for the driver's exam is a distance vision test. Often, the eye fit for near will fail to see the required distance figures. In this case, a letter or form may be required from the physician, explaining the situation.

43.   b) As a rule, soft lenses (being very flexible) do not provide the crisp, sharp vision of rigid lenses.

44.   b) The soft lens' flexible nature also makes it vulnerable to problems of durability. The lens can be torn easily. (Nondisposable types may also crack or split with age. The life expectancy of a nondisposable soft lens is generally considered to be only about 1 year.) However, there is less lens loss, better oxygen permeability, and a lower risk of injury on insertion because the edges are soft.

45.   b) The soft lens is hydrophilic, which means "loves water." The fact that it absorbs water is responsible for its entire nature. This includes comfort, flexibility, and oxygen transmission. There is very little tear exchange under a soft lens (as opposed to a rigid lens). These lenses are not resistant to deposits. A larger diameter is possible because of oxygen transmissibility, but the diameter in and of itself is not responsible for the lens' advantages and disadvantages.

46.   c) The biggest risk listed is that of infection. The pores of soft lens material generally are too small for bacteria to penetrate. However, once the lens forms deposits, there is a rough surface on which bacteria may grow. In addition, the removal of a deposit may create a pit in the lens large enough to harbor bacteria. While it is true that modifications are impossible, residual astigmatism goes uncorrected, and the lenses can discolor, these hardly qualify as risks.

47.   a) If a hydrophilic lens does not get the water it "wants" from the tear film, its thickness (and, thus, optics) can change, making the patient with dry eye a less-than-ideal contact lens patient. Soft lenses usually correct spherical errors quite well. An infant and a child are good candidates because the soft lens provides more comfort and a low rate of lens loss on impact. Rigid lenses may pop out on impact, which makes the soft lens a good choice for the recreational basketball player as well.

48.   d) As a soft lens dries out, its base curve (not diameter) changes, altering its optical qualities and producing blurred vision. Selected tear supplement drops can be used with soft contact lenses in place. The dry lens moves little if at all.

49.   c) There is no connection between taking blood thinners and wearing contact lenses.

50. c) Anyone who continuously works up close and requires "perfect" near vision all the time (such as a bookkeeper or accountant) probably is not a good candidate for monovision. Monovision involves a trade-off. Both distance and near vision are somewhat compromised, and binocular vision is sacrificed, but the patient does not have to cope with bifocals (glasses or contacts). Those people listed in the other answers do some up-close work, but also need to look frequently at a distance to see his or her audience.

51. b) In the monovision technique, one eye (usually the dominant eye) is fitted for distance and the other eye is fitted for near. In some cases, the dominant eye might be fitted for near, but this is not the routine procedure.

52. a) The lower the soft lens' water content, the more rigid it is and, hence, the more durable. Still, the soft lens does not approach rigidity in the sense that a hard or gas-permeable lens does. A low water content lens is less oxygen transmissible.

53. b) The higher the water content of a soft lens, the more oxygen can be transmitted to the cornea. Unfortunately, these lenses are sensitive to dehydration if the environment changes. They also are heat sensitive, and some types may not be disinfected using thermal methods. Given the same water content, the non-HEMA lenses are more durable.

54. b) The Dk value of a contact lens is a laboratory measurement of the oxygen permeability of a material. That is not to say, however, that the Dk is a measurement of how much oxygen actually reaches the cornea.

55. a) A high Dk value indicates greater oxygen permeability. A thinner lens also increases oxygen transmission to the cornea.

56. c) The power of a spherical soft contact is chosen by the spherical equivalent of the refractometric measurement. The K readings are not used for calculating the power.

57. d) To find the spherical equivalent, add half of the cylinder to the sphere, then drop the cylinder (and axis).

58. d) The spherical equivalent is necessary because you are fitting a soft spherical contact. Half of the cylinder is +0.50. Add this to the sphere power: $-3.00 + 0.50 = -2.50$.

59. c) A small amount of astigmatism in a spherical soft lens wearer is merely tolerated, not eliminated. As long as the patient tolerates it, there is no reason to rush into fitting a toric lens.

60. a) Astigmatism that is "left over" after the eye is fit with a contact lens is called residual astigmatism.

61. c) Residual astigmatism is most often caused by lenticular astigmatism, or irregular curvature of the crystalline lens (which does not show up on K readings).

62. a) As long as the astigmatism is less than one-third of the total refractive error, there is a good chance that the patient can tolerate the vision provided by a spherical soft contact lens.

63. d) When fitting a soft toric, you want the least amount of cylinder correction that the patient will accept, because the lens will rotate a bit on the eye. The higher the amount of cylinder, the more pronounced the visual problems caused by this rotation.

64. b) Keeping the cylinder properly aligned means keeping the lens aligned. A spherical lens is normally pushed around and rotates during blinking. This spells disaster for a toric lens fit.

65. b) Soft toric lenses have etch marks or dots either at the base or at the horizontal meridian. These can be observed with the slit lamp. The examiner looks for lens rotation as the patient blinks.

66. d) Because a PMMA lens is not oxygen permeable, nearly all PMMA lenses cause some degree of corneal anoxia (an- means *without* and -oxia means *oxygen*). This, in turn, is responsible for corneal warpage. Because gas-permeable lenses do allow oxygen to reach the cornea, the incidence (and risk) of corneal warpage is much less. In the absence of corneal complications, both rigid lens types should provide crisp vision, are equally easy to handle, and can be ground to correct astigmatism.

67. b) An exophthalmic (bulging) eye usually is fit better with a soft lens, which is more stable on the eye and does not interfere with the lids. Cases represented by the other answers are good candidates.

68. a) Because a gas-permeable contact lens allows more oxygen to get to the cornea, the eye can tolerate a larger lens. True, it is more comfortable than a PMMA lens, but this is due to the fit (sliding under the upper lid versus bumping into it), not permeability. Lens movement still is important. The properly fit gas-permeable lens does not sit on the lower lid.

69. c) The average life of a rigid gas-permeable contact lens is 18 to 24 months. (The gas-permeable material is not as tough as PMMA.)

70. a) Over-refractometry is used to refine the power of the contact lens and has little application in answers b through d.

71. a) If the patient is presbyopic, find out how the lenses are fit before pulling the refractor forward. Are they monofit? Bifocals? Maybe distance in both eyes with reading glasses? Knowing what to expect before you start will make your job easier.

72. a) While a bandage lens of a specific power may be chosen, correcting the refractive error is not the priority in a bandage lens. In fact, a plano lens usually is preferred because it is thinner (in the center for a plus lens and at the edges for a minus lens) and thus more oxygen permeable.

73. c) Getting oxygen to the cornea is the key in selecting a bandage lens. A bandage lens is generally not handled by the patient. K readings may be taken and used, but not in every case.

74. b) See answer 72.

75. c) A high water content lens versus a low water content lens is preferred because it is more oxygen permeable.

Chapter 4

Equipment Maintenance and Repair

Ledford JK.
*Certified Ophthalmic Assistant: Exam
Review Manual, Third Edition* (pp. 39-52).
© 2012 Taylor & Francis Group.

Clean and Lubricate[1]

1. **Acuity projector slides can be cleaned by:**
   a) washing with soap and water
   b) spraying with commercial cleaner
   c) wiping with a dry lens wipe
   d) wiping with a wet lens wipe

2. **Which of the following will help prevent dust build-up on the lenses of a direct ophthalmoscope?**
   a) the direct ophthalmoscope has no built-in lenses
   b) cleaning daily with cleanser
   c) removing the instrument facing for direct access to the lenses
   d) storing the instrument with the lens setting on zero

3. **Which of the following is *not* appropriate when cleaning an indirect ophthalmoscope?**
   a) cleaning the front surface mirror with a brush
   b) rubbing debris off the bulb with the finger
   c) cleaning the bulb contacts by scraping with a file
   d) wiping the headband with an alcohol wipe

4. **Unless the manufacturer's instructions indicate otherwise, the perimeter bowl surface may be cleaned with:**
   a) mild detergent and water
   b) lighter fluid
   c) contact lens solution
   d) lens cleaner

5. **When brushing or wiping the perimeter bowl surface, it is important to avoid:**
   a) any moisture at all
   b) excessive pressure/friction
   c) fibrous cotton balls
   d) using a soft brush or cloth

6. **Dirty tangent screen test objects should be cleaned with:**
   a) cleanser
   b) an alcohol wipe
   c) soap and water
   d) acetone

7. **Discolored tangent screen white test objects should be:**
   a) replaced
   b) painted with correction liquid
   c) used as is
   d) wiped with an alcohol wipe

[1]For cleaning of Goldmann tonometer, see Chapter 17; for lensometer, Chapter 5; and for keratometer, Chapter 6.

8. **The tangent screen itself can be cleaned:**
   a) by gentle whisking with a very soft brush
   b) by brushing with a wire brush
   c) with a commercial dry-cleaning product
   d) with soap and water

9. **To prevent dirt from collecting on the back surface of the refractor/phoroptor lenses:**
   a) use the widest pupillary distance possible
   b) adjust the forehead rest to avoid lash/lens contact
   c) make sure the refractor is level
   d) request that patients remove mascara before refractometry

10. **If the internal lenses of the refractor are dirty:**
    a) spray them through the aperture with lens cleaner
    b) open the refractor and clean the lenses one at a time
    c) add one line of acuity to everyone's measurement
    d) have the instrument professionally cleaned

11. **To clean the friction plate under the joystick:**
    a) wipe with an alcohol wipe
    b) remove the plate, and put it in the autoclave
    c) rub with bathroom cleanser
    d) spray with lens cleaner

12. **To lubricate the friction plate under the joystick:**
    a) lightly coat with cooking oil and wipe it almost dry
    b) lightly coat with automotive oil and wipe it almost dry
    c) lightly coat with silicone oil and wipe it almost dry
    d) lightly sprinkle with graphite

13. **Solid ultrasound probes should be cleaned:**
    a) only if an infectious disease is suspected
    b) once each week
    c) once each day
    d) between each patient exam

14. **All of the following tend to loosen the glue of a mounted lens** *except*:
    a) drying out over time
    b) heat
    c) cool water
    d) alcohol or acetone

15. **Unless the manufacturer's instructions state otherwise, a glass lens (nonbloomed) may be cleaned by any of the following** *except*:
    a) 4:1 ratio of ether and alcohol
    b) commercial chrome cleaner
    c) 1:1 ratio of ammonia and isopropyl alcohol
    d) commercial glass or lens cleaner

16. **Do not use commercial glass cleaner on plastic lenses because:**
    a) this can scratch the surface
    b) this can remove lens coatings
    c) this can cloud the lens
    d) this can cause crazing

17. **Besides soap and cool water, which of the following can be used to clean plastic lenses?**
    a) contact lens solution
    b) lighter fluid
    c) bathroom cleanser
    d) baking soda

18. **Which of the following will remove the coating on a bloomed lens (such as the indirect ophthalmoscope lens)?**
    a) gently wiping the dry lens with a tissue
    b) wiping the lens with ethyl or methyl alcohol
    c) blowing the lens with compressed air
    d) heavily rubbing the lens to remove fingerprints

19. **When cleaning a lens that is fixed into an instrument:**
    a) spray lens cleaner on the lens in the instrument
    b) use a stream bottle to irrigate the lens in the instrument
    c) spray lens cleaner on a wipe, and clean the lens with the wipe
    d) fixed lenses cannot be cleaned

20. **The best way to remove dust from a fundus camera lens is to first:**
    a) dust it with a camel's hair brush
    b) blow off dust with air
    c) wipe dust off with a dry cloth
    d) clean dust off with isopropyl alcohol

21. **Which surface of an exophthalmometer might require disinfection?**
    a) the mirrors
    b) the gauges
    c) the prisms
    d) the points of patient contact

22. **Which surface of an ophthalmodynamometer might require disinfection?**
    a) the tip
    b) the gauge
    c) the lens
    d) the watch glass

23. **Which of the following is *untrue* regarding front surface mirrors?**
    a) The silver coating can be rubbed off over time.
    b) The coating can be scratched by mishandling.
    c) They produce a faint double image of the reflection.
    d) They reflect 100% light transmission.

24. **Prior to cleaning a front surface mirror, one should:**
    a) rub with a cotton ball to remove loose dust
    b) use canned air to remove loose dust
    c) blow on it to remove loose dust
    d) spray it with water

25. **Which of the following can be used to clean a front surface mirror?**
    a) a paper towel and commercial glass cleaner
    b) a cotton-tipped applicator and dry baking soda
    c) a fingertip to rub off smudges
    d) a lens wipe with a 4:1 ratio of ether and alcohol

26. **A mirror surface should be dried by:**
    a) patting with a lint-free lens wipe
    b) wiping with a lint-free lens wipe
    c) rubbing with a tissue or cotton ball
    d) patting with a paper towel

27. **Which surface is *not* affected by friction during cleaning?**
    a) front surface mirrors
    b) bloomed lenses
    c) projector screens
    d) glass trial lenses

28. **A projector screen is cleaned by:**
    a) wiping with an alcohol wipe
    b) scrubbing with cleanser
    c) a solution of mild detergent
    d) commercial glass cleaner

29. **One of the easiest and least expensive ways to prolong the life of ophthalmic/optometric equipment is to:**
    a) wipe it daily with an alcohol wipe
    b) have it serviced every 6 months
    c) change bulbs and batteries every 6 months
    d) cover or store it when not in use

Tighten Screws

30. **Turning a screw counterclockwise (to the left) will cause it to:**
    a) tighten
    b) loosen
    c) strip out
    d) fall out

31.   **The first several turns of inserting a screw are difficult. You should:**
   a) force it
   b) use a hammer
   c) stop and try resetting the screw
   d) spray lubricant on the instrument

Replace Parts

32.   **To extend the life of a slit-lamp bulb:**
   a) use the lowest voltage setting as much as possible
   b) scrape the contact points weekly
   c) turn it 180 degrees weekly
   d) use the lowest illumination as much as possible

33.   **If the filament of a bulb is aligned incorrectly in the housing:**
   a) the bulb will blow out
   b) chromatic aberration will occur in the light field
   c) the light will be deviated from prismatic power
   d) the projected light will not illuminate the entire field

34.   **If the light in a piece of electrical equipment begins to flicker or does not come on, the first and easiest thing to check is:**
   a) the filament
   b) the bulb's seating
   c) the instrument's plug
   d) the instrument's fuse

35.   **When changing light bulbs in a piece of equipment, all of the following are important *except*:**
   a) turn off and unplug the instrument
   b) allow the old bulb to cool, if it is hot
   c) remove the old bulb with pliers
   d) do not touch the glass of the new bulb

36.   **If the bulb contacts become corroded, one may remedy this problem by unplugging the instrument and:**
   a) replacing the contacts
   b) wiping the contacts with alcohol
   c) scraping with a metal file
   d) blowing with compressed air

37. **The projector bulb has a build-up of oxidation on one side, decreasing its illumination. You should:**
a) replace the bulb
b) turn the bulb 180 degrees to use the other side (without the build-up)
c) remember that nothing needs to be done as long as all patients are checked in the same illumination
d) scrape off the contacts in the bulb housing

38. **Which is true of rechargeable batteries and recharging units?**
a) the battery will last 10 years or more
b) the rechargers cannot be left on indefinitely
c) batteries can lose the ability to recharge
d) all batteries can be installed in either direction

39. **An instrument operating on rechargeable NiCad batteries:**
a) should be placed in the charger after each use during the day
b) should be placed in the charger only at the end of the day
c) will not operate if more than 25 feet away from the charger
d) works best if the batteries are cooler than room temperature

40. **Regular cell batteries should be stored:**
a) in a heated room
b) in the refrigerator
c) in the freezer
d) at room temperature

41. **If a particular fuse repeatedly burns out, one should:**
a) replace the fuse as needed
b) use a fuse with a lower ampere (AMP) rating
c) get professional assistance
d) replace the instrument

Other[2]

42. **Match the instrument image on the following pages with its name:**

direct ophthalmoscope	slit lamp (biomicroscope)
indirect ophthalmoscope	ultrasound (A-scan)
retinoscope	keratometer (ophthalmometer)
lensmeter (lensometer)	trial lens set
perimeter	Schiøtz tonometer
tangent screen	Goldmann tonometer
phoroptor (refractor)	muscle light

[2]While the current JCAHPO® COA® criteria do not have a listing to which these questions apply, they are from the first and second editions of the *Certified Ophthalmic Assistant Exam Review Manual* and I did not feel comfortable leaving them out.

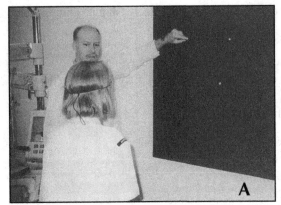

Figure 4-1. Reprinted with permission of Choplin N, Edwards E. *Visual Fields*. SLACK Incorporated; 1998.

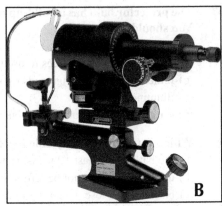

Figure 4-2. Reprinted with permission of Marco.

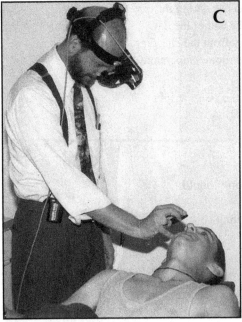

Figure 4-3. Reprinted with permission of Jim Ledford, PA-C, PhD.

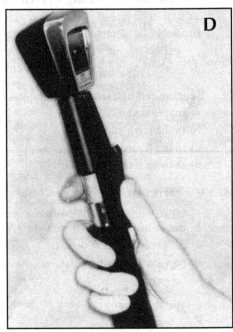

Figure 4-4. Reprinted with permission of Jim Ledford, PA-C, PhD.

Figure 4-5. Reprinted with permission of Herrin MP. *Ophthalmic Examination and Basic Skills*. SLACK Incorporated; 1990.

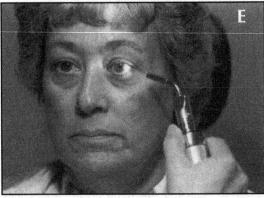

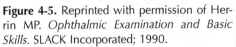

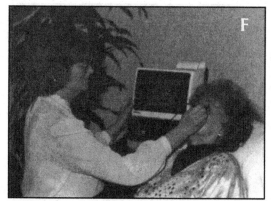

Figure 4-6. Reprinted with permission of Kendall CJ. *Ophthalmic Echography.* SLACK Incorporated; 1990.

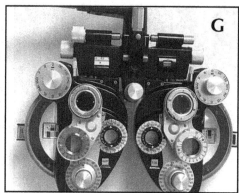

Figure 4-7.

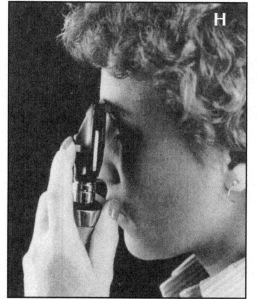

Figure 4-8. Reprinted with permission of Herrin MP. *Ophthalmic Examination and Basic Skills.* SLACK Incorporated; 1990.

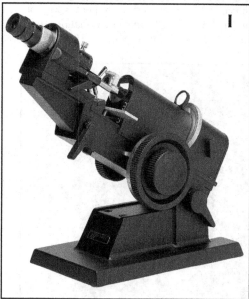

Figure 4-9. Reprinted with permission of Marco.

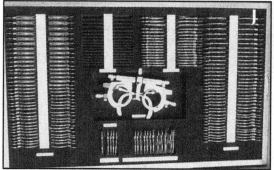

Figure 4-10. Reprinted with permission of Herrin MP. *Ophthalmic Examination and Basic Skills.* SLACK Incorporated; 1990.

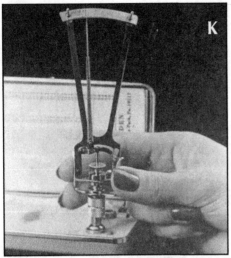

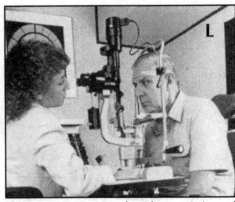

Figure 4-12. Reprinted with permission of Herrin MP. *Ophthalmic Examination and Basic Skills.* SLACK Incorporated; 1990.

Figure 4-11. Reprinted with permission of Herrin MP. *Ophthalmic Examination and Basic Skills.* SLACK Incorporated; 1990.

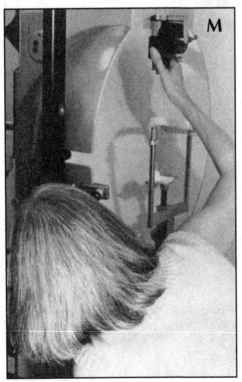

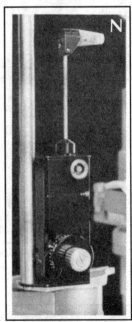

Figure 4-14. Reprinted with permission of Herrin MP. *Ophthalmic Examination and Basic Skills.* SLACK Incorporated; 1990.

Figure 4-13. Reprinted with permission of Garber N. *Visual Field Examination.* SLACK Incorporated; 1988.

43. **One might adjust the concave mirror in an acuity projector in order to:**
     a) change the size of the letters to fit a shorter room
     b) increase the clarity of the letters
     c) improve faulty illumination
     d) change the place where the target is projected

44. **To calibrate the size of the target of an acuity projector, one must:**
     a) have a 20-foot test distance
     b) use a template and adjust the projection tube until the letter fits into the correct bracket
     c) use a table to convert every patient's measurement if the test distance is not 20 feet
     d) use a template, and adjust the concave mirror until the letter fits into the correct bracket

45. **If the vertical alignment of an indirect ophthalmoscope is misaligned:**
     a) adjust the headband
     b) make sure the mirror is clean
     c) adjust the mirror
     d) have the instrument professionally serviced

46. **A bent, or C-shaped streak in a streak retinoscope is caused by:**
     a) a weak bulb
     b) a bent bulb filament
     c) a weak battery
     d) using it with the sleeve down

47. **During a normal workday, when not in immediate use, the retinoscope should be stored:**
     a) by lying it on its side on the table
     b) by leaving it turned on
     c) by placing it upright
     d) by lying it in a protected drawer

48. **If the retinoscope light flickers and the bulb placement is solid, the flickering is probably due to:**
     a) a loose bulb filament
     b) inadequate charge
     c) internal wiring problems
     d) weak batteries

49. **Which of the following is *not* true regarding fluid-filled ultrasound probes?**
     a) the membrane tip is fragile and lasts only a few days
     b) the probe is filled with sterile saline solution
     c) air bubbles must be removed from the probe before use
     d) the crystal in the probe can lose sensitivity over time

50. **Ultrasound units are calibrated by:**
     a) touching the probe to a test block specific for that machine
     b) touching the probe to a flat surface
     c) routinely measuring the same person's eye as a standard
     d) pressing the calibration button on the instrument

51. **Care of the noncontact tonometer includes all of the following *except*:**
    a) firing it at the beginning of each day to blow dust from the air nozzle
    b) checking calibration by firing the air burst against your finger
    c) covering it when not in use
    d) cleaning the objective lens and aperture

52. **The muscle light (transilluminator) might require the following maintenance:**
    a) brightness calibration
    b) bulb and battery replacement
    c) sterilization
    d) tip and casing replacement

Explanatory Answers

1. c) Use a dry lens wipe to clean acuity projector slides. Liquids can dissolve the paint and ruin the slides.
2. d) With the setting on zero, there are no exposed lenses in the instrument's aperture.
3. b) Oil from the fingers is transferred to the bulb if you touch it. (The front surface mirror may also be cleaned with a lens wipe moistened with ether and alcohol in a ratio of 1:4.)
4. a) A mild detergent and water are appropriate for cleaning the perimeter bowl surface.
5. b) Putting too much pressure on an area inside the bowl might change the reflective properties of the bowl in that area or scratch the finish.
6. c) Mild soap and water are the choice for cleaning dirty test objects.
7. a) If the test objects are discolored, they should be replaced, not "repaired." If they are too dingy, they can affect the accuracy of the test.
8. a) Answers b through d are too aggressive. A gentle whisking is appropriate.
9. b) Oil and makeup can accumulate on the lenses when there is contact between the lids and lenses. Adjust the forehead rest to push the patient back a little. (But keep in mind that this also increases the vertex distance.)
10. d) The refractor (phoroptor) is a complicated instrument and should be cleaned only by a trained professional. Never spray anything into the instrument.
11. a) The slit lamp will not move smoothly if the friction plate is dirty. Clean it with an alcohol wipe.
12. c) Alcohol will dissolve oil and grease, so lubricate the clean friction plate with silicone oil or WD-40 (The WD-40 Company, San Diego, CA).
13. d) Because the probe makes direct contact with the eye tissues, it should be cleaned between patients.
14. c) Cool water does not affect the glue of a mounted lens. The other items listed can cause the glue to loosen.
15. b) Chrome cleaner is not appropriate for use on glass lenses. "Blooming" refers to a special coating on the lens.
16. c) A plastic lens may cloud if cleaned with commercial glass cleaner.
17. a) Because contact lenses are plastic, it makes sense that you can use contact lens solution to clean plastic lenses. The other items are too abrasive or caustic.
18. d) Friction can remove the coating on a bloomed lens. Be gentle!

19.   c) Never spray cleaner into an instrument. If you want to use cleaner, spray it on a wipe first. Then, use the wipe on the instrument.

20.   b) The order of cleaning for a camera lens is blow using a bulb syringe (*not* your breath!), brush, and wipe.

21.   d) Any part of the exophthalmometer (or any instrument) that touches the patient should be cleaned between patients.

22.   a) See answer 21. The tip of the instrument touches the eye and therefore must be disinfected after every use.

23.   c) Front surface mirrors do not produce a double image. That is why they are used in optical situations.

24.   b) Prior to cleaning the mirror, use canned air or an air bulb to remove loose debris, which could scratch the mirror when it is being wiped. If you use canned air, be sure it is approved for use on mirrors and lenses; the type usually used for general office use sometimes has a liquid additive that can coat the surface.

25.   d) A front surface mirror can be scratched easily, and a little bit of the silver is rubbed off every time it is cleaned. Clean it with a lens wipe moistened with ether and alcohol, gently moving the wipe in down-strokes. Do not rub the mirror. (Alternately, in Stein, Stein, and Freeman's *The Ophthalmic Assistant, 8th Edition*, the authors suggest using small spritzes of commercial glass cleaner and cotton balls.)

26.   a) To avoid scratching, do not rub the mirror, and do not use an abrasive wipe. If necessary, pat dry with a lint-free lens wipe or cotton ball.

27.   d) The items in answers a through c can all be ruined by hard rubbing.

28.   c) The projector screen is designed to be highly reflective. Clean it gently with mild detergent.

29.   d) Covering or storing equipment prevents dust build-up and reduces breakage.

30.   b) Remember the little ditty, "Righty tighty, lefty loosey." Turning a screw to the left, or counterclockwise, will loosen it.

31.   c) Forcing a screw may strip it, making it nearly impossible to remove later. It could also cause the instrument housing to crack at that point.

32.   a) Use the lowest voltage setting of the slit lamp or any other instrument to prolong the bulb life.

33.   d) If the bulb filament is not lined up, then the field will not be entirely lit.

34.   c) The golden rule in troubleshooting electrical equipment is always check the plug first!

35.   c) If you try to remove the bulb with pliers, the bulb may break. Then, you will have a problem trying to get the housing out. Let the bulb cool, then use your fingers or a special bulb remover.

36.   c) The only way to remove corrosion is to scrape it off. Alcohol or air will not work.

37.   b) Turn the bulb around to the side that does not have oxidation on it—this is certainly more cost-effective than changing the bulb. Of course, you can only do this once! When the other half gets grimy, you will have to replace the bulb.

38.   c) Rechargeable NiCad batteries have a "memory" and can lose their rechargeable attribute. This is not a problem with lithium ion batteries. The other answers are false.

39.   b) Because of the NiCad battery's "memory" (mentioned in answer 38), a rechargeable instrument should be placed in the charger only at the end of the working day, not after each use.

40. d) Store extra batteries at room temperature. Chilling them used to be recommended, but that no longer applies to modern batteries.

41. c) An instrument that continuously blows fuses is in need of professional repair.

42. Matching:

direct ophthalmoscope	h)	slit lamp (biomicroscope)	l)
indirect ophthalmoscope	c)	ultrasound (A-scan)	f)
retinoscope	d)	keratometer (ophthalmometer)	b)
lensmeter (lensometer)	i)	trial lens set	j)
perimeter	m)	Schiøtz tonometer	k)
tangent screen	a)	Goldmann tonometer	n)
phoroptor (refractor)	g)	muscle light	e)

43. c) Adjust the mirror to improve illumination. The other 3 items are done by adjusting the lens or location of the projector.

44. b) A template is available to adjust the target to the appropriate size. Move the projection tube until the letter fits the template.

45. d) Improper vertical alignment in an indirect ophthalmoscope must be adjusted by a professional. If the vertical alignment is off, the examiner will have double vision or trouble fusing the images.

46. b) A bent bulb filament will cause the retinoscope streak to be distorted. (This is caused by lying the instrument on its side.)

47. c) The retinoscope should be placed upright to prevent the filament from distorting.

48. c) A flickering light, when the bulb is seated properly, is usually due to internal wiring problems.

49. b) Water-filled probes contain distilled water, not saline solution.

50. a) The test block supplied with an ultrasound unit is specific for that instrument.

51. b) Calibration in the noncontact tonometer is done by simply firing the machine. No finger necessary!

52. b) The muscle light usually runs on batteries (often rechargeable) and will occasionally blow a bulb. The tip might require disinfection (not sterilization) with an alcohol swab (if applied directly to the sclera for transillumination, for example).

Chapter 5

Lensometry

Ledford JK.
*Certified Ophthalmic Assistant: Exam
Review Manual, Third Edition* (pp. 53-64).
© 2012 Taylor & Francis Group.

1. **The prescription of a lens is written in the following order:**
   a) cylinder power, sphere power, sphere axis
   b) sphere power, cylinder axis, cylinder power
   c) sphere power, cylinder power, cylinder axis
   d) sphere power, sphere axis, cylinder axis

2. **In a glasses prescription reading +1.25 – 3.75 × 082, the –3.75 refers to:**
   a) sphere power
   b) cylinder power
   c) cylinder axis
   d) add power

3. **In a glasses prescription reading –2.25 + 1.50 × 173, which of the following is *true*?**
   a) The prescription is written in minus cylinder.
   b) The sphere power is "plus."
   c) The cylinder power is written as "plus."
   d) The cylinder axis is a multiplier.

4. **In a glasses prescription reading +1.00 + 1.00 × 180 | 1.25/2.50, the number 1.25 refers to:**
   a) the trifocal power
   b) the bifocal power
   c) the total add power
   d) the cylinder power

5. **Which of the following glasses prescriptions would definitely be questioned by an optician?**
   a) +1.50 + 2.25 × 181
   b) Plano – 9.25 × 072
   c) +11.75 – 1.75 × 175
   d) –2.50 + 6.50 × 018

Automated Lensometry

6. **When using an automated lensometer, it is important to designate:**
   a) lens material
   b) lens manufacturer
   c) desired cylinder type
   d) desired base curve type

7. **An advantage of the automated lensometer is the ease with which it:**
   a) detects Fresnel prism
   b) reads progressive add lenses
   c) identifies lens material
   d) identifies polarized lenses

8. **An automated lensometer may be disadvantageous in identifying:**
   a) optical centers
   b) add powers
   c) prisms
   d) warped lenses

9. **A key advantage of the automated lensometer is that it:**
   a) eliminates math errors
   b) converts the glasses prescription to a contact lens prescription
   c) takes vertex distance into account
   d) identifies photosensitive lenses

10. **All of the following are true regarding automated lensometers *except*:**
    a) they should be set on an antistatic mat
    b) they should not be placed and used in direct sunlight
    c) the internal lenses and mirrors can be cleaned by removing the instrument housing
    d) the computer components are sensitive to dust

Manual Lensometry

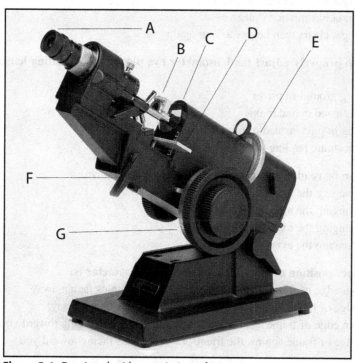

Figure 5-1. Reprinted with permission of Marco.

11. **Label the parts of the lensmeter[1] (Figure 5-1):**

    | axis wheel | lens holder | frame stage |
    | eye piece | lens stop | power wheel |
    | table control lever | | |

[1]*Lensmeter* is, technically, the name of the instrument. *Lensometer* was a trade name introduced by Bausch + Lomb that has since become a commonly used generic term (much like "phoropter").

12. **The first step in reading a pair of glasses with the manual lensometer is to:**
    a) position the glasses in the holder with the temples away from you
    b) position the glasses in the holder with the temples toward you
    c) clean the lenses before reading
    d) adjust the eye piece of the instrument

13. **When adjusting the lensometer eye piece:**
    a) you should wear your own habitual correction
    b) the lensometer's power dial should be set to your prescription
    c) the lensometer's axis indicator should be set to 180
    d) the lensometer's axis indicator should be set to match your own astigmatism

14. **Before adjusting the lensometer eye piece:**
    a) turn the eye piece to the most minus position
    b) turn the eye piece to the most plus position
    c) turn the eye piece to an axis of 180
    d) turn the eye piece to the axis of your astigmatism

15. **When adjusting the lensometer eye piece, the eye piece is slowly rotated until:**
    a) the target just begins to blur
    b) the target is first seen to be clear
    c) the target has turned 90 degrees
    d) the target clears then begins to blur again

16. **Failure to properly adjust the lensometer eye piece before reading lenses may result in:**
    a) missing ground-in prism
    b) a misaligned cylinder axis
    c) reading in plus instead of minus cylinder
    d) an inaccurate reading

17. **A lens can be read in a lensometer in plus or minus form:**
    a) by changing the axis 180 degrees
    b) by changing the axis 90 degrees
    c) by changing the axis 360 degrees
    d) by changing the axis 45 degrees

18. **The proper position of glasses on the manual lensometer is:**
    a) bottom edge of frame against the frame stage, temples facing away
    b) top edge of frame against the frame stage, temples facing away
    c) bottom edge of frame against the frame stage, temples facing toward you
    d) top edge of frame against the frame stage, temples facing toward you

19. **When beginning to read the right lens, the first step is to:**
    a) try to center the target by moving the stage
    b) move the stage so the target is in the uppermost part of the field
    c) move the stage so the target is in the lower part of the field
    d) change the eye piece again to refocus

20. **Which target is analyzed first?**
    a) the instrument makes this selection
    b) the circular mires
    c) the wide/triple lines
    d) the narrow/single lines

21. **If all the lines of the lensometer target clear at the same time, the lens is:**
    a) monocentric
    b) spherical
    c) cylindrical
    d) spherocylindrical

22. **If the narrow/single line and wide/triple lines of the lensometer target do not clear at the same time, the lens is:**
    a) bicentric
    b) spherical
    c) plano
    d) spherocylindrical

23. **If the lens is determined to be spherocylindrical, one can deduce that the patient has:**
    a) myopia
    b) hyperopia
    c) astigmatism
    d) presbyopia

24. **You are reading the right lens, and the narrow lines appear broken. This means you need to adjust the:**
    a) eye piece
    b) lens table
    c) axis wheel
    d) power wheel

25. **If the narrow/single lines are clear and you wish to read the lens in minus cylinder form, you should:**
    a) turn the power-focusing wheel toward yourself
    b) turn the power-focusing wheel away from yourself
    c) change the axis 90 degrees
    d) focus the triple lines first instead

26. **The narrow/single lines are clear. You wish to read the glasses in plus cylinder. Turning the power wheel toward yourself does not bring the wide/triple lines into focus. What should you do?**
    a) read the lenses in minus cylinder instead
    b) subtract the reading for the narrow/single lines from the reading for the wide/triple lines
    c) add the reading for the narrow/single lines to the reading for the wide/triple lines
    d) rotate the axis 90 degrees

27. **You have taken the following lensometer reading: The narrow/single line clears at –2.00. The wide/triple lines clear at –3.00. Axis is on 083. The prescription is:**
   a) –2.00 – 3.00 × 083
   b) –2.00 – 1.00 × 083
   c) –2.00 – 1.00 × 173
   d) –3.00 + 1.00 × 083

28. **You have taken the following lensometer reading: The narrow/single line clears at +6.25. The wide/triple lines clear at +8.00. Axis is on 132. The prescription is:**
   a) +8.00 – 6.28 × 042
   b) +6.25 + 8.00 × 132
   c) +6.25 + 1.75 × 042
   d) +6.25 + 1.75 × 132

29. **You have taken the following lensometer reading: The narrow/single line clears at –1.50. The wide/triple lines clear at +1.25. The axis is on 097. The prescription is:**
   a) –1.50 + 1.25 × 097
   b) –1.50 + 2.75 × 007
   c) –1.50 + 2.75 × 097
   d) –0.25 – 1.25 × 097

30. **You have taken the following lensometer reading: The narrow/single line clears at +2.25. The wide/triple lines clear at –0.25. The axis is on 178. The prescription is:**
   a) +2.25 – 0.25 × 178
   b) +2.00 – 0.25 × 178
   c) –0.25 + 2.50 × 088
   d) +2.25 – 2.50 × 088

31. **You have centered and read the distant portion of the right lens of a pair of bifocals. What is the next step?**
   a) move the stage up to read the bifocal segment
   b) switch to the left lens, center, and read its distant portion
   c) switch to the left lens and note the position of the target
   d) turn the glasses over and read the front power of the right lens

32. **To read the power of bifocal or trifocal segments, you should:**
   a) move the frame table upward until the segment mires appear in the center
   b) slide the glasses down until the segment mires appear in the center
   c) slide the glasses up and hold them there by hand
   d) always turn the glasses around to read the back of the lens

33. **The power of a bifocal will be the difference between:**
   a) the axes of the distant and bifocal portions of the lens
   b) the point where the wide lines clear on the distant part of the lens and where the thin lines clear on the bifocal
   c) the point where the narrow/single lines clear on the distant part of the lens and where they clear on the bifocal
   d) the point where the narrow/single lines clear on the distant part of the lens and where the wide lines clear on the bifocal

34. The distance portion of the lens prescription is –1.25 sphere. You are now reading the bifocal add, and the lensometer dial reads +1.50. The add should be recorded as:
     a) +1.50
     b) +0.25
     c) +0.75
     d) +2.75

35. The distant portion of the lens prescription is +1.25 (narrow/single lines) – 1.25 (wide/triple lines) × 180. You are now reading the bifocal add, and the narrow lines clear at +3.00. The add should be recorded as:
     a) +3.00
     b) plano
     c) +1.75
     d) +4.25

36. The distance portion of the lens is –2.00 + 2.00 × 072. You are now reading the bifocal add, and the wide lines clear at +3.00. The add is:
     a) plano
     b) +1.00
     c) +2.00
     d) +3.00

37. The best method for reading the add on a no-line progressive lens using a manual lensometer is to:
     a) mark the lens first using the template from that manufacturer
     b) use the least plus reading for the distance and the most plus reading for the add
     c) take the distant lensometry reading at a point between the laser marks on the lens
     d) center the target in the lensometer

38. To read the bifocal portion of an aphakic spectacle lens:
     a) the distance and bifocal spherical power should be read with the temples toward the technician
     b) the distance and bifocal spherical power should be read with the temples away from the technician
     c) one need only read the distance spherical power, because all aphakic lenses have a +3.50 add
     d) one must adjust the eye piece to compensate for the high amount of plus power

39. Regarding the power of the midlevel trifocal lens segment:
     a) it is impossible to read the power on the lensometer
     b) it is always half the power of the bifocal
     c) it is always twice the power of the bifocal
     d) it can be read using the lensometer

40. Lenses that are not correctly centered on the visual axis result in:
     a) off-axis prescriptions
     b) extra edge thickness
     c) unwanted prism
     d) accurate prescriptions

41. **Prism diopters are measured using a lensometer by:**
    a) the rings in the reticle
    b) the number of lines in the target
    c) the position of the target
    d) the position of the glasses on the stage

42. **Prism direction is indicated in the lensometer by:**
    a) the rings in the reticle
    b) the number of lines in the target
    c) the position of the target
    d) the position of the glasses on the stage

43. **If the target *can* be centered in the lensometer, how does one determine whether or not there is induced prism due to decentration?**
    a) by marking the centers
    b) by marking the centers and measuring the distance between them
    c) by marking the centers and observing the glasses on the patient
    d) decentered lenses cannot be centered in the lensometer

44. **The target of the right lens is displaced to the right, and the lines cross at the third ring. The prism power and direction is:**
    a) 3 prism diopters base-out
    b) 3 prism diopters base-in
    c) 1.5 prism diopters base-out
    d) 1.5 prism diopters base-in

45. **The target of the left lens is displaced to the right, and the lines cross between the first and second rings. The prism power and direction is:**
    a) 1 prism diopter base-in
    b) 2 prism diopters base-out
    c) 1.5 prism diopters base-in
    d) 1.5 prism diopters base-out

46. **Base-out prism is induced when:**
    a) the optical center separation is greater than the pupillary distance with minus lenses
    b) the optical center separation is less than the pupillary distance with minus lenses
    c) the optical center separation is less than the pupillary distance with plus lenses
    d) the optical separation is offset vertically with plus or minus lenses

47. **To check a manual lensometer for accuracy:**
    a) adjust the eye piece then read a trial lens
    b) set the target lines for your refractive error, then see if they are clear
    c) set the eye piece at zero, then read a trial lens
    d) set the eye piece at zero, and see if the target lines clear at plano

48. **All of the following pertain to maintenance of a manual lensometer *except*:**
    a) reset the eye piece to zero after each use
    b) turn off the instrument when not being used
    c) cover the instrument when not in use
    d) do not put too much ink on the ink pad

Explanatory Answers

1. c) By convention, a lens prescription is written sphere power, cylinder power, cylinder axis. (By the way, there is no such thing as sphere axis!)

2. b) See answer 1.

3. c) The second number in the prescription (1.50) is the cylinder power, and it is written as plus.

4. a) The prescription is written as a trifocal. The 1.25 will be the trifocal (intermediate distance), and the 2.50 will be the bifocal (closest distance). In the case of a trifocal, one might speak of the add as being 1.25/2.50, but not refer to the 1.25 alone as being the add.

5. a) While any of the prescriptions might earn a phone call from the optician to verify the numbers, the first one would undoubtedly earn a phone query because of the axis. There is no axis at 181; the axis designation goes from 001 to 180 and not beyond.

6. c) An automated lensometer can be set to read in plus or minus cylinder.

7. b) The most modern automated lensometers make reading a progressive add lens a snap. Fresnel prism is obvious without a lensometer because of the ridges on the lens. Lens material and polarized lenses are not detected with any lensometer.

8. d) The automated lensometer is not very useful in identifying a warped lens. Characteristics of the lens itself (aside from the numerical measurements) are better identified with a manual lensometer.

9. a) Because you can set the automatic lensometer for plus or minus cylinder, any math errors in transposition are eliminated, as are errors in reading the numbers off the wheel of a manual lensometer and figuring the cylinder power, axis, and add power. No lensometer can do the tasks in answers b, c, and d.

10. c) The housing should not be removed by anyone except qualified service personnel. To reduce dust exposure, cover the instrument when not in use.

11. Labeling:

axis wheel	e)	frame stage	d)
eye piece	a)	lens holder	b)
lens stop	c)	power wheel	g)
table control lever	f)		

12. d) Before you can read glasses accurately, you must first adjust the eye piece.

13. a) If you wear glasses or contact lenses during the work day, you should have them on (or in) when you adjust the eye piece.

14. b) The eye piece should be rotated to its most plus position. (Minus will trigger your accommodative reflex.)

15. b) Stop turning the eye piece when the target first becomes clear. If you continue to turn it, you will add unneeded minus, and your own accommodation will interfere.

16. d) If you do not adjust the eye piece, you may get inaccurate readings.

17. b) You can read any lens in plus or minus form by rotating the axis by 90 degrees.

18. a) Glasses are placed on the frame table with the bottom toward you, and against the frame stage, and the temples pointing away.

19. a) The first step in reading lenses is to attempt to center the target.

20. d) The narrow/single lines are cleared first. *Note:* While different brands of lensmeters may have different targets, this text is using narrow/single and wide/triple target lines.

21. b) In a spherical lens, the target lines will all clear together.
22. d) In a spherocylindrical lens, the narrow/single and wide/triple lines do not clear together.
23. c) Cylinder is used to correct astigmatism. (*Spherocylindrical* means the lens has sphere combined with cylinder.)
24. c) If the lines appear broken, the axis needs to be aligned. Turn the axis wheel until the lines are solid.
25. b) If you want the reading in minus power, you should turn the wheel away from yourself after clearing the narrow/single lines, in order to clear the wide/triple lines.
26. d) If you want to read a lens in plus cylinder, after clearing the narrow/single lines, you need to be able to clear the triple/wide lines by turning the power wheel toward yourself. If you cannot do this, rotate the axis by 90 degrees and start again by clearing the narrow/single lines.
27. b) The single line clears at –2.00, so the spherical power is –2.00. There is a –1.00 step between –2.00 and –3.00, so the cylinder power is –1.00. The axis is given as 083. Thus, the prescription is –2.00 – 1.00 × 083.
28. d) The single line clears at +6.25, which is your sphere power. There is a +1.75 step between +6.25 and + 8.00 so the cylinder power is +1.75. The axis is given as 132. The prescription is +6.25 + 1.75 × 132.
29. c) The single line clears at –1.50, which is your spherical power. There is a +2.75 step from –1.50 to +1.25 so the cylinder power is +2.75. The axis is given as 097. The prescription is –1.50 + 2.75 × 097.
30. c) The single line clears at +2.25, which is your spherical power. There is a –2.50 step from +2.25 to –0.25, making this the cylinder power. The axis is given as 178. The prescription is +2.25 – 2.50 × 178. However, this is not given as an answer, which is your cue to transpose.[2] Add the sphere and cylinder powers together algebraically: +2.25 + (–2.50) = –0.25, your spherical power. Change the sign on the cylinder power: + 2.50. Rotate the axis by 90 degrees (178 – 90): 088. The answer is –0.25 + 2.50 × 088.
31. c) It is very important to go from distant, right lens, to distant, left lens, without moving the stage. Otherwise, you could miss induced vertical prism.
32. a) To read the segments, move the frame table up. This will stabilize the lenses in proper alignment (versus moving the glasses up without using the frame table). Sliding the glasses up and holding them there can introduce error.
33. c) The bifocal power is the difference between the reading where the narrow/single lines clear on the lens' distant portion and where they clear on the lens' bifocal (or bottom segment of a trifocal). Alternately, it is *also* the difference between the reading where the *wide/triple* lines clear on the lens' distant portion and where *they* clear on the lens' bifocal (or bottom segment of a trifocal). This works because the proportions are the same in both the distant and near parts of the lens. The main thing is to use the same lines (eg, both narrow or both wide) when moving from the distant to the near part of the lens.[3] For example, in the distant lens reading, narrow lines clear at +1.00 and wide lines clear at +2.00 × 180. In the bifocal reading, if the narrow lines clear at +3.00, the wide lines will clear at +4.00, keeping that 1.00 diopter of cylinder.

[2]See Chapter 15, Spectacle Skills for more on transposition.
[3]Of note, Stein, Stein, and Freeman, in *The Ophthalmic Assistant, 8th edition,* mention clearing the *triple/wide* lines of distant and add portions of the lens to get the add power. In Cassin's *Fundamentals for Ophthalmic Technical Personnel*, clearing the *single/narrow* lines is used.

34. d) It may be helpful to remember that the power wheel is actually a number line. Each mark on the wheel represents 0.25 D. Ask yourself: how many lines/units did I move to get from −1.25 to +1.50? The answer is 11 lines; 11 × 0.25 = +2.75.

35. c) The difference between 3.00 and 1.25 is 1.75. (How many lines from +1.25 to +3.00? The answer is 7 lines; 7 × 0.25 = +1.75.)

36. d) This time you were asked to analyze the add by using the wide lines. For the distance portion of the lens, the wide lines would have cleared at plano. (You started at −2.00 with the thin lines clear, then turned the wheel toward you; the wide lines cleared at plano, which gave you the cylinder power of +2.00.) When reading the bifocal, the thin lines would clear at +1.00 and the wide lines at +3.00. Because you are using the wide lines, the add would be the difference between plano and +3.00, which is +3.00.

37. a) Most companies who manufacture no-line progressives have a template for their lens. The lens is laid on the template, and a wax pencil is used to trace the markings onto the lens. A circle indicates where the reading should be taken.

38. a) To accurately read the add on an aphakic lens, you should read the distant and add sphere power on the back of the lens. (Of course, when *recording* the distant portion, you should read the lens front, as usual; you only turn the lens over when calculating the add power.) Some authors recommend reading the add power on every lens by reading the back of the lens (ie, temples toward you).[4] Others apply this technique only to lenses over +3.00 in the distant portion.

39. d) Even though the middle portion of *most* trifocals is half the add power, it's not always so. The lens can be read on a lensometer. (Note the mention of a segment, which lets you know that this is not a progressive add lens.)

40. c) Unwanted prism results when lenses are not aligned with the visual axis. (*Note:* The visual axis is the "line" from the fovea, through the pupil, to the object of regard, not to be confused with the axis of astigmatism.)

41. a) Prism diopters are indicated by the rings in the reticle of the lensometer, with each ring representing one prism diopter. The target position tells you the direction of the base. (Yes, that was rather tricky.)

42. c) See answer 41.

43. c) Looking at the marked lenses on the patient will show if there is induced prism because the centers of the lenses will not line up with the patient's visual axis. Or, measure the distance between the lens centers and then compare this number to the patient's pupillary distance (not given as an option on this question). A decentered lens can often be centered in the lensometer. (A lens with ground-in prism cannot.)

44. b) Because the lines cross at the third ring, you know there are 3 prism diopters. An image displaced to the right in the right lens is displaced nasally, so the base is in.

45. d) Because the lines cross between the first and second rings, there are 1.5 prism diopters. An image displaced to the right in the left lens is displaced temporally, so the base is out.

46. b) This one is tough. Remember that a minus lens is made up of prisms aligned apex-to-apex. If the pupillary distance is wider than the optical center separation, this would place the visual axis temporal to the centers (Figure 5-2). Hence, base-out.

---

[4]Borover WA. *Opticianry: The Practice and the Art*, Vol 1. Chula Vista, CA: Gracie Enterprises, Inc; 1981. Frames 367 to 383 of his excellent programmed text.

Figure 5-2. Schematic showing a minus lens (ie, apex-to-apex prisms) with visual axis decentered out, inducing base-out prism.

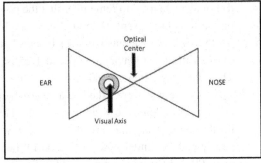

47.   a) An accurate lensometer should read a trial lens exactly. Be sure to adjust the eye piece first, however.

48.   a) It might be convenient for the next user if you set the eye piece to zero, but it makes no difference in the maintenance of the instrument. Be sure to read all questions carefully!

Chapter 6

Keratometry

Ledford JK.
*Certified Ophthalmic Assistant: Exam
Review Manual, Third Edition* (pp. 65-74).
© 2012 Taylor & Francis Group.

Corneal Curvature

1.   **The structure of the eye with the most refractive power is the:**
    a) lens
    b) cornea
    c) vitreous/aqueous
    d) retina

2.   **Corneal curvature is measured (quantified) using the:**
    a) Placido's disk
    b) slit lamp
    c) vertexometer
    d) keratometer

3.   **Corneal curvature can be recorded as:**
    a) millimeters/diopters
    b) milliliters/diopters
    c) millimeters/cylinder
    d) centimeters/decibels

4.   **Unequal corneal curvature where the flattest and steepest curves are 90 degrees apart is known as:**
    a) myopia
    b) presbyopia
    c) astigmatism
    d) hyperopia

5.   **The average power of the human cornea is:**
    a) 30 to 32 D
    b) 35 to 36 D
    c) 43 to 44 D
    d) 45 to 47 D

6.   **Average thickness of the central cornea is:**
    a) 0.8 mm
    b) 0.5 mm
    c) 0.2 mm
    d) 1.0 cm

7.   **The following prescription, Plano – 2.00 × 180, is an example of:**
    a) with-the-rule astigmatism
    b) against-the-rule astigmatism
    c) oblique astigmatism
    d) irregular astigmatism

8. **Which of the following is an example of oblique astigmatism?**
    a) -2.00 + 1.25 × 093
    b) -0.75 - 1.25 × 003
    c) -4.25 + 2.75 × 046
    d) Plano

9. **If the axes of astigmatism are *not* 90 degrees from each other, this is termed:**
    a) irregular astigmatism
    b) compound astigmatism
    c) dry eye syndrome
    d) astigmatism of vitreous face

10. **Of the following, which patient is *most* likely to have irregular astigmatism?**
    a) postoperative cataract
    b) aphakic
    c) surface ocular trauma
    d) postoperative LASIK

11. **The steepest part of the cornea is the:**
    a) periphery
    b) inferior one-fourth
    c) stroma
    d) center

12. **The diameter of the cornea's optic zone, or cap, measures:**
    a) 4.0 mm
    b) 0.5 mm
    c) 20 mm
    d) 3.06 μm

Keratometry[1]

13. **Manual keratometry would *not* be the most appropriate method for reliable measurements in which of the following cases?**
    a) fitting contact lenses
    b) monitoring keratoconus
    c) calculating intraocular lens (IOL) power
    d) evaluating after cataract surgery

14. **Keratometry would be useful in evaluating all of the following *except*:**
    a) keratoconus
    b) preoperative cataract surgery
    c) contact lens fitting
    d) corneal ulcer

[1]Originally the term *keratometer* was a trade name but has fallen into common use. The generic name of the instrument is ophthalmometer.

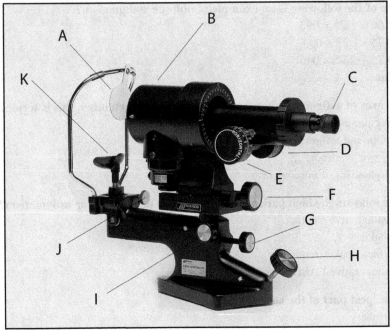

Figure 6-1. Reprinted with permission of Marco.

15. **Label the parts of the keratometer[2]:**

barrel	lock	vertical barrel adjustment
chin rest	occluder	vertical mires adjustment
chin rest adjustment	eye piece	horizontal mires adjustment
focus adjustment	forehead adjustment	

16. **Number the following steps of using a keratometer in chronological order:**

____occlude the eye not being tested

____turn the drum so that the horizontal plus signs are aligned exactly tip-to-tip

____turn the dials to superimpose the horizontal plus and vertical minus signs

____position the patient

____focus the mires, and center the cross-hairs in the lower right hand circle

____focus the eye piece

17. **Occluding the eye not being measured is helpful because it:**

a) reduces reflections

b) aids in fixation

c) eliminates lenticular astigmatism

d) reduces irregular astigmatism

[2]While keratometry itself is listed as a criterion only on the COT® and COMT® levels, my JCAHPO® VOW said that a COA® candidate would be expected to know how to use the instrument.

18.   **You are attempting a K reading and do not see both horizontal plus signs. This might be due to:**
   a) a drooped upper lid
   b) the patient closing his or her eye
   c) a keratometer occluder in the way
   d) improper focusing

19.   **Matching. Select one best answer:**

Probable condition	Keratometer mires appear
flat cornea	a) small
corneal warpage	b) round
keratoconus	c) elliptical
spherical cornea	d) very large
steep cornea	e) clear, then quickly blur
dry eye	f) wavy, blurred, discontinuous
astigmatism	g) distorted, small, cannot superimpose

20.   **If the cross-hairs of the keratometer are not centered during the initial reading for contact lens fitting:**
   a) the fit may be inaccurate
   b) lens diameter may be incorrect
   c) lenses will be difficult to handle
   d) the lens will not transmit oxygen

21.   **K readings in a contact lens-wearing patient may be used to evaluate all of the following *except*:**
   a) progressive corneal steepening
   b) lens fit
   c) lens coverage
   d) corneal warpage

22.   **The patient's keratometry mires are very oval-shaped. This means that there is:**
   a) no astigmatism
   b) high emmetropia
   c) significant astigmatism
   d) inaccurate alignment

23.   **The patient's keratometry mires are squiggly looking and change when the patient blinks. You should try:**
   a) instilling topical anesthetic
   b) instilling artificial tears
   c) re-explaining the procedure
   d) realigning the patient

24.   **No matter how you rotate the keratometer drum, the "plus signs" remain aligned. This indicates that there is:**
   a) irregular astigmatism
   b) poor tear film
   c) poorly focused eye piece
   d) no astigmatism

25. Which of the following types of astigmatism is *not* obvious when measuring with the keratometer?
    a) astigmatism at 180 degrees
    b) irregular astigmatism
    c) lenticular astigmatism
    d) oblique astigmatism

26. You are taking a K reading. The power drum is at 52.00 D (the upper limit of the scale), and the mires are still not aligned. To extend the range of the keratometer, you should:
    a) affix a –1.00 D trial lens over the aperture
    b) affix a +1.25 D trial lens over the aperture
    c) affix a +2.25 D trial lens over the eye piece
    d) it is not possible to extend the range of a keratometer

27. You have taken a K reading by extending the instrument's range. To get the correct value, you can:
    a) use a conversion chart
    b) subtract the power of the extending lens
    c) add the power of the extending lens
    d) simply record the drum reading

28. You are adjusting the keratometer eye piece by looking at the occluder through the ocular. The mires are distorted. You should:
    a) calibrate with metal balls
    b) spray cleaner into the instrument
    c) clean the instrument with compressed air
    d) return to the manufacturer for cleaning

29. When calibrating the keratometer with the metal balls, all of the following are done *except*:
    a) using chrome balls of known radius
    b) placing holder on the headrest
    c) setting the eye piece for your refractive error
    d) placing the chrome ball in the holder with your fingers

30. If calibration of the keratometer reveals a discrepancy:
    a) adjust the drums
    b) tighten the headrest
    c) loosen the top screw
    d) have the manufacturer repair it

31. If the keratometer's occluder is loose:
    a) simply remove it
    b) rebend or replace the washer
    c) tape it up out of the way
    d) adjust the headrest appropriately

Explanatory Answers

1.   b) While the lens, cornea, and vitreous/aqueous each have refractive power, and in spite of the fact that the lens can adjust and focus, the cornea is the strongest refracting structure of the eye.

2.   d) The keratometer is the only device listed that measures corneal curvature. Placido's disk is used to evaluate corneal shape and topography, but it does not give a measurement. The vertexometer is used to measure vertex distance, the distance between a corrective lens and the front surface of the cornea.

3.   a) Corneal curvature can be designated in both millimeters and diopters. (Did you notice that answer b was in microliters?)

4.   c) Astigmatism occurs when the cornea is more curved in one direction and less in the other. Think of the back of a spoon or the surface of an eggshell; these curves are almost always 90 degrees from each other.

5.   c) The average refractive power of the cornea is 43 to 44 D.

6.   b) The average thickness of the central cornea is 0.5 mm. (***Note:*** Be sure to pay attention to measurement designations: Answer d was in centimeters.)

7.   a) In with-the-rule astigmatism, the strongest corneal axis is vertical; this translates to approximately 180 degrees in minus cylinder and approximately 90 degrees in plus cylinder. Against-the-rule astigmatism is the opposite, with the strongest corneal axis in the horizontal, approximately 90 degrees in minus cylinder and approximately 180 degrees in plus. Irregular astigmatism does not have a single axis because the flattest and steepest meridians are not at 90 degree angles from each other.

8.   c) Oblique astigmatism means the axes are not vertical (eg, 093) or horizontal (eg, 003), but at an angle in between (eg, 046). Note that the axes do not have to be "on the dot" at 90, 180, 45, or 135 to qualify.

9.   a) Irregular astigmatism occurs when the steepest and flattest curves are not 90 degrees from each other. Compound astigmatism is a type of regular astigmatism. Answer d is bogus.

10.   c) The most common cause of irregular astigmatism is trauma to the ocular surface. While ocular surgery can cause irregular astigmatism, it is not the most likely of those listed.

11.   d) The cornea is steepest in the center, then flattens out toward the periphery. (Remember, the *stroma* is a layer of the corneal tissue.)

12.   a) By definition, the corneal cap or optic zone is the central 4.0 mm of the cornea. (Did you notice that answer d was in micrometers?)

13.   b) This was a tough one; did you catch the phrase "most appropriate"? Because the keratometer evaluates only a tiny section of the cornea (3 mm), it would be more accurate to follow keratoconus using corneal topography. This is not to say that one cannot use manual keratometry in this case, but the question asked for "most appropriate."

14.   d) The keratometer is definitely useful in measuring the curvature of the central cornea for contact lens fitting and IOL calculations. Keratoconus is better followed by corneal topography although one can use the keratometer. The best answer is d, corneal ulcer, which would cause irregular keratometry mires and is best evaluated at the slit lamp.

15.   Labeling:
barrel	b)
chin rest	k)
chin rest adjustment	g)
eye piece	c)
focus adjustment	f)
forehead adjustment	j)
horizontal mires adjustment	e)
lock	i)
occluder	a)
vertical barrel adjustment	h)
vertical mires adjustment	d)

16.   Order:

      <u>3</u> occlude the eye not being tested

      <u>5</u> turn the drum so that the horizontal plus signs are aligned exactly tip-to-tip

      <u>6</u> turn the dials to superimpose the horizontal plus and vertical minus signs

      <u>2</u> position the patient

      <u>4</u> focus the mires and center the cross-hairs in the lower right hand circle

      <u>1</u> focus the eye piece

      (*Note:* Steps 5 and 6 may be reversed, but most examiners prefer to set the axis before completing alignment. In addition, some keratometers have plus sign mires at both horizontal AND vertical, rather than plus at horizontal and minus at vertical.)

17.   b) The occluder forces the patient to fixate with the eye being measured. This helps hold that eye steady for an accurate reading.

18.   c) The plus sign is projected on the side, and the main thing that might obstruct the mires from the side is the occluder on the keratometer. A common vertical obstruction (which would obstruct the minus signs) is the patient's upper lid.

19.   Matching:
flat cornea	d) very large
corneal warpage	f) wavy, blurred, discontinuous
keratoconus	g) distorted, small, cannot superimpose
spherical cornea	b) round
steep cornea	a) small
dry eye	e) clear, then quickly blur
astigmatism	c) elliptical

20.   a) If the cross-hairs are not centered, you are not reading the corneal apex. Because the corneal periphery is flatter, the resulting fit will be too loose when placed on the steeper corneal apex.

21.   c) The keratometer can be used to evaluate corneal steepening by taking a series of readings over time. Corneal warpage is evident by distorted mires. By using the keratometer to look at a patient while actually wearing his or her contacts, the fit can be evaluated by the appearance of the mires and whether they clear/blur before or after a blink. (Of course, a slit-lamp exam is still required to complete the evaluation.) Lens coverage of the cornea is evaluated at the slit lamp, not with the keratometer.

22. c) Oval mires indicate the presence of significant astigmatism. Actually, this makes the reading easier, as even a tiny turn of barrel or dial makes an obvious difference. An eye with no astigmatism would have very round mires. Emmetropia is lack of refractive error, so it cannot be classified as high, low, or in between. Inaccurate alignment is evident when the cross-hair is not centered in the lower right circle.

23. b) "Squiggly" mires that change when the patient blinks indicate a problem with the tear film. Instill some artificial tears, have the patient blink a lot, and blot gently with a tissue. Then, try the readings again. There is no need to use an anesthetic.

24. d) If the corneal surface is spherical (ie, no astigmatism), the "plus signs" will stay aligned no matter where the barrel is positioned, because the curve is the same in every meridian.

25. c) Answers a and d are evident by the axis readings on the keratometer. Irregular astigmatism can be detected by the fact that the sections of the mires do not focus together, and there seems to be several "axes," although a measurement is not possible. Lenticular astigmatism is caused by the crystalline lens, which is not detected with the keratometer, but rather by noting a difference in the amount of astigmatism found on keratometry and that found on refractometry.

26. b) If the keratometer reading is past the upper range (52.00 D), affix a +1.25 D trial lens to the aperture. (If the reading is below the lower range, then a -1.00 D trial lens is used.)

27. a) If a trial lens is used to extend the range of the keratometer, the new reading is most conveniently interpreted using a conversion chart. If you are aching to do the math and you have extended the range upward, multiply the reading by 1.1659. If you have extended the range downward, divide by 1.1659.

28. d) Distorted mires are caused by problems with the internal filters and lenses. Only the manufacturer can handle that.

29. d) Do not handle the chrome balls with your fingers. Use a tissue or magnet. Oils from the fingers can cause the chrome to corrode, changing the readings.

30. d) If you test the keratometer and the readings are not true, the manufacturer will have to repair it.

31. b) A loose occluder can be rebent, or you can replace the washer. It is important to use the occluder, however, because it helps keeps the eye centered for the reading.

Chapter 7

Medical Ethics, Legal, and Regulatory Issues

Ledford JK.
Certified Ophthalmic Assistant: Exam
Review Manual, Third Edition (pp. 75-86).
© 2012 Taylor & Francis Group.

Third-Party Coding

1.   **Current procedural terminology (CPT) codes are used to:**
     a) communicate between providers
     b) communicate with insurance companies
     c) provide legal documentation
     d) inform patients regarding their health care

2.   **CPT has a direct impact on:**
     a) clinical certification
     b) presenting evidence in court
     c) patient feedback
     d) reimbursement

3.   **A procedure might carry a different charge, depending on who performs it. This may mean that the procedure code needs an additional code called a(n):**
     a) service number
     b) qualifier
     c) modifier
     d) HIPAA code

4.   **The International Classification of Diseases (ICD) codes of *nuclear cataract 366.16* and *astigmatism 367.21* are examples of:**
     a) AMA codes
     b) procedure codes
     c) diagnosis codes
     d) encounter codes

5.   **A reviewer is looking over an encounter form for a patient visit to your practice to make sure that diagnosis codes and procedure codes match up. Which of the following would be marked as unacceptable?**
     a) CPT: incise and drain ICD: chalazion
     b) CPT: epilation ICD: trichiasis
     c) CPT: probe and irrigation ICD: cataract
     d) CPT: biopsy ICD: lesion of the eyelid

Government and Institutional Rules and Regulations[1]

6.   **A patient who had a blepharoplasty is upset because now she has dry eyes. The court determined that the patient was not told about this risk prior to surgery. This is an example of:**
     a) failure to disclose
     b) breach of promise
     c) failure to perform
     d) intentional harm

[1]See also sections *Ethical and Legal Standards*, *Confidentiality*, and *Informed Consent* in this chapter.

7. **A patient who is moving to another state has stopped by the office requesting his records. He would like you to hand over the chart so he can take it with him. Your response to this is to:**
    a) make copies for the office and give him the original
    b) tell the patient you will mail the original to his new provider
    c) give the patient lab work reports from his chart
    d) make copies for the patient and keep the original for the office

8. **Which of the following is a legal regulation?**
    a) An eye care practitioner must fit any patient who desires it with contact lenses.
    b) The patient who has a refractive eye exam must be provided with a copy of the glasses prescription.
    c) A prescription for glasses is only good for 6 months.
    d) K readings must be included on every glasses prescription in case the patient decides to get contact lenses.

9. **An ophthalmic assistant who measures a patient's refractive error and then writes the patient a glasses prescription, where the physician does not see the patient or review the record, is:**
    a) breaking the law
    b) violating patient privacy
    c) doing the patient a favor
    d) in accordance with current practice

10. **The right of a patient to protection of his or her personal health information is a federal law known as:**
    a) Health Insurance Portability and Accountability Act (HIPAA)
    b) Occupational Safety and Health Administration (OSHA)
    c) Joint Commission on Accreditation of Health Care Organizations (JCAHO)
    d) American Academy of Ophthalmology (AAO)

11. **OSHA has developed laws regarding:**
    a) standards for safety lenses
    b) eye protection in the workplace
    c) privacy laws
    d) scope of practice

12. **Which of the following is *true*?**
    a) An eye care practitioner may charge a fee to release a patient's glasses prescription.
    b) An eye care practitioner may restrict eye exams only to those who agree to purchase eyewear from the practice's optical shop.
    c) An eye care practitioner may refuse to release a patient's glasses prescription until the patient has paid for the eye exam, if it is customary to require payment at the time of service.
    d) An eye care practitioner who has fit a patient for contacts may require that the patient buy the first year's supply of lenses from the practitioner's practice.

13. **The Federal Trade Commission (FTC) has regulations affecting all of the following** *except*:
    a) the "intraocular lens implant rule"
    b) advertising for refractive surgery
    c) the "eyeglass rule"
    d) the "contact lens rule"

14. **OSHA regulations regarding medical practices require all of the following** *except*:
    a) every new hire is to be trained in infection control practices
    b) all contact lenses must be fit by a licensed eye care practitioner
    c) the employer must provide personal protective equipment to employees
    d) OSHA regulations must be posted in the workplace

15. **The "Red Flags Rule" was developed by the FTC in order to prevent:**
    a) employee injuries
    b) identity theft
    c) insurance fraud
    d) sexual harassment in the workplace

16. **All the following are** *true* **regarding the Patient Protection and Affordable Care Act (PPACA)** *except*:
    a) It affects insurance coverage for pre-existing conditions.
    b) It is concerned with health insurance reform.
    c) It enforces health care privacy laws.
    d) It was signed into law by President Barack Obama.

Quality Assurance[2]

17. **Quality assurance (QA) depends upon:**
    a) opinions of caregivers
    b) patient compliance
    c) being able to measure something
    d) having favorable surgical results

18. **Which of the following does** *not* **apply to QA?**
    a) One characteristic of QA is to minimize problems and poor outcomes.
    b) One characteristic of QA is to identify procedures that need to be changed.
    c) One characteristic of QA is to be a once-and-done procedure.
    d) One characteristic of QA is that it can lead to better patient care.

19. **An example of data collected for QA purposes regarding outcomes would be:**
    a) employee turnover
    b) visual acuity after cataract surgery
    c) number of patients seen daily
    d) number of referral patients

[2]See also questions 29 through 32 regarding ANSI standards.

20. **Which of the following is *true*?**
    a) QA is the responsibility only of the practitioner.
    b) QA helps hold health care workers accountable.
    c) QA is only an issue if the practice is to be inspected.
    d) QA is not concerned with access to health care.

21. **Your practice is developing a QA program. One area to be addressed is strabismus surgery. Which of the following would *not* fit into the list of the logical assessments?**
    a) preoperative and postoperative prism measurements of the deviation
    b) patient or parental survey of satisfaction with the process as a whole
    c) data concerning postoperative complications
    d) putting strategies into place that will prevent alterations to the process

Ethical and Legal Standards[3]

22. **The standards that govern moral conduct, especially of a person/group with some type of power in issues regarding conduct, rights, and actions is:**
    a) informed consent
    b) patient rights
    c) ethics
    d) medicolegal code

23. **The basis for medical ethics is:**
    a) The Oath of Hammurabi
    b) The Hippocratic Oath
    c) The Mayflower Compact
    d) The Constitution of the United States

24. **You have just seated your patient and ask if she's having any problems with her eyes. She states that she would like to discuss that only with the physician. You explain your role in gathering information and assure her of confidentiality, but she insists that she will speak only to the doctor. You should:**
    a) explain that it is office policy that she speak to you first
    b) offer to appoint her for another day when she may feel more cooperative
    c) affirm her right to speak only to the physician and acquiesce
    d) recommend that the physician dismiss her from the practice

25. **The physician is out of the office, and a patient comes by on his way to an optical shop. He has broken his glasses and asks you to "test me for glasses" and give him a new, updated prescription to take to the optician. For you, as an ophthalmic assistant, this is a question of:**
    a) patient rights
    b) scope of practice
    c) confidentiality
    d) moral obligation

[3]See also sections *Confidentiality* and *Informed Consent* in this chapter.

26. **Your new patient had cataract surgery at another practice in town 6 months ago and is unhappy with her vision. She states that she was nearsighted before, but now she cannot read anything up close without glasses. Your refractometric measurement of the eye is +3.75 sphere for distance, with a +2.25 add for near. Which of the following is a potentially libelous thing to say?**
    a) "You're the second patient in a month from that practice who has this problem!"
    b) "We'll know more after Dr. Davis looks at you."
    c) "Unfortunately, measuring for the power of an implant is an inexact science."
    d) "Has the surgeon suggested anything that might help?"

27. **Which of the following does *not* carry with it the "duty to report?"**
    a) incompetence
    b) child abuse
    c) data collection
    d) impaired eye care professional

28. **Which of the following is *true* regarding certifications for eye care paraprofessionals?**
    a) Certification is required in order to be employed.
    b) Certification acknowledges that a person has attained specific professional standards.
    c) Certification legally permits the individual to evaluate and interact with patients.
    d) Certification is required in order to perform certain functions, such as refractions.

29. **Compliance with the American National Standards Institute (ANSI) standards is:**
    a) required by federal law
    b) required by state statutes
    c) relative to the type of industry involved
    d) voluntary

30. **Which of the following is *true* regarding the ANSI standards concerning eyeglasses?**
    a) The ANSI standards apply only to prescription eyewear.
    b) The ANSI standards designate allowable variance between the power of the lenses ordered and the lenses dispensed.
    c) The ANSI standards apply to safety lenses, but not to any type of lens coating.
    d) The ANSI standards apply only to safety lenses and frames.

31. **Which of the following is *true* regarding the ANSI standards concerning contact lenses?**
    a) The ANSI standards apply to contact lens materials but not to care products.
    b) The ANSI standards apply to rigid contact lenses, but not to soft contact lenses.
    c) The ANSI standards dictate what information must appear on the contact lens label.
    d) The ANSI standards do not mention disinfection of multiuse trial contact lenses.

32. **Regarding intraocular lens implants, which of the following is *not* covered by the ANSI standards?**
    a) phakic IOLs
    b) optical properties and biocompatibility
    c) sterility and shelf-life
    d) patient selection

Scribing

33. **At its most basic, the duty of a scribe is:**
    a) personal assistant to the practitioner
    b) patient educator and advocate
    c) coding and charting coordinator
    d) patient flow coordinator

34. **Which of the following is *not* a function of scribing?**
    a) documenting what the practitioner tells the patient about his or her diagnosis
    b) writing and signing a prescription for the patient's glaucoma drops
    c) remaining after the physician and teaching the patient how to do lid scrubs
    d) recording exam findings as the doctor dictates them

35. **You are scribing for the physician, and he tells the patient that while he expects her vision to improve, it will not be 20/20 after cataract surgery because of macular degeneration. Which of the following notations *best* illustrates the scribe's function as a witness in this case?**
    a) that cataract surgery has been recommended
    b) that the patient has cataracts and macular degeneration
    c) that the physician told the patient that cataract surgery would improve vision
    d) that the physician explained the effects of macular degeneration on postoperative vision

36. **You are functioning as a scribe in a practice that uses paper charts. At first, the doctor describes a cataract as 3+. You write this in the chart. Later, the physician changes that rating to 2+. Which of the following is the right way to make the correction?**
    a) scratching out the first entry so it cannot be read
    b) using a commercial product that covers errors
    c) completely erasing the first entry
    d) drawing one line through the error and writing the correction above it

Confidentiality

37. **You may discuss a patient's case with another technician if:**
    a) you do so only in front of the patient
    b) it is pertinent to the patient's care
    c) the patient was difficult to handle and you need to unload
    d) the patient has symptoms of communicable disease

38. **It is permissible to ask a patient questions related to his or her health:**
    a) in the reception area, if all the exam rooms are full and you are running behind
    b) in a group if everyone has gathered for the same purpose, such as surgical counseling
    c) in front of someone whom the patient has brought into the exam room
    d) in a multipurpose room where other patients are having tests run

39. **Which of the following is a breach of confidentiality?**
    a) Leaning across the front desk and saying, "Here are your glaucoma drops, Mrs. Smith."
    b) Discussing the exam results of a minor child with a parent over the phone.
    c) Telling the operating room nurse what a surgery patient's drug allergies are.
    d) Telling your boss that the patient has recently lost her spouse and is very upset today.

Informed Consent

40. **Regarding minor surgery and informed consent:**
    a) informed consent is not required if the procedure has minimal risk
    b) informed consent is not required if general anesthesia is not used
    c) informed consent is not required if intravenous injection is not used
    d) informed consent is required prior to any surgical procedure

41. **Each of the following is a key element of informed consent *except*:**
    a) potential risks and benefits
    b) description of procedure
    c) watching a video about the procedure
    d) optional treatments

42. **Which of the following statements regarding informed consent is *true*?**
    a) The physician may have a technician do the patient education.
    b) It only involves having the patient sign papers.
    c) It is necessary only if the patient is a minor.
    d) Only the patient can sign.

43. **You have just finished counseling an alert 87-year-old man who needs cataract surgery, and you ask him to sign the informed consent. "I understand what you've told me," he says, "but I'm just not sure." His 62-year-old daughter has accompanied him and says, "Oh, come on, Dad! Just sign it and let's go!" An appropriate response from you would be:**
    a) "You'll be very happy with your vision after surgery."
    b) "Why don't you discuss this at home and give me a call later?"
    c) "Dr. Snyder thinks this is the best thing for you."
    d) "This is a very common surgery, nothing bad ever happens."

44. **Which of the following is appropriate wording on an informed consent regarding the description of the procedure?**
    a) "The recommended procedure is a lateral rectus recession."
    b) "The recommended procedure is laser trabeculoplasty."
    c) "The recommended procedure is removal of redundant skin from both upper lids."
    d) "The recommended procedure is CE with IOL."

45. **Which of the following is *not* appropriate when explaining the risks of cataract surgery?**

a) "A person is more likely to be in a car accident than to go blind from having a cataract removed."

b) "The risk of developing glaucoma after surgery is so miniscule that you don't have to worry about it."

c) "While very unlikely, you do run a slightly higher risk of retinal detachment because you're so nearsighted."

d) "The chances of developing a severe infection after cataract surgery are less than one-fourth of 1%."

46. **Which of the following would *not* be allowed due to informed consent?**

a) A vitrectomy when vitreous suddenly comes forward during cataract surgery.

b) An unplanned arcuate keratectomy during cataract surgery to reduce the patient's astigmatism.

c) Cryotherapy to seal a scleral hole caused inadvertently during extraocular muscle surgery.

d) Exploratory surgery to locate a "dropped" extraocular muscle during strabismus surgery.

Explanatory Answers

1. b) The purpose of CPT codes is to communicate with insurance companies, or "third-party payers," regarding health care services rendered.

2. d) Coding, be it proper or improper, directly affects the reimbursement that the practice gets from third-party payers.

3. c) Modifiers provide more explicit information about a procedure. Thus, a modifier might be called for when a procedure carries an additional element, such as being performed by a technician or by a mid-level practitioner.

4. c) ICD codes are numeric codes that identify disorders, diseases, conditions, etc. The current edition is 9 (ie, ICD-9), but version 10 is already in use and will eventually be mandatory (ie, ICD-10).

5. c) It is vital that procedure codes have an appropriate diagnosis code to justify them. One would expect a CPT code indicating that a probe and irrigation had been done would be coupled with a diagnosis code of nasolacrimal duct obstruction (or some other associated lacrimal problem).

6. a) "Failure to disclose" occurs when a patient has not been informed about the risks of a particular procedure. This "duty of disclosure" is part of the informed consent process. See the section titled *Informed Consent*.

7. d) The physical chart belongs to the practice; the information belongs to the patient. That means that choices a, b, and c are incorrect. Of course, prior to providing the copies, you must get a signed release of information form. Some clinics have further rules that govern how medical records are to be handled.

8. b) A patient has a right to a copy of the glasses prescription. The expiration of glasses prescriptions varies from state to state, but the minimum will be 1 year.

9. a) The procedure described is a *refraction*, which involves clinical judgment allowed only to a licensed professional. A technician who performs refractions is practicing medicine without a license, which is illegal. Ophthalmic technicians may, however, perform *refractometry*, where the refractive error is measured but the prescribing/clinical judgment is left to the licensed practitioner.

10. a) HIPAA establishes the rights of a patient to protection of his or her health information.

11. b) OSHA deals with employee safety and has rules regarding eye protection in the workplace (such as safety goggles worn when assisting with laser surgery).[4]

12. c) The FTC has determined that if it is customary to ask any patient to pay when services are rendered, then the prescription may be withheld until payment is made.[5] The scenarios in the other answers are strictly forbidden.

13. a) For more information on marketing refractive surgery, see the FTC's *Marketing of Refractive Eye Care Surgery: Guidance for Eye Care Providers.*[6] For more information on the Eyeglass Rule and the Contact Lens Rule, see the FTC's *Q&A: The Contact Lens Rule and the Eyeglass Rule.*[7]

14. b) OSHA does not legislate prescribing or dispensing of medical devices.[8]

15. b) The Red Flags Rule was developed by the FTC in order to detect identity theft. The rule requires businesses (including medical practices) to develop a plan of identifying "relevant patterns, practices, and specific forms of activity—the 'red flags'—that signal possible identity theft."[9]

16. c) PPACA does not deal with health care privacy. The other statements are true.[10]

17. c) QA requires that something be measured, regardless of whether the data come from a patient survey, patient records, checklists, etc.

18. c) The intent of QA is to monitor routine procedures so that problems can be identified and corrected, resulting in better patient care. To be effective, QA is an ongoing process, not something done once to qualify for a certification or to pass an inspection.

19. b) A formal QA program collects data that give an indication of the quality of the service rendered in part by evaluating outcomes. Simply counting the number of patients does not really yield data that reflect quality. But, evaluating the postoperative vision of the practice's cataract surgery patients helps monitor treatment outcome.

20. b) A practice's QA system helps to set minimum standards to which all in the clinic (not just the practitioner) are held. QA is generally focused on outcome (eg, vision after cataract surgery), the relationship of cost to benefit (eg, time, money, and effort put into patient care versus benefit to the patient), and access to care (eg, availability of the services needed by the patient). While a viable QA system may be required for certain clinical certifications, every practice needs to have such a system.

21. d) One of the main goals of QA is to identify problems (which could be revealed by items in answers a, b, and c) and implement the change that is needed to improve outcome.

[4] Available at: www.osha.gov/SLTC/eyefaceprotection/index.html. Accessed 7/30/11.

[5] Available at: www.oaa.org/files/StateRegulatoryInformation/Federal/FEDEyeglassesOne.pdf. Accessed 7/30/11.

[6] Available at: www.ftc.gov/bcp/guides/eyecare2.shtm. Accessed 7/30/11.

[7] Available at: www.ftc.gov/opa/2004/10/BUS63-contactfaq.pdf. Accessed 7/30/11.

[8] Available at: www.ncbi.nlm.nih.gov/pubmed/1469738. Accessed 7/30/11.

[9] "Fighting Fraud with the Red Flags Rule." Available at: www.ftc.gov/bcp/edu/microsites/redflagsrule/index.shtml. Accessed 8/17/11.

[10] Available at: www.oig.dol.gov/public/reports/oa/2011/09-11-003-12-121b.pdf. Accessed 4/15/12.

22. c) Ethics are the standards that govern our personal and professional behavior. In medicine, these are the standards that help us make moral judgments regarding such things as how we treat our patients (both personally and medically), how we treat our peers, what kind of employee we are, and much more. It includes providing the best and most intelligent care of which we are capable and maintaining honest relationships with others.

23. b) Hippocrates lived in the fifth century BC. He was a Greek physician who held himself to a strict code of behavior and quality of care, which included conduct, confidentiality, and scope of practice. From this grew the concept of medical ethics, and the Hippocratic Oath (which speaks to those same virtues) is named after him.

24. c) It is the patient's right to discuss her case with the physician only; be sure to document in the chart that the patient has made this choice. You might ask if you can go ahead and do a "few tests" so that the doctor will have some information when she speaks to the patient, such as visual acuity, lensometry, pupil evaluation, slit-lamp evaluation, and perhaps noncontact tonometry. Without a history, it is inadvisable to instill drops or perform any type of contact test (tonometry, Schirmer's, etc). In addition, while the patient may not wish to discuss his or her eye problems, he or she may be willing to give other information about his or her history.

25. b) "Scope of practice" relates to what you are allowed to do in the performance of your job. Because ophthalmic/optometric technicians are not permitted to "refract" (ie, measure refractive error and then apply clinical judgment to write the prescription), this request would be beyond your scope of practice.

26. a) The comment in answer a suggests that there is a problem with the surgeon, who has made the same mistake twice in just a few weeks. Discussing another doctor, practice, or even someone in your own clinic in a negative fashion is not good ethics...even if they are at fault.

27. c) In QA, data are collected and compared; there is no duty to report. Accusations of a health care worker's incompetence or impairment needs to be evaluated with caution, but evaluated nonetheless. And even the *suspicion* of child abuse must be reported.

28. b) Certification attests to a person's ability to meet a specific professional standard. It is not required in order to work in the field of eye care, but it is a statement to patients, to other professionals, and to the community at large that a person has attained those standards. It is not licensure, a legal instrument that allows the bearer certain privileges. It is not legal for any eye care paraprofessional (certified or not) to "refract" patients. See answer 9.

29. d) Were you surprised to learn that compliance with ANSI standards is voluntary? It is!

30. b) The ANSI standards allow for a slight amount of difference in lens power between the lenses ordered and those that are actually dispensed. The stronger the lens power, the smaller the allowable variance.[11]

31. c) The ANSI standards detail specific information that must appear on the labels of contact lenses. In addition, the standards apply to contact lens materials, rigid and soft lenses, contact lens care products, and disinfection of multiuse trial sets.

32. d) The ANSI standards do not apply to patient selection.

33. a) Scribing is essentially being the practitioner's right hand. While the main duty may be documentation, the scribe also performs other duties at the physician's discretion, including patient education, coordinating patient flow, and overseeing billing forms and chart work.

---

[11]A summary of the standard is available at www.opticampus.com/tools/ansi.php. Accessed 7/30/11.

34.   b) A scribe may write out a prescription for medication as directed by the practitioner, but may not sign it. A scribe generally documents the physician's findings as dictated during the patient exam and during the patient briefing. A scribe may also remain after the doctor has left the exam room, providing patient education as necessary.

35.   d) Charting for this patient's visit will not be complete unless there is a statement indicating the physician specifically explained that cataract surgery will not restore "perfect" vision because of the macular degeneration. If the case went to court, the scribe would be able to say he or she was in the room at the time and heard the surgeon explicitly tell the patient that macular degeneration will prevent 20/20 vision even after the cataract is removed.

36.   d) Never eliminate a written chart entry or render it unreadable. The only proper way to make corrections in a written record is to draw one line through the mistake, write the correction above it, and initial.

37.   b) Discussing a patient with another assistant is permissible if it is pertinent to the patient's care (eg, you need advice on what testing needs to be done).

38.   c) Privacy is the key in taking a history. If others can hear, it is not private enough. However, if a patient has someone accompany him or her, it is implied that the guest has the patient's permission to hear the history.

39.   a) In answer a, you just announced to the entire waiting room (which may be filled with Mrs. Smith's peers) that she has glaucoma (a disease). This is a breach of confidentiality. The other situations are acceptable.

40.   d) Any procedure requires an informed consent regardless of risk, anesthesia type, or use of an IV.

41.   c) Watching a video may be part of the practice's patient education routine, but there are numerous ways in which a patient may be "advised" regarding the risks, benefits, procedure, and optional treatments.

42.   a) It is permissible for the physician to have someone else do the patient education. The key is that the information be presented in a way that the patient (or parent/guardian) can understand. Informed consent consists of more than signed papers (which in some cases *must* be signed by someone else [parent, power of attorney, etc]) and is necessary regardless of the patient's age.

43.   b) Of the answers offered, b is the best. The others sound too much like guarantees or even coercion. If the patient is mentally competent to make the decision, he must be allowed to make it. Other options are to ask the patient what his specific concerns are, if he has more questions, or if he would like to speak to the doctor again.

44.   c) The informed consent must contain the information in lay terms that someone with a sixth to eighth grade reading level can understand. Also, abbreviations are not acceptable.

45.   b) Telling a patient that the risk is so small he or she "does not have to worry about it" is discounting a viable risk and suggests a guarantee that it will not happen. The other answers appropriately acknowledge the risk involved.

46.   b) A surgeon may not simply "decide" to do an extra procedure. Unforeseen difficulties during surgery, as in answers a, c, and d may necessitate procedures that are not specifically spelled out in the informed consent, however. In such cases, the surgeon must respond in the way that most other surgeons would reasonably respond given the same circumstances.

Chapter 8

Microbiology

Ledford JK.
*Certified Ophthalmic Assistant: Exam
Review Manual, Third Edition* (pp. 87-92).
© 2012 Taylor & Francis Group.

Office Antisepsis[1]

1.   **Prior to disinfection or sterilization, contaminated instruments must be:**
   a) soaked in instrument milk
   b) boiled
   c) cleaned
   d) wiped with ether

2.   **Disinfection involves:**
   a) the reduction of microorganisms on inanimate surfaces
   b) the destruction of microorganisms on inanimate surfaces
   c) the destruction and inhibition of microorganisms on any surface
   d) the reduction of microorganisms on any surface

3.   **Sterilization involves:**
   a) the reduction of microorganisms on inanimate surfaces
   b) the destruction of microorganisms on inanimate surfaces
   c) the destruction and inhibition of microorganisms on any surface
   d) the reduction of microorganisms on any surface

4.   **The effectiveness of a sterilization method is based on:**
   a) temperature
   b) destruction of bacteria
   c) destruction of bacterial spores
   d) destruction of viral spores

5.   **Sanitation can be described as:**
   a) destruction of bacteria and bacterial spores
   b) reduction of bacteria and bacterial spores
   c) destruction of viruses and viral spores
   d) "clean enough to be healthy"

6.   **If a sterile package falls to the floor:**
   a) it may be wiped with alcohol and used
   b) it must be removed from use
   c) it may be used if the floor is clean
   d) it may be used if the wrapping is linen

7.   **The presence of even one bacterium on an object in the sterile field means that the object is:**
   a) bactericidal
   b) antiseptic
   c) contaminated
   d) bacteriostatic

[1]For aseptic technique related to minor surgery, see section *Aseptic Technique*; for sterilization techniques regarding major ocular surgery, see section *Sterilization*, both in Chapter 11.

8. **A chemical used to disinfect inanimate objects is a(n):**
    a) germicide
    b) antiseptic
    c) antibiotic
    d) ester

9. **A chemical used to disinfect living tissue is a(n):**
    a) germicide
    b) antiseptic
    c) antibiotic
    d) alcohol

10. **To test the effectiveness of any sterilization method, one may:**
    a) attempt to culture bacteria from "sterilized" instruments
    b) visually inspect the "sterilized" instruments
    c) use heat-activated testing tape
    d) keep records of any ensuing patient infections

11. **The organism that may contaminate ophthalmic solutions, including fluorescein, and can destroy an eye in 48 hours is:**
    a) Herpes simplex
    b) *Haemophilus influenzae*
    c) *Mycobacterium tuberculosis*
    d) *Pseudomonas aeruginosa*

12. **Which of the following might be *least* susceptible to contracting an eye infection?**
    a) A patient with human immunodeficiency virus (HIV).
    b) A patient with recurrent erosion syndrome.
    c) A patient wearing contact lenses.
    d) A patient working in the public sector.

Universal Precautions

13. **The organization involved with ensuring employee health and safety is:**
    a) JCAHPO®
    b) EOE
    c) OSHA
    d) HIPAA

14. **The Bloodborne Pathogens Standard involves all of the following *except*:**
    a) use and disposal of sharps
    b) one-time employee education
    c) provision of personal protective equipment
    d) provision of hepatitis B vaccines

15.   **Universal precautions are:**
    a) a method of infection control regulated by OSHA
    b) a set of standards regulated by ANSI
    c) a set of safety standards set by each clinic
    d) a method of evaluating infection control

16.   **Universal precautions would include all of the following *except*:**
    a) use of personal protective equipment
    b) method of cleaning contaminated spills
    c) method of disposing contaminated materials
    d) regarding some body fluids as always "safe"

17.   **Examples of bloodborne pathogens include all of the following *except*:**
    a) hepatitis B virus
    b) HIV
    c) herpes simplex virus
    d) hepatitis C virus

18.   **Which of the following is *true*?**
    a) one need not wash hands after removing gloves
    b) gloves may be washed and reused if not contaminated
    c) hand washing is necessary only if there is visible soil
    d) hand washing protocol is 15 to 20 seconds with soap and water

19.   **The single most effective method of preventing the spread of germs is:**
    a) use of a mask
    b) hand washing
    c) disinfection of surfaces
    d) covering coughs and sneezes

20.   **Personal protective equipment would include all of the following *except*:**
    a) eye shields
    b) gloves and masks
    c) TonoPen covers (Reichert Technologies, Depew, NY)
    d) gowns

21.   **Universal precautions generally apply to tears (lacrimal secretions):**
    a) in every case
    b) if they are bloody
    c) if the patient is known to have tuberculosis
    d) if the patient has glaucoma

Explanatory Answers

1.   c) Prior to being disinfected or sterilized, instruments must be cleaned to remove soil. This will ensure that all surfaces of the instrument are exposed to the disinfecting or sterilizing agent.

2.   c) Disinfection destroys and inhibits microorganisms on any surface, living or inanimate.

3. b) Only inanimate objects can be sterilized, which kills microorganisms. (Living tissue can be disinfected but not sterilized.)

4. c) A sterilization method is judged effective if bacterial spores are destroyed. (Spores are tougher to kill than the organisms themselves.) Viruses do not produce spores.

5. d) Sanitation is cleanliness, not the destruction or reduction of spores. It may involve something as simple as disposing of paper wrappers. Health is the issue here.

6. b) If a sterile package contacts something outside the sterile field (such as the floor), it is considered contaminated and may not be used.

7. c) Contamination is a matter of the presence or absence of bacteria, not how much or how many.

8. a) Germicides are used to disinfect nonliving objects. Antibiotics are medications used to treat infection.

9. b) If a living tissue is to be disinfected, then an antiseptic is used.

10. a) If bacteria can be cultured from instruments that have supposedly been sterilized, the method of sterilization is ineffective. The indicator tape or bags only testify that the required temperature occurred, not that sterilization has necessarily been achieved.

11. d) *Pseudomonas aeruginosa* is a bacterium known to contaminate eye drops. It is particularly destructive.

12. d) Patients whose immune systems are compromised (such as those with HIV) are more susceptible to any kind of infection. The person with recurrent erosion syndrome has a break in the corneal epithelium, which creates an opening for infectious microbes. Wearing contact lenses increases a person's chances of contracting ocular infections by the mere presence of a foreign body in the eye. Working with the public (versus never going out!) increases the chances of contracting an infection, but of the four listed is the least susceptible.

13. c) OSHA is part of the United States Department of Labor. It was created in 1970 for the purpose of ensuring safety (including health safety) in the workplace.

14. b) Annual training is required.

15. a) Universal precautions (previously known as *standard precautions*) were developed and are regulated by OSHA. The universal precautions mindset considers body fluids (notably blood, semen, vaginal secretions, vitreous, and wound exudates) as potentially infectious.

16. d) The word "always" should have helped clue you in that this was the correct answer.

17. c) The herpes simplex virus is not a bloodborne pathogen.

18. d) Washing hands with soap and water for 15 to 20 seconds (about the length of time it takes to sing "Happy Birthday" twice) is the current recommended protocol.

19. b) Hand washing is the most effective method of preventing the spread of infection, hands down! (Pun, of course, intended!)

20. c) A TonoPen tip cover is barrier protection, but it is for the patient rather than the examiner (the person in "personal"). The other items are used by the examiner as protection against any bloodborne pathogens harbored by the patient.

21. b) Certain fluids always fall under universal precautions procedures, such as blood, semen, vaginal secretions, vitreous, and wound exudates. Fluids that become of concern only when blood is visible in them include tears, sweat, feces, and urine.[2] While HIV has been isolated in human tears, it is not considered to be in high enough concentration to spread the disease.

[2]Carr T (ed). Ophthalmic medical assisting: An independent study course. 3rd ed, revised. The American Academy of Ophthalmology; 2002; San Francisco. In: Stein HA, Stein RM, Freeman MI. *The Ophthalmic Assistant.* 8th ed. Philadelphia, PA: Elsevier Mosby; 2006.

Chapter 9

Pharmacology

Ledford JK.
*Certified Ophthalmic Assistant: Exam
Review Manual, Third Edition* (pp. 93-102).
© 2012 Taylor & Francis Group.

Ocular Medicines (Instilling and Identifying)

1. **Use of eye drops would be advantageous:**
    a) if the drug needs to stay on the eye for a long time
    b) if exterior parts of the eye are being treated
    c) in case of a systemic infection
    d) if the condition being treated is not very serious

2. **A disadvantage of eye drops is that:**
    a) they are expensive
    b) they do not have prolonged contact with the eye
    c) they must be refrigerated
    d) they penetrate too deeply into the eye's structures

3. **Use of eye ointments is advantageous because:**
    a) they are less expensive than drops
    b) they penetrate more quickly than drops
    c) they are easier to apply than drops
    d) they remain in contact with the eye longer than drops

4. **A patient might complain about using eye ointment because:**
    a) it has to be used more often than drops
    b) it is more expensive than drops
    c) it blurs the vision
    d) it is less effective than drops

5. **All of the following are characteristics of locally injected drugs *except*:**
    a) a greater concentration of the drug can be given versus topical
    b) the drug can be delivered directly to the site where it is needed
    c) the drug takes effect quickly
    d) the drug is absorbed through the digestive tract

6. **Systemic drugs are those administered by:**
    a) applying the drug to the surface
    b) injection or mouth
    c) mouth only
    d) injection only

7. **All of the following are examples of systemically administered drugs *except*:**
    a) acetazolamide pills for glaucoma
    b) glycerol liquid drink to reduce intraocular pressure
    c) mannitol intravenous injection to reduce intraocular pressure
    d) timolol eye drops for glaucoma

8. **When a child is to be given anesthetic drops, the assistant should:**
    a) give the drops without warning to avoid hassles
    b) tell the child that the drops will not sting
    c) let the physician do it
    d) briefly explain what is to be done, then do it quickly

9. **A topical ophthalmic drug preparation is considered unsterile:**
    a) once it is opened
    b) only if it touches the lashes or lids
    c) only if bacteria can be cultured from it
    d) none of the above

10. **The physician has asked you to dilate a patient's eyes. The drops used to do this will have:**
    a) a purple cap
    b) a green cap
    c) a white cap
    d) a red cap

11. **Having the patient look down when you instill topical anesthetics might be advantageous because:**
    a) the drop will sting less
    b) the drop will be distributed over the cornea
    c) the drop will stay on the eye longer
    d) the tears will not dilute the solution

12. **Dilating and medicinal topical drops/ointments are most easily instilled by:**
    a) having the patient look to one side
    b) dropping directly on the cornea
    c) using a cotton-tipped applicator
    d) having the patient look up

13. **You are instilling cycloplegic drops, and the dropper tip touches the patient's eyelashes. You should:**
    a) wipe the dropper tip with alcohol
    b) soak the tip in bleach solution
    c) cap the bottle
    d) discard the bottle and drops

14. **Regarding the recapping of multiple-use ophthalmic drops:**
    a) it is unnecessary and inconvenient
    b) it helps to prevent contamination
    c) it needs to be done only at the end of the day
    d) only single-use dispensers should be used

15. **All of the following should be done prior to pupil dilation *except*:**
    a) swinging flashlight test
    b) keratometry
    c) refractometry in a patient over the age of 45
    d) pressure check

16. **Which of the following bottle cap colors are coded for glaucoma medications?**
    a) yellow, blue, red
    b) purple, blue, yellow, green
    c) yellow, white, red, purple
    d) green, yellow, purple, white

Educate Patients on Medications[1]

17. **After instillation of topical anesthetic, the patient should be told:**
   a) "Be sure to wear sunglasses when you go outside."
   b) "Your vision may be blurry for several hours."
   c) "Do not rub your eyes."
   d) "Do not drive until it has worn off."

18. **A patient who has undergone routine dilation for an eye exam can expect:**
   a) better night vision
   b) better vision in bright light
   c) blurred near vision
   d) light sensitivity for 24 hours

19. **A disadvantage of drops used to reverse routine office dilation is:**
   a) it takes a long time to act
   b) the patient is still light-sensitive
   c) it clears near but blurs distant vision
   d) it can cause headaches

20. **Home use of anesthetic eye drops is never prescribed because:**
   a) it causes a breakdown of the corneal surface
   b) a patient in pain will schedule a return visit
   c) it decreases the efficacy of other drugs
   d) it is too expensive to justify home use

21. **A patient has had a piece of metal removed from his cornea one morning. That afternoon he calls the office and asks the doctor to prescribing numbing drops. You tell him:**
   a) the doctor will call it in as soon as possible
   b) come by the office and pick some up
   c) that medication is not prescribed because it interferes with healing
   d) that medication is not prescribed because it can elevate eye pressure

22. **Patients who use nonpreserved artificial tears supplied in "bullets" should be told to:**
   a) use them only once a day
   b) discard the leftover solution at the end of the day
   c) use them only at night
   d) make their own saline because it is cheaper

23. **Dry eye patients should be told to use artificial tears:**
   a) morning and night
   b) only when the eyes water
   c) four times daily
   d) as often as needed to control symptoms

---

[1]See also Chapter 12, section *Patient Instruction—Medication*, for patient instruction regarding use of ophthalmic medications in general.

24.   **The first choice of medicinal treatment for open-angle glaucoma is usually:**
a) oral
b) topical
c) subconjunctival injection
d) intravenous

25.   **The patient should be told that his or her glaucoma medications:**
a) need not be used on the day of the appointment
b) will cure the condition
c) do not need to be refilled
d) should be continued until told otherwise

26.   **Reasons that a patient fails to take his or her glaucoma medications properly include all of the following** *except*:
a) lack of symptoms suggesting the patient has a disease
b) side effects of glaucoma medications
c) he or she understands the serious nature of the disease
d) lack of visual improvement from the medication

27.   **If the patient is given oral antibiotics following surgery, he or she should be told to:**
a) discontinue the pills once the danger of infection is over
b) take half of the prescription, then discontinue if no infection develops
c) take all of the medication until it is gone
d) take the pills only if infection seems to be developing

28.   **The patient is going to be using an ophthalmic medication that is labeled "suspension." You tell the patient to:**
a) keep the bottle refrigerated
b) shake the bottle prior to using
c) use twice the prescribed dose
d) warm the drops prior to using

29.   **The doctor has diagnosed iritis and has asked you to explain the use of cyclopentolate drops to the patient. You tell the patient:**
a) "This will numb your eye and make you more comfortable."
b) "This will dilate your pupil to make your eye more comfortable."
c) "Don't miss a single dose or your eye pressure may go up."
d) "This will minify your pupil to make you more comfortable."

Drug Reactions[2]

30.   **All of the following can be complications of eye drop use** *except*:
a) the patient may have an allergic reaction
b) the patient may develop irritation of the eye or lids
c) the drops can become contaminated
d) the patient may develop a fever

[2]See also Chapter 1, the section titled *Medication*, where drug reactions are discussed as part of the patient's history.

31. **Abnormal drug reactions may occur:**
    a) in patients who are debilitated
    b) in the presence of other drugs
    c) as toxic or chemical reactions
    d) all of the above

32. **Common signs and symptoms of a topical allergic reaction to ocular medication include:**
    a) rash, itching, redness, and swelling
    b) pain, redness, and discharge
    c) pain, photophobia, and mid-dilated pupil
    d) rash, redness, and anterior chamber reaction

33. **Which of the following suggests a drug allergy in the skin?**
    a) redness and itching
    b) increased perspiration
    c) a feeling of heat in the skin
    d) a prickling sensation

34. **Which of the following suggests a drug allergy in the conjunctiva?**
    a) a deep aching
    b) a pus-like discharge
    c) swelling and redness
    d) decreased tearing

35. **If a patient has a localized allergic reaction to a topical medication instilled in the office, one should:**
    a) irrigate the eye immediately
    b) call 911
    c) administer oxygen, cortisone, and epinephrine
    d) check the pH of the eye and neutralize appropriately

36. **Over a period of time, use of steroid eye drops can cause all of the following *except*:**
    a) an increase in intraocular pressure
    b) accelerated growth of certain organisms
    c) iris cysts
    d) slow wound healing

37. **Which of the following has the highest risk of complications?**
    a) a drug given in drop form
    b) a drug given in ointment form
    c) a drug given in topical sustained-release form
    d) a drug given via injection or oral form

38. **All of the following have potentially serious side effects or may cause allergy with *long-term* usage *except*:**
    a) topical anesthetic
    b) topical steroid
    c) topical neomycin
    d) topical preservative-free lubricant

39. **Severe drug reaction may include:**
a) nausea
b) dizziness
c) airway obstruction
d) rash

40. **A patient having an allergic reaction involving shallow respiration should be given:**
a) mouth-to-mouth resuscitation
b) mouth-to-nose resuscitation
c) oxygen from a portable unit
d) resuscitation through a mask

Explanatory Answers

1. b) Topical drops are best used to treat external eye problems. (That is not to say that they do not have a place in treating intraocular problems, of course!)
2. b) Eye medications in drop form are prone to run out the lacrimal drainage system. Many drops are expensive, but this is not the best answer.
3. d) Because ointments are in a petroleum-type base, they do not drain off the eye as rapidly as drops.
4. c) Ointment creates a film in the tears, causing blurry vision. Ointment is generally used less often (ie, fewer doses) than drops.
5. d) Locally injected drugs have all the advantages listed except being absorbed through the digestive tract (which would describe medication given orally, not injected).
6. b) Systemic drugs are "introduced into the system" by intravenous injection or by mouth.
7. d) Eye drops are topical, not systemic.
8. d) You could tell the child that the drops might sting for a second, but do not lie, and do not drag it out. Surprises are unpleasant, too. The physician needs a good rapport with the child in order to complete the exam and render treatment, so it is better if the doctor does not give the drops.
9. a) While the drug may be uncontaminated (ie, no bacteria or other organisms have gotten into it), it is no longer considered sterile once opened.
10. d) Eye drops that dilate (via mydriasis or cycloplegia) all have red caps.
11. b) The theory is that if the patient looks down when the drop is instilled, afterwards when he or she blinks, the eye will automatically roll up, giving better coverage over the cornea. This would be true for most topical dyes (eg, rose bengal) as well. Otherwise, having the patient look *up* during instillation is easier; see answer 12.
12. d) Have the patient look up, and gently pull down the lower lid. The medication is then instilled in the lower cul-de-sac (pocket between the lid and eyeball).
13. d) If the tip of a multiple-use dropper bottle touches the lids, lashes, conjunctiva, or skin, it should be discarded.
14. b) Immediate recapping of dilating and other drops used in the eye clinic helps to prevent contamination of the medication via airborne dust and germs.

15. b) Dilation makes no difference in keratometry readings. (What could make a difference in K readings is if you have applanated the cornea prior to keratometry, but that was not one of the choices.) The swinging flashlight test checks pupillary reaction and, thus, must be done prior to dilating. Patients over the age of 45 are probably going to need a reading add, which needs to be measured prior to "freezing" accommodation by dilating. A check of IOP is also needed before dilation to make sure the patient is not sitting on high pressure readings.

16. b) Red is for cycloplegics/mydriatics, and white can be most anything (tears, anesthetic, steroids, and antibiotics).

17. c) Because of the numbness induced by topical anesthetics, the patient should be reminded not to rub his or her eyes. The danger is that he or she will accidentally rub and abrade the cornea while it cannot feel anything.

18. c) Routine dilation "freezes" accommodation, so, of the choices offered, the patient can expect to be blurred at near. There is generally some light sensitivity, too, but not for a full 24 hours.

19. d) The dilating reversal drops are miotics and can cause headaches.

20. a) Repeated use of topical anesthetic causes corneal melting, which can interfere with healing.

21. c) See answer 20.

22. b) Because there is no preservative to retard bacterial growth, any solution remaining in the bullet at the end of the day should be discarded. These drops may be used many times throughout the day. No one should use homemade saline in the eye because of the risk of contamination.

23. d) Dry eye is a condition that cannot be cured, only controlled. Thus, patients are advised to use the drops as often as needed.

24. b) Topical medications are usually the treatment of choice in open-angle glaucoma.

25. d) Patient education is key to successful treatment of glaucoma using medications. The patient should be told to continue the medication (including refilling it before it runs out) until instructed otherwise. In addition, the medication should be used on schedule, even (especially) when the patient has an appointment that day; otherwise, it is more difficult to assess the treatment's efficacy.

26. c) If the patient understands the gravity of the disease, he or she will be more motivated to use the medication. Answers a, b, and d are common reasons for noncompliance.

27. c) An oral antibiotic should be taken until gone; otherwise, its effectiveness may be reduced or nil.

28. b) A suspension means that the actual medication is in the form of particles, which may settle to the bottom of the bottle. Mixing is necessary to "suspend" the particles throughout the carrier solution. Otherwise, the patient may instill a drop full of "carrier" that has no medication in it.

29. b) Dilating/cyclopleging an eye with inflammation decreases discomfort by temporarily paralyzing accommodation and iris movement. This is analogous to putting a splint on a sprained wrist to limit movement. It also helps to prevent the iris from adhering to the corneal endothelium or to the lens.

30. d) Fever is a sign of infection, not allergy or drug reaction.

31. d) All of the answers list possible scenarios for an abnormal drug reaction. In addition to patients whose general health is compromised, the action of a drug may also not be what is anticipated if the patient is very old or very young. If more than one drug is being used, the medications may interact with one another. This could cause a chemical reaction, or it could accentuate or decrease the effect of one or both drugs. Some drugs can have a toxic effect on the body. (An example is the effect of chloroquine on the retinal cones.) Finally, a chemical reaction could cause toxicity, unexpected interactions, or other effects (such as forming deposits in tissues).

32. a) A local allergic reaction to a topical ocular medication can include rash (of the eyelids), itching, redness (conjunctival and lids), and swelling (conjunctiva and lids).

33. a) A drug allergy affecting the skin is often seen as a rash: swelling, redness, scaling, itching, and oozing can occur.

34. c) Conjunctival swelling (edema or chemosis) and redness may be seen in drug allergy.

35. a) A localized reaction is limited to one area, generally the area of drug administration. In the eye, this would usually be evidenced by redness, swelling, watering, and itching. Irrigation is the first aid action you should take. It is also important to note the allergy in the patient's chart so that the drug is avoided in the future. The items in answer c apply to anaphylactic shock and would be administered by the physician.

36. c) Iris cysts are associated with miotics, not steroids. The other items can occur when using steroid drops; thus, steroids are usually prescribed for short-term use.

37. d) A drug given in systemic form enters the entire body; thus, there is a greater risk of complications.

38. d) Topical lubricants are not dangerous, and preservative-free preparations do not cause an allergic response. Long-term use of topical anesthetic can cause corneal melt, steroids can cause glaucoma, and neomycin is noted for its allergic response.

39. c) Any of the answers could be a drug reaction, but airway obstruction is the most severe reaction listed.

40. c) If the patient is breathing, give him or her oxygen. Do not give artificial respiration to a person who is breathing on his or her own.

Chapter 10

Ocular Motility

Ledford JK.
*Certified Ophthalmic Assistant: Exam
Review Manual, Third Edition* (pp. 103-116).
© 2012 Taylor & Francis Group.

Versions and Ductions

Functions

1. **Positioning the eyes so that an object's image is placed on the macula is known as:**
    a) fixation
    b) binocular vision
    c) stereo vision
    d) depth perception

2. **The coordinating process by which the two images (one received by each eye) are blended into a single image is known as:**
    a) stereo vision
    b) depth perception
    c) binocular vision
    d) fusion

3. **Coordinated movement of both eyes in the same direction is known as:**
    a) ductions
    b) versions
    c) rotations
    d) saccades

4. **Which of the following are *not* considered cardinal positions of gaze?**
    a) down and left, or up and left
    b) up and right, or down and right
    c) straight ahead, or straight up or down
    d) directly left, or directly right

5. **When testing a patient's versions, it is important to:**
    a) test in dim lighting
    b) keep the patient's head still
    c) use an opaque occluder to break fusion
    d) keep the patient's eyes in primary position

6. **Versional movements are those that:**
    a) result in fusion
    b) move one eye
    c) move both eyes in the same direction
    d) move both eyes in a different direction

7. **If the eyes have normal version movements, all of the following will exist *except*:**
    a) each eye will move with equal speed
    b) each eye will move smoothly
    c) the eyes will diverge equally
    d) each eye will be in the same position relative to the other

8. **To test the right inferior rectus (RIR) and the left superior oblique (LSO) muscles, the patient must look:**
    a) directly right
    b) down and to the right
    c) up and to the right
    d) down and to the left

9. **Your patient is looking down and to the left. Which muscles are pulling the eyes into this position?**
    a) RIR and LSO
    b) Right superior oblique (RSO) and left inferior rectus (LIR)
    c) Right superior rectus (RSR) and left inferior oblique (LIO)
    d) Right inferior oblique (RIO) and left superior rectus (LSR)

10. **You want to check the action of the right lateral rectus (RLR) muscle. Where do you direct the patient to look?**
    a) to the left
    b) to the right
    c) down and right
    d) up and left

11. **You want to check the action of the LIO muscle. Where do you direct the patient to look?**
    a) to the left
    b) down and right
    c) up and left
    d) up and right

12. **Ductions refer to:**
    a) muscles that work against each other during eye movements
    b) movements of one eye
    c) movements of both eyes in the same direction
    d) movements of both eyes in the opposite direction

13. **Testing ductions is useful in differentiating cases of:**
    a) restrictive strabismus
    b) accommodative strabismus
    c) congenital esotropia
    d) pseudostrabismus

Anomalies

14. **If one eye is obviously turned in, out, up, or down when you perform a simple external evaluation of the patient, this deviation is a:**
    a) ptosis
    b) phoria
    c) tropia
    d) vergence

15. **A phoria is exhibited when:**
    a) the patient is malingering
    b) fusion is disrupted
    c) the patient is fusing
    d) the patient has diplopia

16. **The difference between a phoria and an intermittent tropia is:**
    a) the patient experiences diplopia with the phoria but not with the intermittent tropia
    b) the phoria rarely is controlled, and the intermittent tropia always is controlled
    c) the phoria usually is controlled, and the intermittent tropia always is uncontrolled
    d) the phoria usually is controlled, and the intermittent tropia sometimes is controlled

17. **An adult patient with a tropia has either:**
    a) amblyopia or anisometropia
    b) prism or slab-off lenses
    c) diplopia or suppression
    d) fusion or stereopsis

18. **Label the following on Figure 10-1:**
    esotropia
    hypotropia
    exotropia
    orthophoria
    hypertropia

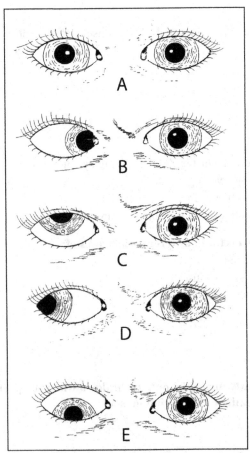

Figure 10-1. Drawing by Holly Hess Smith. Reprinted with permission of Gayton JL, Ledford JK. *The Crystal Clear Guide to Sight for Life.* Starburst Publishers; 1996.

19. **An intermittent horizontal tropia might be aggravated by all of the following *except*:**
    a) inattention
    b) dry eye
    c) illness
    d) fatigue

20. **Vertical deviations are conventionally described by indicating:**
    a) the higher (up-turned) eye
    b) the lower (down-turned) eye
    c) the preferred eye
    d) the eye with best vision

21. **In pseudostrabismus:**
    a) the eye turns only if fusion is disrupted
    b) the eyes are straight, but there is amblyopia
    c) the eyes are straight, but the patient has diplopia
    d) the eyes look crossed, but actually are straight

22. **Pseudostrabismus usually is seen in:**
    a) boys
    b) girls
    c) infants
    d) adults

23. **The most common patient complaint in a *new* nerve palsy is:**
    a) decreased vision
    b) diplopia
    c) an ache in the affected muscle(s)
    d) an inability to read at near

24. **Nerve palsies cause the affected muscle(s) to become:**
    a) overactive
    b) underactive
    c) spasmodic
    d) responsive

Cover Tests

25. **The purpose of covering one eye with an occluder for strabismus screening is to:**
    a) determine if the patient is suppressing
    b) perform monocular testing
    c) disrupt fusion
    d) determine if the patient is malingering

26. **Cover testing can be performed even on an infant because:**
    a) it is nonthreatening
    b) it is painless
    c) it is objective
    d) it is brief

27. **Cover testing can be useful in all of the following patients *except*:**
    a) bilateral aphake
    b) bilateral pseudophake
    c) the patient with suppression
    d) the monocular patient

28. **The cover/uncover test is used to determine the presence of:**
    a) phoria versus tropia
    b) amblyopia
    c) suppression
    d) stereopsis

29. **The cover/uncover test can also reveal the presence of:**
    a) esotropia versus exotropia
    b) vergence insufficiency
    c) depth perception
    d) visual acuity

30. **You have covered the patient's right eye. When you uncover it, the right eye moves inward. Now, you cover the left eye. When you uncover it, the left eye moves inward. At this point, you can only deduce that the patient has an:**
    a) exophoria
    b) exotropia
    c) exodeviation
    d) esodeviation

31. **The patient's vision is 20/20 in both eyes. You cover the patient's right eye and note that when you do so, the left eye moves outward. When you uncover the right eye, neither eye moves. When you cover the left eye, the right eye moves outward. When you uncover the left eye, neither eye moves. This indicates:**
    a) alternating exotropia
    b) esophoria
    c) intermittent esotropia
    d) alternating esotropia

32. **During the cover/uncover test, if a patient has a phoria, the response of the eye that is *not* covered is to:**
    a) take up fixation
    b) move in the same direction as the covered eye
    c) remain straight
    d) deviate in or out

33. **The alternate (cross) cover test does *not* reveal:**
    a) exodeviations
    b) esodeviations
    c) hyper deviations
    d) a phoria versus a tropia

34. **When performing the alternate (cross) cover test, it is important to:**
    a) momentarily remove the cover from one eye before covering the other
    b) move the cover rapidly from one eye to the other
    c) allow the patient to look at the target with both eyes before covering again
    d) move the cover from one eye to the next every half-second

35. **If there is no movement of either eye during any part of the alternate (cross) cover test, one has determined that:**
    a) the patient is amblyopic in one eye
    b) the eyes are orthophoric
    c) the patient has stereo vision
    d) the patient has equal vision in both eyes

36. **You have performed the alternate (cross) cover test and notice that each eye moves inward when uncovered. What is your next step?**
    a) record exodeviation in the chart
    b) record exotropia in the chart
    c) record esodeviation in the chart
    d) perform a cover/uncover test

37. **The alternate (cross) cover test can be used to measure the size of a deviation if:**
    a) the patient can fuse
    b) the corneal reflex can be seen
    c) it is combined with prisms
    d) polarized glasses are used

Stereopsis

38. **Which of the following is *not* a component of binocular vision?**
    a) clear vision in each eye
    b) alignment of the eyes
    c) overlapping visual fields
    d) identical images on each retina

39. **Depth perception:**
    a) requires two eyes
    b) requires overlapping visual fields
    c) is absent in monocular patients
    d) uses environmental "clues"

40. **Stereopsis is recorded in:**
    a) Snellen fractions
    b) degrees of arc
    c) seconds of arc
    d) degrees of field

41. **Which of the following indicates the better stereo vision?**
    a) 50 degrees of arc
    b) 25 degrees of arc
    c) 50 seconds of arc
    d) 25 seconds of arc

42. **Stereopsis can be elicited and measured in which of the following patients?**
    a) 60 diopter esotropia
    b) 45 diopter exotropia
    c) 8 diopter intermittent exotropia
    d) monocular

43. **Stereopsis differs from depth perception in that:**
    a) depth perception is monocular or binocular
    b) stereo vision involves judging spatial relationships
    c) depth perception involves seeing in three dimensions
    d) stereopsis is a learned experience

44. **While it does not give a measurement, a simple stereo test that can be done at bedside is the:**
    a) Hirschberg test
    b) confrontation stereo test
    c) pencil point to pencil point test
    d) Amsler grid stereo test

45. **The Titmus/Wirt test, Randot test, and fly test all use:**
    a) polarized glasses
    b) glasses with one red and one green lens
    c) dissociating prisms
    d) a red filter

46. **You ask a cooperative 3-year-old girl to touch the wings of the Titmus fly. She recoils and refuses. You can assume that most likely:**
    a) she is tired and cranky
    b) she has impaired mental ability
    c) she has at least gross fusion
    d) she has an intermittent deviation

47. **You are testing an intelligent 12-year-old boy with the Titmus/Wirt circles and suspect that he is either a good guesser or a cheater. You should:**
    a) turn the test 90 degrees
    b) turn the test 180 degrees
    c) switch the glasses around
    d) record the patient's responses regardless

48. **An advantage of the Random Dot E test over the Titmus test is that the Random Dot E:**
    a) does not require special glasses
    b) offers monocular clues
    c) does not offer monocular clues
    d) does not require color vision

Nystagmus

49. Rhythmic jerking motions of the eyes are known as:
a) versions
b) ductions
c) nystagmus
d) end-point/gaze-induced

50. When evaluating congenital nystagmus, all of the following might be noted *except*:
a) binocular or monocular
b) direction
c) magnitude
d) head position

51. A patient with nystagmus might find that which of the following decreases the magnitude of the jerking?
a) closing/covering one eye
b) squinting
c) positioning the head
d) wearing sunglasses

52. A head position in which the nystagmus is quietest (least) is known as the:
a) null point
b) near point
c) angle of deviation
d) cyclic amplitude

53. During visual acuity testing and refractometry, it is important to remember that which of the following might cause a worsening of nystagmus?
a) fogging
b) occluding one eye
c) cross cylinder
d) astigmatic dial

54. Your physician plans to prescribe glasses for a patient with nystagmus. Which method will give her the best information?
a) autorefractor alone
b) retinoscopy alone
c) phoroptor measurement
d) trial frames and lenses

55. A type of nystagmus that a normal patient might exhibit in far right or far left gaze is:
a) ductional nystagmus
b) versional nystagmus
c) acquired nystagmus
d) gaze-induced nystagmus

56. **Adult-onset nystagmus will frequently cause the patient to complain of:**
a) diplopia
b) "vibrating" vision
c) photophobia
d) extraocular muscle pain

57. **Which of the following is *not* true regarding congenital nystagmus?**
a) It is often associated with maternal infections.
b) The child may adopt a specific head position.
c) The child will frequently outgrow the condition.
d) It is often associated with visual impairment.

Explanatory Answers

1. a) In fixation, the eyes are positioned so that each macula is receiving the same image (albeit at a slightly different angle).

2. d) The brain merges the slightly different images coming from each eye to create a single three-dimensional image. This is known as fusion.

3. b) Versions are movements of both eyes in the same direction. Ductions are movements of one eye alone.

4. c) Straight ahead (primary gaze), straight up, and straight down are not cardinal positions of gaze. In any of these positions, the action of one muscle can be masked by the action of another, so these positions are not considered diagnostic.

5. b) When testing versions (range of motion), it is important that the patient keep his or her head still. If the patient moves the head to follow the target, you are not able to test the full motion of the eyes, but rather the range of motion of the neck! The test is done in room light so you can see the eyes as they move. An occluder is not used when testing versions. If the eyes remained in primary position, they would not move at all.

6. c) Versions move both eyes in the same direction. Fusion does not necessarily occur; for example, the muscles in a blind eye are still innervated and linked to those of the other (seeing) eye.

7. c) Divergence is when the eyes move in opposite directions, away from each other. In versions, the eyes are moving together in the same direction. (Be sure to read questions carefully—there is a difference between *versions* and *vergences*.)

8. b) Looking down and right (from the patient's perspective) requires the RIR and LSO. Straight ahead (primary gaze) is not diagnostic. RSR and LIO are up and right. RSO and LIR are down and left (Figure 10-2).

9. b) In down and left gaze, the RSO and LIR are being used. RIR and LSO would be down and right. RSR and LIO are up and right. RIO and LSR are up and left.

10. b) The RLR has its primary action in right gaze. Left gaze would be the RMR. Down and right would be RIR, and up and left would be RIO.

11. d) To check the action of the LIO, have the patient look up and right. Left gaze would check the LLR. Down and right would be the LSO, and up and left would be the LSR.

12. b) Ductions refer to movements of one eye. Muscles that work against each other in the same eye are antagonists. Movements of both eyes in the same direction are versions. Movements of both eyes in opposite directions are vergences.

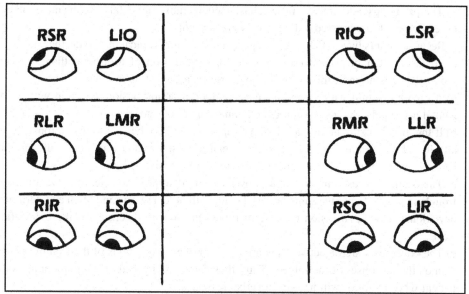

Figure 10-2. Pairs of yoke muscles responsible for moving eyes into various positions of gaze. Reprinted with permission of Karlsson VC. *A Systematic Approach to Strabismus, Second Edition.* SLACK Incorporated; 2009.

13. a) Testing ductions is useful when one eye is at fault for a deviation, as in restrictive strabismus. In answers b through d, it would be more helpful to test versions.
14. c) Unless it is intermittent, a tropia is there all the time. If you can look at the patient and see that one eye is turned, it is a tropia. A phoria is evident only when you cover one eye or otherwise disrupt fusion. Ptosis is a drooped eyelid.
15. b) A phoria is evident only when you disrupt fusion. (***Note:*** Some phorias "break down" when the patient is tired. This is actually an intermittent deviation.)
16. d) A phoria usually is controlled unless fusion is disrupted. When the disruption is removed, the eyes will fuse again. An intermittent tropia comes and goes; sometimes the patient is fusing, and sometimes he or she is not. When the patient is not fusing, the deviation appears.
17. c) An adult with a crossed eye either has learned to suppress the image from the eye that is not fixating or has double vision. Usually, suppression is learned in childhood as the visual system is developing; the brain learns to ignore the image from a crossed eye. In cases where the strabismus occurs as an adult, diplopia occurs because the brain does not know how to suppress a second image. It is not a given that amblyopia or anisometropia exist, although they might. Fusion and stereopsis can occur only when both eyes are working together, looking at the same object.
18. Labeling on Figure 10-1:
     esotropia b)   hypotropia   e)   hypertropia   c)
     exotropia d)   orthophoria   a)
19. b) In the other 3 cases, there is simply not enough effort/strength to maintain fusion.
20. a) Conventionally, vertical deviations are described as a hypertropia of the higher eye. Thus, if the patient was fixating with the right eye and the left eye was deviated downward, the right eye is higher. So this situation would be designated as a right hypertropia (RHT).

21. d) The prefix "pseudo" means false. Thus, pseudostrabismus is false strabismus; the eyes falsely appear to be crossed although they are straight.

22. c) Because infants have a flat nasal bridge and (sometimes) epicanthal folds, they are implicated more often in pseudostrabismus (an optical illusion of esotropia) than any other group. There is no indication whether boys or girls are most often affected.

23. b) An adult or child with a new nerve palsy notices double vision. (A child with a congenital nerve palsy learns to suppress one image and does not see double.)

24. b) If the muscle is not getting a full nerve supply, it will not be able to react properly (if at all). It will thus be underactive. This might manifest itself as an overaction of the muscle's antagonist (the muscle in the same eye that has the opposite action).

25. c) The occluder is used in strabismus cover tests to disrupt fusion (ie, to prevent the eyes from being locked onto the same target). Fusion will hold a phoria and often an intermittent deviation in check, so fusion must be disrupted in order to determine if these deviations exist.

26. c) The cover tests are objective; they are based on the observations of the examiner rather than on the responses of the subject. Thus, they can be performed on an infant or any other patient who cannot or will not give a verbal response.

27. d) There is no point in doing cover tests on a monocular patient because there is no vision in the second eye with which to fuse. The patient must always fixate with the single, seeing eye.

28. a) The cover/uncover test differentiates between a phoria and a tropia.

29. a) The cover/uncover test also indicates the direction of any deviation (ie, eso-, exo-, or vertical deviation).

30. c) The eyes must have drifted out (ie, toward the temple) under the cover if they make inward movements when uncovered, so an exodeviation is present. You were not given enough information to differentiate between a phoria and tropia. For that, you need to know what the uncovered eye is doing, as well.

31. d) An outward motion upon uncovering indicates that the eye has drifted in, denoting an esodeviation. In this case, regardless of which eye is covered, the covered eye drifts in. When the eye is uncovered, it does not move to take up fixation (indicating a tropia). This further indicates that the patient is willing to use either eye to fix, revealing an alternating esotropia.

32. c) In a phoria, the eye under the cover drifts. The eye that is not covered is fixating. When you remove the cover, the resulting diplopia causes the deviated eye to move in order to pick up fixation. The eye that was not covered is fixating already, so it does not need to move. Be sure to read the questions carefully; the answer would have been different if this had been a *cross cover* test.

33. d) The alternate (or cross) cover test will reveal horizontal and vertical deviations, but does not differentiate between a phoria and a tropia.

34. b) When performing the alternate (cross) cover test, move the cover rapidly from one eye to the other, but every half-second is too fast. The important thing is to prevent the patient from seeing with both eyes at once and thus regaining fusion.

35. b) If no motion is seen during the alternate (cross) cover test, it is logical to assume that the patient is orthophoric. You cannot, however, assume that amblyopia does or does not exist, that the patient has stereopsis, or that vision is equal in both eyes.

36. d) The only thing you know at this point is that there is some type of exodeviation. (For the eye to move inward when it is uncovered, it must have drifted outward under the cover.) Once you have found movement on the alternate (cross) cover test, use the cover/uncover test to determine if it is a tropia or a phoria.

37. c) The alternate (cross) cover test combined with prisms to measure the size of a deviation (phoria or tropia) becomes the "prism and cover test." The deviation can be measured in a patient with fusion because the test itself disrupts fusion. The corneal reflex and polarized glasses are not used in the prism and cover test.

38. d) Binocular vision depends on slightly different images coming from each retina. (That was tricky!)

39. d) Depth perception is not the same as binocular, or stereo, vision. A person with one eye can develop depth perception by learning to use "clues" from the environment, such as overlap, grayness, or merging.

40. c) Stereopsis is measured in seconds of arc.

41. d) Twenty-five seconds of arc indicates finer stereo discrimination than 50 seconds of arc. Stereo vision is not measured in degrees of arc as given in answers a and b.

42. c) A patient with a constant esotropia or exotropia over 10 degrees will not have stereo vision, nor will a monocular patient. A binocular patient with an intermittent deviation, a phoria, or a deviation of 10 degrees or less should have a stereo acuity test performed.

43. a) Stereopsis is present only in binocular individuals. Depth perception, however, exists in binocular and monocular patients. Answers b and c are backwards: stereo vision involves seeing in three dimensions, and depth perception involves judging spatial relationships. Stereopsis is not learned; depth perception is.

44. c) Having the patient touch one pencil point to another is an indicator of gross stereopsis. (Try it on yourself: once with both eyes opened and once with one eye closed.) The Hirschberg estimates the size of a deviation, not stereopsis. Answers b and d are contrived.

45. a) Each of the tests listed used polarized glasses.

46. c) The fly was chosen as a test object because it is repulsive. An otherwise cooperative child may refuse to touch the fly because it is ugly and appears to be real. When the child sees it, the huge fly seems to be standing on the page. Refusal is generally considered a positive indication that gross stereopsis exists, but further testing is indicated.

47. b) Turning the test around 180 degrees will change the location of the stereo rings and make them appear sunken instead of elevated. If you turn the test 90 degrees, it will not be stereopic. Polarized glasses are usually designed to be worn only one way. It is in the patient's best interest to get the most accurate measurement possible.

48. c) The first 3 rings of the Titmus/Wirt test can be guessed correctly by a nonfussing patient because the dots look off-center. The Random Dot E test offers no such clues. Neither test requires accurate color vision.

49. c) Nystagmus is rhythmic jerking of the eyes. This movement may be horizontal, vertical, or torsional.

50. a) Because of the laws of extraocular muscle innervation, the eyes of a patient with congenital nystagmus will both jerk. The direction of the jerking should be noted (see answer 49) as well as the magnitude (eg, small, fine movements versus large ones). In some patients, the jerking is lessened when the eyes are in a specific position, so the patient may adopt a head tilt or turn to quiet the eyes.

51. c) See answer 50. In some cases, occluding one eye makes the nystagmus worse.

52. a) The null point is when the head is in a position where the jerking is "most nullified" or lessened (ie, quieter).

53. b) Occluding one eye can make the nystagmus worse. Use a +6.00 to "occlude" (fog) the eye not being examined in visual acuity testing and refractometry.

54. d) Using a trial frame for refractometry will allow the patient to easily adopt his or her null-point head position. This is not as easily done using the phoroptor. Subjective refractometry (versus autorefractor or retinoscopy alone) will provide the best information from which the practitioner might prescribe.

55. d) Gaze-induced nystagmus (also called *end-gaze* and *end-point nystagmus*) sometimes appears when the patient moves the eyes out of primary position, usually to the right or left.

56. b) Vibrating vision (properly termed *oscillopsia*) is where objects of regard seem to move, jerk, or wiggle when the patient concentrates on them. This phenomenon occurs only in acquired nystagmus; patients with congenital nystagmus do not have this symptom.

57. c) In some cases, the nystagmus will resolve as the child grows; however, that is not the case with most types of nystagmus. The other statements are true. The head position is adopted in order to move the eyes into a position where the jerking is quieter or stopped, called the "null point," giving the patient clearer vision. The patient "finds" this position (which varies from patient to patient) at an early age, generally when beginning to sit up or stand. In addition, congenital nystagmus is often associated with lesions in the optic system.

Chapter 11

Assisting in Surgical Procedures

Ledford JK.
*Certified Ophthalmic Assistant: Exam
Review Manual, Third Edition* (pp. 117-136).
© 2012 Taylor & Francis Group.

General[1]

1. **The term *minor surgery* can be defined as:**
   a) a simple procedure with minimal risk
   b) any surgery that is done using only local anesthetic
   c) any surgery that is not required to be performed in a hospital
   d) a simple procedure that can be performed by an assistant

2. **Which of the following could be considered minor surgery?**
   a) cataract extraction
   b) corneal transplant
   c) chalazion removal
   d) enucleation

3. **"Incision" refers to:**
   a) cutting out tissue
   b) cutting into tissue
   c) suturing tissue
   d) giving an injection

4. **"Excision" is defined as:**
   a) cutting out tissue
   b) cutting into tissue
   c) suturing tissue
   d) giving an injection

5. **The procedure that corrects the inversion of the lower eyelid is:**
   a) chalazion removal
   b) ptosis correction
   c) entropion repair
   d) ectropion repair

6. **A surgical schedule would describe the procedure to correct drooping of the upper eyelid as:**
   a) ptosis correction
   b) chalazion removal
   c) scleral buckling
   d) trabeculectomy

7. **The procedure for removal of a fleshy encroachment onto the cornea is a/an:**
   a) ectropion repair
   b) pterygium excision
   c) hordeolum excision
   d) scleral buckling

[1]While this is not listed as a criteria, it seemed prudent to include.

8. **All of the following might be done after the excision of a possible skin cancer *except*:**
   a) placing disposable needles and blades in an approved sharps container
   b) placing the removed tissue in a specimen bottle for biopsy
   c) proper disposal of contaminated disposables
   d) proper disposal of all removed tissue

Instrument Preparation[2]

9. **An ungloved person sets up a sterile tray by carefully "dumping" sterile instruments and materials onto the tray without contacting them. This preparation is known as:**
   a) the "no touch" method
   b) unacceptable, as it is not sterile technique
   c) standard precautions
   d) the sterile method

10. **A sterile tray for a chalazion removal might include:**
    a) chalazion clamp, blade, forceps, and curette
    b) eyelid speculum, blade, and forceps
    c) chalazion clamp, needle holder, and cannula
    d) eyelid speculum, blade, forceps, and curette

11. **A sterile tray for a lacrimal evaluation might include:**
    a) lid speculum, punctal dilator, and lacrimal stint
    b) clamp, needle holder, and curette
    c) forceps, punctal dilator, curette, and lacrimal cannula
    d) medicine glass, punctal dilator, syringe, and lacrimal cannula

12. **In addition to the sterile tray for a lacrimal evaluation, the setup for a procedure to open a blocked tear duct would include:**
    a) blunt needle
    b) set of probes
    c) cautery unit
    d) electrolysis unit

13. **A sterile tray for any growth removal will probably include:**
    a) lid speculum, forceps, curette, and suture material
    b) scalpel, scissors, forceps, needle holder, and sutures
    c) curette, chalazion clamp, forceps, and scalpel
    d) probe, forceps, scissors, and needle holder

14. **Match the following:**
cryo	a) uses focused amplified light
cautery	b) uses electrical impulses
electrolysis	c) uses cold
laser	d) uses heat

[2]For instrument sterilization, see section *Sterilization* in this chapter.

15. **All of the following can cause stains on surgical instruments *except*:**
    a) failure to rinse off detergents
    b) residue from sutures
    c) minerals in the water source
    d) dried blood

16. **Surgical instruments should be lubricated:**
    a) only when they seem to stick
    b) only if cleaned in an ultrasonic unit
    c) after every use
    d) after every fifth use

17. **Which of the following is true regarding ultrasonic cleaners?**
    a) They effectively sterilize surgical instruments.
    b) Scrub instruments before placing them in the unit.
    c) Instruments should not touch while in the unit.
    d) Glass cannot be placed in the unit.

Refractive Surgery[3]

18. **The premise behind refractive surgery is to change the refractive power of the eye by:**
    a) changing the eye's refractive index
    b) eliminating astigmatism
    c) altering the eye's focal length
    d) transposing the refractive error

19. **Laser refractive surgery seeks to correct a refractive error by:**
    a) altering the shape of the cornea
    b) altering the shape of the retina
    c) improving the tear film
    d) inserting a retinal implant

20. **To correct myopia with laser refractive surgery, the goal is to:**
    a) steepen the corneal center
    b) flatten the corneal center
    c) eliminate minus power in the eye
    d) eliminate astigmatism

21. **In which of the following refractive procedures is a corneal flap created and laser used to sculpt the underlying tissue?**
    a) intrastromal rings
    b) radial keratotomy (RK)
    c) laser-assisted in-situ keratomileusis (LASIK)
    d) photorefractive keratectomy (PRK)

[3]Cataract surgery/IOL insertion and corneal transplantation will not be considered in this particular discussion of refractive surgery.

22. **Laser refractive surgery is performed with which type of laser?**
    a) argon
    b) excimer
    c) YAG
    d) krypton

23. **All of the following are forms of laser refractive surgery *except*:**
    a) RK
    b) PRK
    c) LASIK
    d) laser-assisted subepithelial keratomileusis (LASEK)

24. **In LASIK, which corneal layers are excised as part of the flap?**
    a) epithelium
    b) epithelium and Bowman's layer
    c) epithelium and Descemet's membrane
    d) endothelium and stroma

25. **Which of the following allows the surgeon to customize laser refractive surgery during the procedure?**
    a) wavefront LASIK
    b) aberration-free LASIK
    c) LASIK IOLMaster (Carl Zeiss, Jena, Germany) software
    d) LASIK corneal keratometry

26. **Postoperative instructions following LASIK surgery would include all of the following *except*:**
    a) do not bend over
    b) shower from the neck down
    c) wear a shield over the operated eye at bedtime
    d) do not rub the eye

27. **Matching: Match the procedure to the description; items may be used more than once:**

used to treat corneal scars	a) PRK
involves use of a keratome	b) LASIK
corneal epithelium removed	c) LASEK
corneal flap	d) Phototherapeutic keratectomy
very thin corneal flap	(PTK)
treats some types of corneal dystrophy	
corneal flap includes some stroma	
routine use of a postoperative bandage contact lens	

Sterile Fields

28. **The sterile field is an area that is considered to be:**
   a) disinfected
   b) free of chemicals
   c) free of microbes
   d) sanitized

29. **The sterile field would include all of the following *except*:**
   a) sterile, gloved hands
   b) eye drop bottles
   c) the drape around the surgical site
   d) the instrument tray

30. **If an unsterile object touches anything in the sterile field, the field is:**
   a) immediately covered with another drape
   b) immediately rescrubbed
   c) considered contaminated
   d) still adequate and surgery may continue

Aseptic Technique

31. **Techniques used to prevent preoperative, intraoperative, and postoperative microbial infection are collectively termed:**
   a) clean
   b) aseptic
   c) sanitary
   d) health standard

32. **The purpose of aseptic technique is to:**
   a) reduce the number of chemicals present
   b) ensure proper safety measures
   c) reduce the chances of wound infection
   d) ensure proper ventilation

33. **Steps in a minor surgery procedure include all of the following *except*:**
   a) disinfection of the patient's skin
   b) setting up a sterile tray
   c) administering topical or local anesthetic
   d) sterile gowning of surgical personnel

34. **In minor surgery, the assistant might remain ungloved. In this case he or she:**
   a) must not disinfect the patient's skin
   b) must not touch any nonsterile area
   c) must not touch the sterile field
   d) must not apply eye drops

Nonrefractive Laser Therapy[4]

35. **"Laser" stands for:**
    a) light amplification to stimulate emission of radioactivity
    b) light amplification to stimulate emergence of radiation
    c) light absorption to simulate effective radiation
    d) light amplification by stimulated emission of radiation

36. **The basic function of any laser is:**
    a) tissue destruction
    b) tissue sculpting
    c) creation of an opening
    d) to decrease pressure

37. **Which laser is commonly used to remove a cloudy capsule following cataract surgery?**
    a) argon
    b) CO_2
    c) YAG
    d) microendolaser

38. **Phototherapeutic keratectomy (PTK) might be performed on which of the following?**
    a) high myopia
    b) presbyopia
    c) corneal scar
    d) pterygium

39. **The argon laser is commonly used in all of the following disease states *except*:**
    a) diabetic retinopathy
    b) hypertensive retinopathy
    c) cataract
    d) glaucoma

40. **Laser surgery for open-angle glaucoma mainly involves:**
    a) treating the trabecular meshwork
    b) treating the ciliary body
    c) treating the canal of Schlemm
    d) sealing the puncta

41. **In angle-closure glaucoma, a laser is used to create a(n):**
    a) iridotomy
    b) peripheral iridectomy
    c) sector iridectomy
    d) iris ablation

[4]See also *YAG Laser* and *Laser Safety* in this chapter.

42. **Laser treatment of diabetics might include which of the following?**
    a) sealing blood vessels
    b) opening blood vessels
    c) preventing secondary glaucoma
    d) preventing retinal detachment

43. **Panretinal photocoagulation might be used in the treatment of which of the following?**
    a) hypertensive retinopathy
    b) retinal detachment
    c) diabetic retinopathy
    d) retinitis pigmentosa

44. **Which of the following is a laser procedure that would be used to treat a specific area of the retina?**
    a) focal
    b) panretinal
    c) maculectomy
    d) epiretinal

Intraocular Injections

45. **Intraocular injections might be used to treat any of the following *except*:**
    a) wet macular degeneration
    b) diabetic retinopathy
    c) retinal vein occlusion
    d) retinal detachment

46. **Which of the following is not a medication used in intraocular injections?**
    a) Macugen (Eyetech Inc, Palm Beach Gardens, FL)
    b) Pilopine (Alcon Laboratories, Fort Worth, TX)
    c) Kenalog (Squibb, New York City, NY)
    d) Lucentis (Genentech, Inc, South San Francisco, CA)

47. **The tray set-up for an intraocular injection would include all of the following *except*:**
    a) blunt-ended cannula
    b) lid speculum
    c) fine-toothed forceps
    d) calipers

48. **The prep for an intraocular injection involves:**
    a) vigorous scrubbing of the lids and lashes
    b) use of povidone iodine directly on the ocular surface
    c) retrobulbar anesthetic injection
    d) instillation of miotic eye drops

49. **The actual intraocular injection takes about:**
    a) 5 seconds
    b) 30 seconds
    c) 60 seconds
    d) 90 seconds

50. **As soon as the surgeon removes the needle from the eye following an intraocular injection, the assistant must immediately:**
    a) instill a miotic to reverse pupil dilation
    b) check the intraocular pressure
    c) apply a cotton-tipped applicator to the site
    d) check the patient's vision with a near card

51. **Which of the following is a common postoperative occurrence in a patient who has had an intraocular injection?**
    a) floaters
    b) hyphema
    c) increasing pain
    d) marked pressure sensation

YAG Laser

52. **YAG stands for:**
    a) yellow-aqua-green
    b) yttrium-aluminum-garnet
    c) yrinium-angle-geodesic
    d) ystridium-alum-glaucoma

53. **The laser procedure to make a hole in the iris to prevent aqueous blockage is called:**
    a) sector iridectomy
    b) peripheral iridectomy
    c) iridotomy
    d) trabeculectomy

54. **The YAG laser might commonly be used for which of the following procedures?**
    a) Sealing a retinal hole.
    b) Sealing a bleeding retinal blood vessel.
    c) Opening the trabeculum in glaucoma.
    d) Cutting through vitreous adhesions.

55. **A possible complication of a YAG capsulotomy laser procedure is:**
    a) loss of corneal endothelial cells
    b) rise in intraocular pressure
    c) decrease in vision
    d) corneal scarring

56. **The YAG laser is mainly used in which of the following ways?**
    a) photodisruption
    b) photocoagulation
    c) heat
    d) ultraviolet radiation

Sterilization

57. **All of the following are acceptable sterilizing procedures *except*:**
    a) boiling
    b) moist heat (autoclave)
    c) chemical disinfectants (germicides)
    d) infrared radiation

58. **Prior to sterilization, surgical instruments should be:**
    a) boiled in water
    b) cleaned to remove blood and debris
    c) soaked in chemical disinfectant
    d) wrapped in linen

59. **Which statement regarding autoclave sterilizing procedures for ophthalmic instruments is *false*?**
    a) Instruments should be closed when sterilizing.
    b) All detachable parts must be dissembled.
    c) Heavier instruments are placed on bottom.
    d) Preheat instruments in the autoclave before beginning the steam cycle.

60. **The autoclave (moist heat) employs which of the following to accomplish sterilization?**
    a) Steam for an allotted time.
    b) Boiling water under pressure for an allotted time.
    c) Steam under pressure for an allotted time.
    d) Ultrasonic heat for an allotted time.

61. **Disadvantages of boiling to sterilize include all of the following *except*:**
    a) sharp instruments can be dulled
    b) some instruments will rust
    c) only saline solution should be used
    d) it may take several hours to kill certain spores

62. **The temperature and time required to sterilize instruments with dry heat is:**
    a) 320° F for 60 minutes
    b) 320° F for 30 minutes
    c) 250° F for 15 minutes
    d) 120° F for 60 minutes

63. **The minimum time for instrument sterilization in a cold chemical bath is:**
    a) 5 minutes
    b) 20 minutes
    c) 60 minutes
    d) 90 minutes

64. **All of the following are commonly used for chemical sterilization *except*:**
    a) phenol derivatives
    b) ethyl alcohol 70%
    c) formaldehyde
    d) iodine

65. **All of the following are advantages of ethylene oxide sterilization *except*:**
    a) it is inexpensive
    b) it can be used on most materials
    c) its effectiveness
    d) its ability to penetrate

66. **The effectiveness of any procedure used to sterilize instruments may be tested by:**
    a) trying to culture organisms from the instruments after sterilization
    b) trying to culture organisms from the instruments prior to sterilization
    c) periodically documenting the readings on the temperature gauge
    d) whether or not the indicator tape turns color

Site Identification

67. **The surgical time-out refers to:**
    a) guided meditation to calm the patient prior to the procedure
    b) roll call of surgical personnel
    c) a pause during which staff correlates procedure and patient information
    d) removal of an impaired staff member

68. **The surgical time-out is done:**
    a) as soon as the patient arrives
    b) while the patient is being prepped
    c) right before the procedure begins
    d) right after the procedure has been completed

69. **Site identification can be accomplished by all of the following *except*:**
    a) performing a surgical time-out
    b) asking the patient to confirm
    c) consulting the patient's record
    d) marking the skin with a wax pencil

Laser Safety

70. **One of the primary safety procedures regarding laser use is:**
    a) proper disposal of biohazardous tissue
    b) proper disposal of sharps
    c) posting a warning sign regarding laser radiation
    d) use of lead-lined covers

71. **Safety precautions to be taken during ophthalmic laser treatment include:**
    a) containment
    b) eye protection
    c) warning signs/lights
    d) all of the above

72. **Except for the physician performing the procedure and the patient receiving it, everyone in the room when laser is being performed must:**
    a) wear polarized sunglasses
    b) close their eyes when the laser is fired
    c) use artificial tears afterwards
    d) wear eye protection specific to the type of laser used

73. **The organization requiring employers to provide the proper eye protection for workers assisting in laser surgery is:**
    a) The American National Safety Institute (ANSI)
    b) The Food and Drug Administration (FDA)
    c) Occupational Safety and Health Administration (OSHA)
    d) Federal Trade Commission (FTA)

74. **The physician performing the laser treatment is protected from laser exposure by:**
    a) built-in filters in the instrument's oculars
    b) being at least 15 feet away from the patient
    c) closing his or her eyes when firing the laser beam
    d) wearing appropriate eye protection

75. **Your practice has installed an observation ocular to the existing laser unit. Which of the following is also necessary?**
    a) Proper focusing to better direct the laser beam.
    b) A filter to prevent laser damage to the observer.
    c) A second joystick for dual control.
    d) A diffuser for general viewing.

76. **Any time the laser unit is moved, one must be sure to:**
    a) update the computer software
    b) realign the beam
    c) rinse off the laser media
    d) realign the filters

77. **Your employer finished the last laser treatment of the morning at 11:45 AM. The next laser patient is due to come in at 2:00 PM. According to OSHA safety standards, what should be done?**
    a) The door to the laser room should be locked.
    b) The laser must be capped.
    c) The laser must be turned off.
    d) Someone must check the laser hourly.

Assist With Procedures[5,6]

78. **Which of the following is *not* true regarding ambulatory surgical centers (ASCs)?**
    a) Any ophthalmic clinic can set up its own ASC.
    b) Physicians at an ASC must maintain hospital privileges.
    c) ASCs are held to state and federal standards.
    d) An ASC must have periodic inspections and assessments.

79. **Which of the following members of the surgical team would be unscrubbed?**
    a) surgeon
    b) circulator
    c) surgical assistant
    d) scrub nurse/technician

80. **Which of the following is proper technique when scrubbing?**
    a) Use water as hot as you can stand.
    b) Scrub hands up to point of wrists.
    c) Rinse from hands to elbows, hands up.
    d) Put on a mask after scrubbing.

81. **Which of the following is *not* performed in the OR itself?**
    a) drying of scrubbed hands
    b) donning gown
    c) donning gloves
    d) donning head cover

82. **Which of the following regarding gowning is *not* true?**
    a) The gown may be tied by an unscrubbed person.
    b) Gown cuffs are stretched over the glove cuffs.
    c) The back of the sterile gown is considered unsterile.
    d) The sterile gown below the sterile field is considered unsterile.

---

[5]The COT® criteria include the additional topic of scrub technician duties not present on the COA® list. The difference between assisting and scrub technician duties are not always clear. In Cassin's book, the assistant "provides exposure of the surgical field, cuts sutures, and assists in hemostasis." (See Appendix B for reference.)

[6]For questions regarding types of ophthalmic surgery, see Chapter 12, section *Patient Instruction,* subheadings *Procedure* and *Treatments.* See also the section titled *Surgical Site Identification* earlier in this chapter.

83. **The technique of using the cuffs of one's sterile surgical gown to handle sterile gloves while putting them on is:**
   a) no-touch technique
   b) open gloving technique
   c) closed gloving technique
   d) assisted gloving technique

84. **Once scrubbed and gloved, which of the following is permissible?**
   a) Picking up something that has fallen off the instrument stand.
   b) Keeping the hands above the waist.
   c) Opening suture packets.
   d) Dabbing the surgeon's forehead with a sterile 4 × 4 gauze.

85. **How should members of the scrubbed surgical team move about the OR?**
   a) With their backs to the sterile field.
   b) Passing each other face-to-face.
   c) Only the circulator may move around the OR.
   d) No particular technique is needed.

86. **A common mistake in performing the skin prep prior to ocular surgery is:**
   a) scrubbing back and forth
   b) prepping the lashes
   c) irrigating afterwards
   d) cleansing from inner to outer canthus

87. **Which of the following is *true* regarding draping?**
   a) The entire drape is considered sterile.
   b) A warm blanket may be placed on top of the body drape for patient comfort.
   c) Only the circulator may drape the patient.
   d) The skin prep is performed prior to draping.

88. **The table on which surgical instruments are placed is the:**
   a) prep table
   b) back table
   c) Mayo stand
   d) circulation stand

89. **Which of the following would probably *not* be placed on the instrument (Mayo) stand?**
   a) forceps and needle holders
   b) eye shield and tape
   c) sutures and needles
   d) gem blades and scissors

90. **Hemostasis refers to:**
   a) placing sutures
   b) filtering blood flow
   c) stopping blood flow
   d) opening blood flow

91. **Match (draw a line) from these standard surgical instruments to their purpose[7]:**

Instrument	Purpose
calipers	grasping
cannulas	cutting
clamps	delivering fluids
forceps	isolating tissue/lesion
hooks	measuring
needle holders	separating eyelids
probes/dilators	opening obstructed canals
scissors	identify muscles, grasp IOL loops
speculum	holding suture needles

Explanatory Answers

1. a) Simple procedures that have minimal risk may be considered minor.
2. c) The chalazion excision is a minor procedure. The other procedures listed are not simple and have at least moderate risk.
3. b) Incision refers to cutting into a tissue as compared to tissue removal.
4. a) If tissue is removed, the procedure is an excision.
5. c) An inverted lower eyelid is an entropion. It is corrected to prevent corneal irritation and scarring from constant rubbing by the eyelashes.
6. a) Ptosis is a drooped eyelid. It might be repaired for cosmetic or visual reasons.
7. b) A pterygium is a fleshy growth that extends from the conjunctiva onto the cornea. It is removed because it can grow across the front of the cornea, impeding sight.
8. d) Any tissue that might be cancerous is sent for biopsy, not disposed of.
9. a) The "no touch" method of setting up a sterile tray for minor surgery is acceptable as long as there is strictly no contact with anything that touches the tray.
10. a) A chalazion clamp, blade, forceps, and curette might all be used for a chalazion removal. An eyelid speculum, cannula, and/or needle holder are not generally required.
11. d) A lacrimal setup would include a medicine glass (for saline), punctal dilator, syringe, and cannula for lavage (irrigation).
12. b) A probe is the wire-like instrument that is passed through the punctum and canaliculus, then pushed through the blockage.
13. b) Any growth removal will probably require a scalpel, scissors, forceps, needle holder, and suture material. A lid speculum might be used, but a curette and chalazion clamp are for chalazia and a probe is for lacrimal procedures.
14. Matching

cryo	c) uses cold
cautery	d) uses heat
electrolysis	b) uses electrical impulses
laser	a) uses focused amplified light

15. b) Okay, I confess, I made up answer b. All the rest can cause staining.
16. d) As a general rule, lubricate surgical instruments after every fifth use.

[7]Adapted from Boess-Lott R, Stecik S. *The Ophthalmic Surgical Assistant*. Thorofare, NJ: SLACK Incorporated; 1999.

17. c) Ultrasonic cleaners do not sterilize, you do not have to scrub first, and you can put glass in them. But the instruments should not touch.

18. c) The focal length of the eye (or of any lens/lens system) is the distance from the lens system to the focal point, where light is focused. Refractive surgery seeks to alter this in order to put the focal point directly on the retina (ie, macula).

19. a) The cornea accounts for most of the refractive power of the eye. It is also accessible, as opposed to the other parts of ocular media, except for the tear film. Changing the cornea's shape (flattening or steepening) alters the refractive error.

20. b) Flattening the cornea's center moves the eye's focal point back toward the retina. In myopia, the focal point falls somewhere in the vitreous. (**Note:** Regarding answer c, the myopic eye has too much *plus* power, which is why we neutralize it with *minus*.)

21. c) In LASIK surgery, a microkeratome (a keratome is a surgical knife/blade used to incise the cornea; a microkeratome is small and capable of making very precise incisions) is used to cut a thin flap in the top-most corneal layers. The excimer laser is then used to sculpt the underlying tissue to correct the refractive error. The flap is then put back into place, over the ablated area.

22. b) The name excimer is derived from "excited dimer." This laser uses ultraviolet radiation that breaks or photoevaporates chemical bonds between tissues and is ideally suited for work on the cornea.

23. a) In RK, the surgeon uses a diamond blade to alter the cornea's shape.

24. b) In LASIK, a microkeratome is used to create a flap of the epithelium and Bowman's layer (and, technically, a bit of the stroma). The laser is then used to sculpt the underlying stroma.

25. a) Wavefront technology creates a rough map of the patient's eye, allowing very precise control and treatment during the refractive procedure. The idea is to reduce aberrations, thus reducing side effects such as glare, haloes, and blur. The other answers are bogus.

26. a) There is no restriction on bending over after LASIK surgery. Otherwise, patients are told to avoid water/sweat in the eye, do not rub the eye, wear the shield at bedtime, avoid smoke, and not to wear make-up. The duration of these restrictions varies.

27. Matching:

used to treat corneal scars	d)
involves use of a keratome	b), c)
corneal epithelium removed	a), sometimes d)
corneal flap	b),c)
very thin corneal flap	c)
treats some types of corneal dystrophy	d)
corneal flap includes some stroma	b)
routine use of a postoperative bandage contact lens	a), d)

28. c) The sterile field is considered to be free of microorganisms. Disinfection is not sterility; it does not remove the most resistant microbes. Sanitization means that the number of microbes has been reduced to a "safe" level.

29. b) While many minor ophthalmic procedures would include the use of eye drops before, during, or after the surgery, the bottles are not sterile. The sterile gloved hands of the surgical team, the exterior of the eye drape, and the instrument tray (with sterile instruments on a sterile drape or towel of some sort) are each part of the sterile field.

30. c) There is no such thing as "almost" sterile; if an unsterile item contacts the sterile field, the field is considered contaminated.

31. b) Aseptic technique is used to prevent contamination by infectious microorganisms. The level of asepsis varies according to the procedure, ranging from clean to aseptic to sterile. Clean technique is used for noninvasive procedures such as tonometry. Aseptic technique is applied to minor surgical procedures. Sterile technique is used in major surgery, where exposure of tissues might be more deep and lengthy. (You can see that "aseptic technique" has a rather double meaning; be sure to read questions carefully.)

32. c) The purpose of aseptic technique is to eliminate microorganisms that could potentially cause infection.

33. d) Sterile gowning is not required for minor surgery, as a rule.

34. c) If an ungloved assistant touches the sterile field, the field becomes contaminated.

35. d) Light amplification by stimulated emission of radiation is the basis of the acronym.

36. a) Regardless of laser type, mode of action, or treatment type, a laser is used to destroy tissue. The purpose may be to open (as in laser capsulotomy), cause scarring (the theorized action of laser trabeculectomy), or seal (as in punctoplasty or diabetic retinopathy). Each of these involves tissue destruction, whether by heat (photocoagulation), vaporization, cutting (photodisruption), or breaking down the chemical bonds of tissues (photoablation).

37. c) Laser capsulotomy is usually performed with the YAG laser. The argon is used for photocoagulation, the CO_2 for skin lesions, and the microendolaser for internal treatments.

38. c) PTK is a laser treatment for surface corneal disease such as shallow scars, recurrent erosion, and some types of corneal dystrophy. The goal is to create a smooth corneal surface that will heal evenly.

39. c) A cataract cannot be removed with a laser at this time.

40. a) A laser trabeculoplasty, the current most popular laser treatment for open-angle glaucoma, is directed at the trabecular meshwork in an attempt to increase aqueous drainage.

41. a) A laser iridotomy is used to create an opening in the iris to prevent pressure build-up in angle-closure glaucoma, providing aqueous drainage even if the angle is blocked. Answers b and c require conventional surgery. Answer d would mean destruction of the iris, which is not done.

42. a) In diabetes the blood vessels of the body, including the eye, tend to weaken, which means they can leak blood into surrounding tissues. There can also be the formation of new blood vessels, which tend to bleed. Most laser treatment in diabetics is done in an effort to seal blood vessels in order to stop or prevent leakage.

43. c) Panretinal photocoagulation is used to treat diabetic retinopathy by applying a laser to multiple points of the retina. The Greek prefix *pan-* refers to "all" or "whole."

44. a) The term *focal* refers to a defined, circumscribed area. *Panretinal* refers to treating a broad area, usually for diabetes.

45. d) Intraocular injections are not used to treat retinal detachment. Wet macular degeneration and diabetic retinopathy would be treated with medications aimed at preventing the growth of new, abnormal blood vessels. Treatment for a retinal vein occlusion would be used to alleviate macular swelling.

46. b) Pilopine is a topical miotic gel sometimes used in glaucoma treatment. Macugen and Lucentis are used in treating wet macular degeneration. Kenalog is a steroid used to treat macular edema, or swelling.

47. a) A lid speculum holds the eye open and helps to keep the lashes out of the way. Fine-toothed forceps are used to keep the eye in position by grabbing the conjunctiva. The calipers are used to measure from the limbus to the intended injection site, so as to avoid anterior segment structures.

48. b) Povidone iodine (in drop or wash form) is applied to the ocular surface (as well as lashes and lids) when prepping for an intraocular injection. Vigorous scrubbing is contra-indicated, as this may expulse the bacteria-containing contents of the various glands in the lids. Topical anesthetic, or possibly a local injection just under the conjunctiva, is usually used. The pupil is generally dilated (versus miosis) so that it is easier to evaluate the patient's retina following the procedure.

49. a) The actual injection is a quick affair of 5 seconds or less. (When you are educating the patient beforehand, be sure to tell him this!)

50. c) A cotton-tipped applicator is placed on the injection site immediately after the needle is removed to prevent any medication from leaking out.

51. a) Floaters are common after intraocular injections. Such "spots" may even be bubbles that entered the eye during the procedure.

52. b) YAG stands for yttrium-aluminum-garnet, a reference to the crystals that emit radiation when stimulated by an energy source.

53. c) A laser iridotomy makes a hole in the iris, providing aqueous drainage even if the angle is blocked.

54. d) Procedures a, b, and c require the use of a laser than can fuse tissues rather than the scalpel-like qualities of the YAG. A complication of ocular surgery is where the vitreous pushes out of the posterior segment and into the anterior chamber. In this case there is concern that the vitreous pulling on the retina (to which it is still attached) may cause a retinal detachment. If the vitreous has adhered to a surgical incision, it may also be a con-duit for bacteria to enter the eye. In such a scenario, the YAG laser is used to cut through the vitreous strand in a procedure known as vitreolysis.

55. b) A rise in intraocular pressure, usually temporary, can occur following a YAG capsuloto-my.

56. a) The YAG is generally used as a photodisruptor, destroying tissue in what is sometimes called a "microexplosion." Other types of lasers work by other methods (ie, Argon is a thermal/photocoagulation laser; excimer lasers use ultraviolet light).

57. d) Infrared radiation is not a sterilizing method.

58. b) Always clean instruments before sterilizing them.

59. a) Instruments should be open when sterilizing to expose and sterilize all surfaces.

60. c) The autoclave utilizes steam under pressure for a specific length of time.

61. c) Saline solution is not used to boil or sterilize equipment.

62. a) When dry heat is used, 320° F for an hour is considered adequate.

63. b) Cold chemical sterilization is considered adequate after 20 minutes.

64. d) Iodine is not commonly used to sterilize instruments; it is used to disinfect the skin.

65. a) Ethylene oxide is great, but expensive.

66. a) Any sterilization method can be checked by trying to culture organisms from the instru-ment after it has been supposedly sterilized. Temperature gauges can be wrong, and indica-tor tape only tells whether or not the desired temperature was reached.

67. c) The surgical time-out is a time during which the surgical team "steps back" to be sure they have the right patient, the right procedure, the right site, and the right records/instru-ments/supplies.

68. c) The time-out occurs immediately before the procedure begins (ie, before the "first cut"). The patient has been prepped and is on the table, the team is present, and everyone must concur that they have the right patient, the right procedure, the right site, and the right records/instruments/supplies.

69. d) When marking the skin to identify the surgical site, an indelible marker is used, not a wax pencil.

70. c) A warning sign on the door will advise those in the vicinity that a laser is housed therein.

71. d) Containment (locating the equipment in an enclosed room), eye protection (appropriate to the type of laser being used), and approved warning signs and/or lights are all safety precautions to be in place when an ophthalmic laser is in use.

72. d) Eye protection is the biggest issue with those who are present in the room when laser is being used. The type of filtration lens required depends on the type of laser in use.

73. c) OSHA requires employers to provide appropriate personal protective equipment to those employees performing tasks with potential risk, including assisting in laser surgery. While ANSI does have a set of standards regarding laser exposure, compliance is voluntary. The FDA regulations involving lasers apply to instrument manufacturers.

74. a) The oculars of a laser have built-in safety filters to protect the user from exposure. The filter may be designed to flip into place when the laser is fired, or it may be fixed into place permanently. If an observation ocular is added to existing equipment, it is vital to be sure that the new ocular is filter-protected as well.

75. b) The operator's oculars already have a filter in place to protect the physician. If the laser came with the observation scope already installed, it probably does as well (but you should check). But if extra oculars are added later, you should inquire if they need the filter installed as well.

76. b) After moving the laser, the beam must be realigned prior to use.

77. c) According to OSHA Standard 1926.54,[8] the laser must be turned off if it is not going to be used for a length of time. The examples given in the Standard are lunch break, shift change, or overnight.

78. a) Only a clinic that is in compliance with state and federal standards can establish an ASC.

79. b) The circulator is a nonscrubbed person who generally sees to the patient's comfort, adjusts nonsterile instrumentation, brings in additional supplies when needed, and handles paperwork.

80. c) Scrubbed arms are held hands-up when rinsing so that run-off goes toward the elbows and not back over the hands. The scrub suit, head cover, shoe covers, and mask should all be donned prior to scrubbing. Water should be tolerably warm, and the scrub extends to include the forearms.

81. d) The head cover is put on prior to the scrub, which is done outside the OR.

82. b) Glove cuffs are stretched over the gown cuffs, not vice versa. An unscrubbed person may tie the gown as long as they do not touch the front of the gown or any part of the tie that touches the front. The parts of the gown that are considered unsterile is the neck, the arm pits, the shoulders, the cuffs, the back, and any area that is below the surgical field.

---

[8]Insert available at: www.eyesafety.4ursafety.com/OSHA-Laser-regulations.html. Accessed 03/08/2011.

83. c) The closed gloving technique, also called the closed cuff gloving technique, involves putting the arms through the sterile gown up to the point of the cuffs. The hands, still inside the gown cuffs, are used to manipulate the gloves without touching them directly. In the open gloving technique, the fingers of one hand touch only the edge of the inner cuff of one of the gloves. The second glove is put on with the first gloved hand.

84. b) Everything below the waist is considered nonsterile, so the hands must be kept above waist level. The other answers are incorrect. A nonscrubbed person would perform answer d, holding the gauze with forceps or tongs of some sort.

85. b) Scrubbed team members should move around each other either face-to-face or back-to-back (ie, never face-to-back). In general, everyone in the OR is facing the sterile field. The circulator may move around, of course, but is not scrubbed.

86. a) Cleansing should begin at the lid margin and move outward in widening circles, from the inner to the outer canthus. One should not scrub from cleansed to non-cleansed back onto cleansed again.

87. d) The skin of the surgical site is prepped before the drape is applied. Only the top of a drape is considered sterile; the back (touching the patient) is not, nor is any part of the drape that extends beyond the surgical field (eg, over the table). A blanket would be placed directly on the body prior to draping, not after. The circulator is unscrubbed and therefore would not be handling the sterile drapes.

88. c) The Mayo stand, also called the instrument stand, is a tray covered with a sterile drape on which instruments and other needed materials are placed. The prep table holds items needed to prepare the surgical site. The back table holds gowns, gloves, towels, basins, drapes, and extra supplies.

89. b) Eye shields and tape are not used during the procedure, and are not sterile. This equipment would contaminate the sterile Mayo stand.

90. c) *Hemo-* meaning blood, *-stasis* meaning standing, or still. Hemostasis is stilling the flow of blood. A surgical assistant may be asked to stop blood flow by applying pressure or other means, as directed.

91. Matching:

calipers	→	measuring
cannulas	→	delivering fluids
clamps	→	isolating tissue/lesion
forceps	→	grasping
hooks	→	identify muscles, grasp IOL loops
needle holders	→	holding suture needles
probes/dilators	→	opening obstructed canals
scissors	→	cutting
speculum	→	separating eyelids

Chapter 12

Ophthalmic Patient Services and Education

Ledford, JK.
*Certified Ophthalmic Assistant: Exam
Review Manual, Third Edition* (pp. 137-214).
© 2012 Taylor & Francis Group.

Patient Education[1]

Surgery[2]

Plastics

1. **A patient who has an upper blepharoplasty has been treated for:**
   a) chalazion
   b) epicanthal folds
   c) dermatochalasis
   d) brow ptosis

2. **Ptosis surgery is done to repair which of the following?**
   a) strabismus
   b) drooping upper lid
   c) lax lower lid
   d) redundant skin and fat

3. **The procedure for removing a growth from the eyelid is:**
   a) excision
   b) incision
   c) decompression
   d) biopsy

4. **The most common surgical treatment for a chalazion is:**
   a) cautery
   b) electrolysis
   c) incise and drain
   d) probe and irrigate

5. **A patient wants to have an upper blepharoplasty to improve his looks. This type of surgery is termed:**
   a) functional
   b) cosmetic
   c) mandatory
   d) sight-threatening

6. **The main purpose of a biopsy is to:**
   a) determine the type of lesion
   b) determine the effectiveness of surgery
   c) determine the expected outcome of surgery
   d) identify malingerers

[1]Patient education is one of the top tasks performed by technicians as listed by ophthalmologists. Obviously, a technician must understand ophthalmic surgery, systemic and ocular diseases, and anatomy and physiology (both general and ocular) in order to be able to explain such topics to a patient. For this reason, not all questions are worded as if teaching a patient. However, every effort has been made to be thorough.

[2]For informed consent, see Chapter 7, the section titled *Informed Consent*.

7. **The surgical procedure where skin or other tissue is transplanted from one part of the body to another is a(n):**
   a) flap
   b) incision
   c) graft
   d) implant

8. **The surgery to fix an in-turned eyelid is:**
   a) epilation
   b) frontalis sling
   c) blepharoplasty
   d) entropion repair

9. **The surgery to fix an out-turned eyelid is:**
   a) ptosis repair
   b) trichiasis repair
   c) ectropion repair
   d) iridotomy

Lacrimal

10. **When repairing a lower lid laceration in the area of the punctum, tissue alignment is especially critical because:**
    a) the lacrimal drainage system is involved
    b) the tear-producing ducts are involved
    c) infection may set in
    d) eyelash alignment may be affected

11. **An infant with a blocked nasolacrimal duct might initially need which of the following procedures?**
    a) dacryocystorhinostomy
    b) removal of the tear gland
    c) punctal dilation
    d) probe and irrigation

12. **A patient with dry eyes might have which of the following procedures?**
    a) lacrimectomy
    b) cyclocryo
    c) punctal occlusion
    d) punctal dilation

Cornea[3]

13. **The grafting of corneal tissue from one human eye to another is a(n):**
    a) enucleation
    b) keratoplasty
    c) dacryocystorhinostomy
    d) corneal topography

[3]For more on refractive surgery, see Chapter 11, the section titled *Refractive Surgery*.

14. **Each of the following might be associated with a corneal transplant** *except*:
    a) follow-up radiation treatment
    b) tissue rejection
    c) irregular astigmatism
    d) 12-month recovery time

15. **Which of the following might need to be surgically removed because it is growing across the cornea?**
    a) pingueculum
    b) punctal plug
    c) pterygium
    d) xanthelasma

16. **Recurrent corneal erosion might be treated by:**
    a) corneal scraping
    b) punctal occlusion
    c) enucleation
    d) corneal transplant

17. **Surgery that is performed in order to correct hyperopia, myopia, and/or astigmatism is classified as:**
    a) amniotic membrane transplant
    b) refractive surgery
    c) corneal transplant
    d) corneal endothelial correction

18. **A popular technique for correcting refractive errors using laser technology is:**
    a) laser-assisted in situ keratomileusis (LASIK)
    b) radial keratotomy (RK)
    c) astigmatic keratotomy (AK)
    d) corneal implants

19. **Which of the following refractive surgeries does *not* involve creating a corneal flap?**
    a) epi-LASIK
    b) photorefractive keratectomy (PRK)
    c) laser-assisted subepithelial keratomileusis (LASEK)
    d) LASIK

20. **Which laser is most commonly used in refractive surgery?**
    a) yttrium-aluminum-garnet (YAG)
    b) argon
    c) krypton
    d) excimer

21. **Anesthesia for laser refractive surgery is usually:**
    a) local
    b) general
    c) topical
    d) not needed

Strabismus/Extraocular Muscle

22. A person with esotropia might have what kind of surgery?
   a) trabeculectomy
   b) recession and resection
   c) blepharoplasty
   d) ptosis repair

23. The purpose of extraocular muscle (EOM) surgery as a child might include all of the following *except*:
   a) prevention/resolution of amblyopia
   b) cosmesis
   c) correction of anisometropia
   d) establish stereo vision

Cataracts

24. A cataract is a:
   a) growth on the lens
   b) clouding of the cornea
   c) lens opacity
   d) growth on the retina

25. Symptoms of cataract include:
   a) halos
   b) floaters
   c) flashes
   d) foreign-body sensation

26. Symptoms of cataract include:
   a) becoming more nearsighted
   b) becoming more farsighted
   c) early presbyopia
   d) discharge

27. Symptoms of cataract include:
   a) ghost image
   b) vertical diplopia
   c) stabbing pains
   d) lid twitch

28. Symptoms of cataract include:
   a) tearing
   b) ptosis
   c) increased contrast sensitivity
   d) change in color vision

29. Symptoms of cataract include:
   a) granulated eyelids
   b) looking through a fog
   c) dull ache
   d) pressure sensation

30. **The most common cause of cataract is:**
    a) smoking
    b) aging
    c) hypertension
    d) eye strain

31. **Cataracts can be caused by all of the following *except*:**
    a) exposure to ultraviolet light
    b) injury
    c) open-angle glaucoma
    d) diabetes

32. **A cataract that occurs due to some other condition or medication is known as:**
    a) secondary
    b) subcapsular
    c) congenital
    d) lenticular

33. **Current, accepted treatment of a cataract is:**
    a) "eye vitamins"
    b) laser ablation
    c) homeopathic eye drops
    d) surgical extraction

34. **Your patient says his neighbor had her cataracts removed with laser and wants to know if his will be taken off in the same way. You tell him:**
    a) "Yes, we use only the latest technology."
    b) "No, she's probably referring to the way we use ultrasound to break the cataract into tiny pieces. It's not actually a laser."
    c) "Yes, it's called the YAG laser."
    d) "No, she doesn't know what she's talking about."

35. **The vision a patient may have after cataract surgery can be estimated with:**
    a) potential acuity meter (PAM; Marco Technologies Inc, Jacksonville, FL)
    b) brightness acuity tester (BAT)
    c) pinhole
    d) accurate refractometry

36. **Postoperative cataract surgery vision might not be substantially improved in a patient with:**
    a) ptosis
    b) small pupils
    c) macular degeneration
    d) strabismus

37. **A preoperative B-scan might be required in which cataract patient?**
    a) diabetic retinopathy
    b) macular degeneration
    c) extremely dense cataract
    d) pterygium

38. Prior to cataract surgery, an A-scan is used to:
a) measure the length of the eye
b) establish postoperative vision
c) evaluated the corneal endothelium
d) evaluate retinal health

39. Specular microscopy ("cell count") might be needed prior to cataract surgery if the patient has:
a) corneal dystrophy
b) Graves' disease
c) astigmatism
d) dry eye

40. Which gives the most accurate idea of a cataract patient's visual disability?
a) pinhole vision
b) standard Snellen vision chart
c) PAM
d) BAT

41. A cataract is often removed when:
a) vision is reduced below 20/200
b) the cataract is "ripe"
c) the patient fails a color vision test
d) the patient notes impairment of daily living

42. Preoperative cataract surgery measurement of a patient's corneal curvature is known as:
a) keratometry ("K reading")
b) exophthalmometry
c) interferometry
d) tonometry

43. Each of the following is used in intraocular lens implant (IOL) calculation *except*:
a) K reading
b) desired postoperative refraction
c) A-scan
d) intraocular pressure

44. Medications of concern for the preoperative cataract patient include all of the following *except*:
a) those containing aspirin
b) those for erectile dysfunction
c) estrogen-based hormones
d) blood thinners

45. Your patient wants to know if she will have stitches in her eye after cataract surgery. You tell her:
a) "No, cataract surgery is always 'stitchless' now."
b) "No, cataract surgery is done with laser."
c) "No, unless something changes during surgery."
d) "Yes, stitches are a safeguard against wound gape."

46. **Currently, the most commonly used type of anesthesia for cataract surgery is:**
    a) topical
    b) retrobulbar injection
    c) intravitreal injection
    d) general

47. **Reducing a cataract into small pieces by use of ultrasonic energy is termed:**
    a) can-opener method
    b) open sky technique
    c) phacoemulsification
    d) intracapsular extraction

48. **Your patient asks if he will still need glasses after cataract surgery. You tell him:**
    a) "No, the intraocular lens implant will allow you to see normally."
    b) "No, everyone gets specialty implants now so you don't need glasses."
    c) "Probably, just to fine-tune either distance or near vision."
    d) "No, all patients having cataract surgery see 20/20 after the procedure."

49. **Which of the following are general restrictions immediately following cataract surgery?**
    a) No bathing.
    b) Do not bend over or lift anything heavy.
    c) Keep the eye patched at all times.
    d) Keep the head elevated when reclining.

50. **Symptoms of a posterior subcapsular opacity:**
    a) mimic those of a cataract
    b) mimic those of angle-closure glaucoma
    c) include flashes and floaters
    d) can be alleviated with artificial tears

51. **The term "secondary cataract" is a misnomer because:**
    a) most cataracts are congenital
    b) once removed, a cataract cannot grow back
    c) it actually occurs in the IOL implant
    d) it is actually an opacity of the cornea

52. **A posterior capsule opacity is treated by performing a:**
    a) cryo-capsulotomy
    b) laser iridotomy
    c) surgical capsulotomy
    d) laser capsulotomy

53. **Insertion of a phakic IOL would be done for the purpose of:**
    a) cataract removal
    b) correction of refractive error
    c) preventing cataracts
    d) intraocular medication

Glaucoma Surgery

54. **In which of the following surgical procedures might a drainage implant be placed in the eye?**
  a) cataract surgery
  b) nasolacrimal surgery
  c) strabismus surgery
  d) glaucoma surgery

55. **The aim of most types of glaucoma surgery is to:**
  a) increase aqueous production
  b) improve optic nerve health
  c) increase aqueous outflow
  d) avoid medication use

56. **Laser treatment for primary/chronic open-angle glaucoma is a(n):**
  a) valve implant
  b) iridotomy
  c) iridectomy
  d) trabeculoplasty

57. **A surgically created, conjunctiva-covered, external opening through which aqueous can drain is a:**
  a) bleb
  b) seton
  c) drainage implant
  d) sebaceous cyst

58. **Angle-closure glaucoma is *most often* treated by performing a:**
  a) surgical trabeculectomy
  b) valve implant
  c) laser iridotomy
  d) surgical iridectomy

Retina/Posterior

59. **The removal of the jelly-like substance in the back of the eye is a(n):**
  a) centesis
  b) vitrectomy
  c) evisceration
  d) enucleation

60. **Laser photocoagulation might commonly be used to treat all of the following *except*:**
  a) hypertensive retinopathy
  b) hyphema
  c) diabetic retinopathy
  d) macular degeneration

61. **Laser, scleral buckle, and intravitreal gas or air bubble are all treatments for:**
    a) diabetic retinopathy
    b) retinal hemorrhage
    c) retinal detachment
    d) macular degeneration

62. **The intent behind intravitreal injections for macular degeneration is to:**
    a) inhibit the growth of new, abnormal retinal blood vessels
    b) seal off leaking blood vessels
    c) reattach the macula
    d) create a drainage bleb

Other Surgery

63. **Removal of the entire eyeball is an:**
    a) evisceration
    b) exenteration
    c) ectropion
    d) enucleation

64. **In the event that the eyeball is removed, an implant is placed into the orbit. The purpose of this implant is to:**
    a) provide an attachment for electronic vision devices
    b) maintain the shape of the orbit
    c) cosmetically look like a natural eye
    d) keep the eye shut

Systemic and Ocular Diseases

65. **Diabetes is a condition resulting from:**
    a) increased thirst and urination
    b) an imbalance in the insulin-glucose levels of the body
    c) an imbalance in the calcium content of the blood
    d) fluctuations in vision

66. **When seeing a diabetic patient for a routine eye exam, it is important to know how stable her sugar level has been recently because fluctuations:**
    a) can change the refractometric measurement
    b) can cause extraocular muscle palsies
    c) can cause diplopia
    d) can cause eye pain

67. **The hallmark of proliferative diabetic retinopathy is:**
    a) fluctuating vision
    b) resistance to dilation
    c) increased intraocular pressure
    d) growth of new retinal blood vessels

68. Diabetic retinopathy is currently treated with:
a) topical medication
b) oral medication
c) insulin injections
d) laser

69. Hypertension mainly affects which eye structure?
a) cornea
b) lens
c) retina
d) optic nerve

70. Hypertension is when, most of the time, the blood pressure is equal to or greater than:
a) 140 systolic and/or 90 diastolic
b) 120 systolic and/or 80 diastolic
c) 180 diastolic and/or 95 systolic
d) 200 systolic and/or 100 diastolic

71. Which of the following is most commonly used in the treatment of retinal disease caused by hypertension?
a) topical medication
b) periodic injections
c) conventional surgery
d) laser surgery

72. The main ocular concern in a patient with cancer is:
a) accelerated presbyopia
b) decreased blood supply to the eye
c) spread of cancer to the eye's tissues
d) decreased nerve response

73. Atherosclerosis is characterized by fatty deposits along the walls of the:
a) arteries
b) veins
c) capillaries
d) atrium

74. Which of the following can occur in the eye as a result of atherosclerosis?
a) posterior vitreous detachment
b) macular edema
c) central retinal artery occlusion
d) corneal dystrophy

75. Leukemia and sickle cell disease both produce abnormal blood cells. These cells can:
a) clump together and clog retinal blood vessels
b) cause retinal detachment
c) cause spasms of the extraocular muscles
d) interfere with nerve transmission

76. **All of the following are infections that can be present at birth _except_:**
    a) toxoplasmosis
    b) herpes simplex
    c) siderosis
    d) gonorrhea

77. **Shingles is a systemic infection that can also affect the eye and is caused by:**
    a) _Toxocara canis_
    b) _Pseudomonas aeruginosa_
    c) herpes simplex
    d) herpes zoster

78. **Herpes zoster occurs in patients:**
    a) who have had malaria
    b) who have had a tetanus booster
    c) who have had tuberculosis
    d) who have had chicken pox

79. **One of the more common viruses seen in acquired immune deficiency syndrome (AIDS) patients is:**
    a) herpes simplex
    b) herpes zoster
    c) _Adenovirus_
    d) _Streptococcus_

80. **All of the following are often seen in the patient with AIDS _except_:**
    a) dry eye
    b) recurrent blepharitis
    c) xanthelasma
    d) optic neuritis

81. **The most likely route of human immunodeficiency virus (HIV) infection from patient to ophthalmic medical personnel would be:**
    a) contaminated tears during applanation tonometry
    b) needle stick during minor surgery
    c) being in the same room with an HIV-positive patient
    d) shaking hands with an HIV-positive patient

82. **Which of the following systemic disorders is _most_ commonly associated with dry eye?**
    a) hypertension
    b) rheumatoid arthritis
    c) osteoporosis
    d) diabetes

83. **Which of the following might be done on a patient with thyroid eye disease?**
    a) exophthalmometry
    b) B-scan ultrasound
    c) glare test
    d) duochrome test

84. **Smoking can cause all of the following *except*:**
    a) dry eye and tobacco amblyopia
    b) ptosis, trichiasis, and retinoblastoma
    c) increased risk of diabetic and hypertensive retinopathy
    d) increased risk of macular degeneration

Ocular Diseases

Lids/Skin

85. **All of the following are usually noncancerous skin and lid growths *except*:**
    a) xanthelasma
    b) molluscum contagiosum
    c) milia (skin tags)
    d) basal cell tumors

86. **Sagging and eversion of the lower eyelid is termed:**
    a) entropion
    b) ectropion
    c) epiphora
    d) trichiasis

87. **Entropion is defined as:**
    a) lids that turn inward
    b) lids that have inward-turned hairs
    c) upper lids that droop
    d) lids that turn outward

88. **Infection of the lash follicle is a:**
    a) chalazion
    b) hordeolum
    c) xanthelasma
    d) blepharitis

89. **A condition in which eyelashes grow inward, toward the eye is:**
    a) lash ptosis
    b) blepharitis
    c) trichiasis
    d) keratitis

90. **An infected meibomian gland causes a(n):**
    a) blepharochalasis
    b) obstructed nasolacrimal duct
    c) chalazion
    d) hordeolum

91. **Blepharitis is a common:**
    a) lid infection
    b) corneal infection
    c) lid droop
    d) retinal disorder

92. **Which of the following refers to a drooped upper lid?**
    a) ptosis
    b) exophthalmos
    c) trachoma
    d) blepharospasm

93. **Redundant skin of the lids is referred to as:**
    a) blepharoptosis
    b) subluxation
    c) ectropion
    d) dermatochalasis

Lacrimal

94. **Infection of the lacrimal sac is termed:**
    a) canaliculitis
    b) lacrimitis
    c) lacrimal cystitis
    d) dacryocystitis

95. **The condition where the lacrimal gland slips down under the conjunctiva is known as a(n):**
    a) obstructed tear gland
    b) conjunctival bleb
    c) prolapse
    d) pinguecula

96. **Which of the following is *not* a symptom of dry eye?**
    a) burning
    b) epiphora (streaming tears)
    c) gritty, foreign-body sensation
    d) extreme itching

97. **The standard test for diagnosis of dry eye is:**
    a) rose bengal test
    b) Schirmer's test
    c) fluorescein
    d) nasolacrimal irrigation

98. **A blockage of the nasolacrimal duct might result in any of the following *except*:**
    a) recurrent erosion syndrome
    b) epiphora
    c) chronic infections
    d) tearing in an infant

External Globe

99. **Your physician has told the patient that she has a subconjunctival hemorrhage (SCH) and has left you to educate the patient. You should:**
    a) warn her that she may later have a retinal detachment
    b) tell her to leave the pressure patch on for 24 hours
    c) reassure her that it will dissipate in 1 to 3 weeks
    d) impress her with the serious nature of the condition

100. **Slit-lamp examination of your patient reveals a yellowish nodule on the conjunctiva just nasal of the cornea. Most likely this is a(n):**
    a) pterygium
    b) xanthelasma
    c) episcleritis
    d) pinguecula

101. **All of the following are common indications of viral conjunctivitis *except*:**
    a) photophobia
    b) recent sore throat
    c) moderate redness
    d) yellow crusting

102. **All of the following are true regarding epidemic keratoconjunctivitis (EKC) *except*:**
    a) it is highly contagious
    b) it is caused by a bacterium
    c) the cornea is usually involved
    d) it is also known as "shipyard eye"

103. **The type of conjunctivitis caused by constant irritation (such as a contact lens) is:**
    a) giant papillary
    b) seasonal
    c) bacterial
    d) viral

104. **An inflammation of the white of the eye that can be very painful is:**
    a) episcleritis
    b) scleritis
    c) uveitis
    d) iritis

105. **Protrusion of the eyeball is known as:**
    a) exophthalmos
    b) keratoconus
    c) buphthalmos
    d) ptosis

Cornea

106. A cream-colored arc in the cornea at the limbus that may be related to cholesterol is:
a) toxic pemphigoid
b) keratoconus
c) drug reaction
d) arcus

107. Neovascularization of the cornea is generally related to:
a) lack of blood supply
b) lack of adequate tears
c) enucleation
d) lack of oxygen

108. Trachoma, a leading cause of world blindness, is seen in populations with poor diet and hygiene. This devastating disease causes:
a) scarring of lids, conjunctiva, and cornea
b) retinal detachment
c) hemorrhagic keratoconjunctivitis
d) sympathetic ophthalmia

109. On slit-lamp examination, a corneal lesion caused by herpes simplex typically appears:
a) as a small, round, ulcerated area
b) as a branched-looking erosion
c) as a raised red nodule
d) as a fleshy encroachment on the cornea

110. Slit-lamp examination of your patient reveals bulging, centrally thinned corneas. Refractometry shows an increase in astigmatism. The patient probably has:
a) pathologic astigmatism
b) keratoconjunctivitis
c) keratoconus
d) exophthalmos

111. Your patient has an abrasion of the corneal epithelium. All of the following are true *except*:
a) the abraded area will be evident with fluorescein and a blue light
b) there will likely be a corneal scar
c) it may heal as quickly as overnight
d) there may continue to be a foreign-body sensation until fully healed

112. When asked about previous eye surgery, your patient says that she once had "a piece of skin removed that was growing onto the clear part of my eye." Most likely she is describing a:
a) pinguecula
b) cataract
c) corneal dystrophy
d) pterygium

113. **You are eliciting the patient's chief complaint, and he says, "I wake up in the middle of the night, and my right eyelid seems stuck shut. Then, when I get it open, it's like it pulled part of my eye with it. My eye hurts, and I can hardly stand the light." An ocular condition that can cause these types of symptoms is:**
     a) recurrent erosion syndrome
     b) keratoconus
     c) corneal dystrophy
     d) chemical splash

Intraocular

114. **Blood in the anterior chamber (AC) of the eye is a(n):**
     a) hypopyon
     b) aqueous humor
     c) rubeosis
     d) hyphema

115. **Which of the following refers to a layer of inflammatory cells/pus in the AC?**
     a) hypopyon
     b) leuko-aqueous
     c) hypophema
     d) eosinophilosis

116. **Prior to dilating a patient, one should evaluate:**
     a) the space between the iris and lens
     b) the iridocorneal angle
     c) for cataracts
     d) the cup-to-disc ratio

117. **An inflammation of the iris (only) is termed:**
     a) posterior uveitis
     b) uveitis
     c) iritis
     d) retinitis

Glaucoma

118. **Which of the following indicates a risk for open-angle glaucoma?**
     a) a pressure sensation in the eyes
     b) red, painful eyes
     c) a family history of glaucoma
     d) halos around lights at night

119. **Glaucoma is classically characterized by increased intraocular pressure, visual field loss, and:**
     a) pigment in the trabecular meshwork
     b) headaches at bedtime
     c) fluctuating visual acuity
     d) optic nerve head damage

120. **Because of elevated intraocular pressure, a child born with glaucoma has:**
    a) buphthalmos
    b) exophthalmos
    c) proptosis
    d) lid lag

121. **What are the symptoms of angle-closure glaucoma?**
    a) redness, pain, blurred vision, and halos around lights
    b) redness, tearing, blurred vision, and pain from bright lights
    c) discharge, redness, and pain from bright lights
    d) redness, small pupil, and halos around lights

122. **Symptoms and signs for acute angle-closure glaucoma include all of the following** *except*:
    a) severe pain
    b) decreased vision
    c) vomiting/nausea
    d) miotic pupil

123. **Secondary glaucoma can be caused by all of the following** *except*:
    a) trauma
    b) extended use of topical steroids
    c) blood in the AC
    d) strabismus

124. **Risk factors for glaucoma include all of the following** *except*:
    a) rheumatoid arthritis
    b) positive family history
    c) African-American heritage
    d) ocular trauma

125. **All of the following are problems common to public glaucoma screening programs** *except*:
    a) air-puff tonometry, commonly used for screening, is not the most accurate method
    b) a single, normal pressure reading does not necessarily indicate the absence of glaucoma
    c) it generates public interest in the disorder and its treatment
    d) some normal pressures register as high and some high pressures read normal

126. **The most common type of glaucoma is:**
    a) congenital
    b) secondary
    c) open-angle
    d) angle-closure

127. **The diagnosis of glaucoma may be based on which set of the following tests?**
    a) tactile pressures, slit-lamp exam, confrontation fields
    b) slit-lamp exam, glare test, A-scan
    c) tonometry, perimetry, ophthalmoscopy, central corneal thickness
    d) slit-lamp exam, gonioscopy, peripheral corneal thickness, cup-to-disc ratio

128. **Vision lost by glaucoma damage:**
    a) can be recovered if the intraocular pressure (IOP) is brought under control
    b) can be recovered if laser treatment is used
    c) can be recovered with certain topical or oral medications
    d) generally cannot be recovered

129. **The appearance of halos around lights during an attack of angle-closure glaucoma is due to:**
    a) lens edema
    b) corneal edema
    c) vitreous hemorrhage
    d) optic nerve damage

130. **All of the following are true regarding open-angle glaucoma *except*:**
    a) the patient generally has no sensation of eye pressure
    b) it can be cured
    c) optic nerve damage cannot be reversed
    d) it might be controlled with a single medication

131. **The dangerous element of open-angle glaucoma is:**
    a) pain
    b) rapid, irreversible visual loss
    c) lack of symptoms
    d) lack of signs

132. **In open-angle glaucoma:**
    a) the iris blocks off the angle structures
    b) the pressure damages the ciliary body
    c) the angle allows too much aqueous to drain out
    d) the angle looks normal

133. **A patient known to have open-angle glaucoma:**
    a) should not be dilated
    b) should have his pressure checked with an air-puff tonometer
    c) should be checked annually with confrontation fields
    d) needs annual dilation, gonioscopy, and formal visual fields

134. **A patient in the end stages of open-angle glaucoma:**
    a) may have a small temporal island of vision
    b) may have a small central island of vision
    c) may have a small nasal island of vision
    d) still has enough peripheral vision to get around

135. **A patient with open-angle glaucoma has missed an appointment for a pressure check. The practice should:**
    a) wait for the patient to call and reschedule, then emphasize the importance of IOP checks
    b) inform the patient's relatives, and stress the importance of having IOP checks
    c) have the pharmacist ask the patient to call the office when medication needs to be refilled
    d) contact the patient to reschedule, emphasizing the importance of IOP checks

Crystalline Lens[4]

136. The total absence of a crystalline lens is termed:
   a) phako-dislocation
   b) pseudophakia
   c) aphakia
   d) phacoemulsification

137. A dislocation of the crystalline lens is termed:
   a) iridodonesis
   b) phako-prolapse
   c) lacrimation
   d) luxated

Posterior Chamber/Retina[5]

138. Signs and symptoms of uveitis include all of the following *except*:
   a) perilimbal redness
   b) sensitivity to light (photophobia)
   c) dizziness and nausea
   d) smaller, sluggish pupil on the affected side

139. Spontaneous retinal detachments are more common in patients with:
   a) myopia
   b) hyperopia
   c) astigmatism
   d) presbyopia

140. Usual symptoms of retinal detachment include all of the following *except*:
   a) curtain over the vision
   b) floaters
   c) pain
   d) light flashes

141. Most cases of floaters and flashes are caused by:
   a) posterior vitreous detachment (PVD)
   b) retinal detachment
   c) retinitis
   d) vitreous hemorrhage

142. A progressive breakdown of the macular tissue usually associated with age is:
   a) retinitis pigmentosa
   b) presumed ocular histoplasmosis
   c) cystic macular edema
   d) macular degeneration

[4]For questions on cataracts, see questions 24 through 53 in this chapter.
[5]For questions on diabetic and hypertensive retinal changes, see questions 65 through 71 in this chapter.

143. **The physician has asked you to educate a patient with macular degeneration regarding home care. This will most likely include:**
    a) instillation of eye drops and punctal occlusion
    b) Amsler grid, UV protection, and vitamin therapy
    c) cleansing techniques and physical therapy
    d) vision exercises and home color vision testing

144. **Intravitreal injections and laser treatments may sometimes be used in which type of macular degeneration?**
    a) wet
    b) dry
    c) congenital
    d) tobacco-related

145. **A patient has had a sudden, painless loss of vision. She should be seen immediately as an emergency because these are the symptoms of a(n):**
    a) intravitreal infection
    b) sympathetic ophthalmia
    c) endophthalmitis
    d) retinal artery occlusion

146. **All of the following are true regarding a retinal vein occlusion *except*:**
    a) the symptoms are easily distinguished from a retinal artery occlusion
    b) it occurs most often in patients with hypertension
    c) there is still blood flow into the retinal tissues
    d) there may be a visual field change

147. **Toxoplasmosis is a protozoan-caused infection that can damage the choroid and retina. It is most often passed to humans by means of:**
    a) contaminated water
    b) heterosexual contact
    c) contaminated drug paraphernalia
    d) cat feces

148. **Histoplasmosis is a fungus-caused infection that can attack the choroid. A human gets histoplasmosis by:**
    a) drinking contaminated water
    b) eating contaminated meat
    c) contact with dog feces
    d) inhaling the spores

149. **Which of the following is commonly seen in open-angle glaucoma?**
    a) optic nerve edema
    b) optic neuritis
    c) optic nerve pinching
    d) optic nerve cupping

150. **An infection of the internal ocular tissues occurring after surgery or penetrating injury is:**
    a) retinitis
    b) orbititis
    c) endophthalmitis
    d) cellulitis

151. **A rare condition in which one eye is injured and the fellow, noninjured eye develops an inflammation that can destroy the eye is:**
    a) endophthalmitis
    b) blow-out
    c) sympathetic ophthalmia
    d) syncope

152. **Treatment for sympathetic ophthalmia is:**
    a) enucleation of the inflamed, uninjured eye
    b) enucleation of the injured eye
    c) enucleation of both eyes
    d) emergency lens extraction

153. **All of the following are hereditary *except*:**
    a) albinism
    b) retinitis pigmentosa
    c) trachoma
    d) coloboma

Anatomy and Physiology (General)

154. **Match the organ or tissue to the correct system:**

    Organ/Tissue   System
    a) pancreas   cardiovascular
    b) auricles and ventricles   respiratory
    c) lungs   endocrine
    d) pituitary gland   nervous
    e) brain
    f) spinal cord
    g) carotid artery
    h) alveoli
    i) aorta
    j) parathyroid
    k) bronchi
    l) thyroid
    m) neuron
    n) capillaries
    o) cerebellum
    p) veins
    q) trachea
    r) cranial nerves I to XII

155. **Which blood cell carries oxygen in the blood?**
    a) platelets
    b) macrophages
    c) white blood cells
    d) red blood cells

156. **Which order represents human circulation?**
    a) capillaries, arteries, heart, lungs, heart, veins, capillaries
    b) capillaries, veins, heart, lungs, heart, arteries, capillaries
    c) veins, arteries, capillaries, heart, lungs, heart, veins
    d) arteries, heart, veins, lungs, capillaries, heart, arteries

157. **Human respiration follows which order?**
    a) pharynx, esophagus, diaphragm, arteries
    b) trachea, bronchus/bronchioles, alveoli, capillaries
    c) trachea, bronchial filaments, gill arch, arterioles, arteries
    d) alveoli, bronchus/bronchioles, trachea, arterioles

158. **What occurs as a result of respiration?**
    a) The blood gives up carbon and takes on dioxide.
    b) The blood gives up ammonia and takes on oxygen.
    c) The blood gives up carbon dioxide and takes on oxygen.
    d) The blood gives up oxygen and takes on carbon dioxide.

159. **Endocrine glands synthesize and release chemicals known as:**
    a) oxidizers
    b) hormones
    c) neurotransmitters
    d) stimulants

160. **Chemicals from the endocrine glands travel to the target organ through the:**
    a) muscle fibers
    b) bone marrow
    c) bloodstream
    d) nerve fibers

161. **Nerve cells release chemicals known as:**
    a) antioxidants
    b) inhibitors
    c) stimulants
    d) neurotransmitters

162. **A predictable, involuntary motor response to a specific stimulus is a(n):**
    a) stimulus
    b) extension
    c) flexion
    d) reflex

163. **The human nervous system is divided into which two structural parts?**
     a) central and peripheral
     b) cardiac and visceral
     c) sensory and motor
     d) cranial and spinal

164. **The human nervous system is divided into which two functional parts?**
     a) central and peripheral
     b) cardiac and visceral
     c) sensory and motor
     d) cranial and spinal

Anatomy and Physiology (Ocular)

165. **Label the following (Figure 12-1):**
     anterior segment
     posterior segment

Figure 12-1. Reprinted with permission of Nemeth SC, Shea CA. *Medical Sciences for the Ophthalmic Assistant.* SLACK Incorporated; 1988.

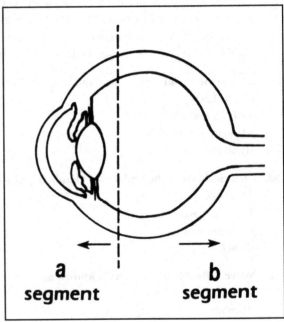

a
segment

b
segment

166. Label the following (Figure 12-2):

bulbar conjunctiva	eyebrow	iris
eyelashes	pupil	palpebral fissure
lateral canthus	plica (semilunaris)	sclera
caruncle	eyelids	medial canthus

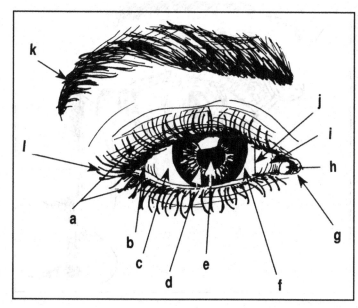

Figure 12-2. Drawing by Holly Hess Smith. Reprinted with permission of Gayton JL, Ledford JK. *The Crystal Clear Guide to Sight for Life.* Starburst Publishers; 1996.

167. Label the following (Figure 12-3):

optic nerve	vitreous
anterior chamber	posterior chamber

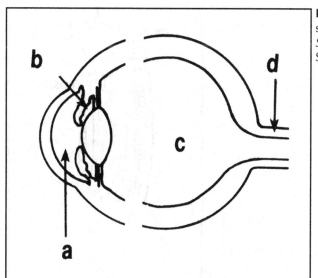

Figure 12-3. Reprinted with permission of Nemeth SC, Shea CA. *Medical Sciences for the Ophthalmic Assistant.* SLACK Incorporated; 1988.

168. Label the following (Figure 12-4):

nasolacrimal duct   nasolacrimal sac

lacrimal gland   punctum

canaliculus

Figure 12-4. Drawing by Holly Hess Smith. Reprinted with permission of Gayton JL, Ledford JK. *The Crystal Clear Guide to Sight for Life.* Starburst Publishers; 1996.

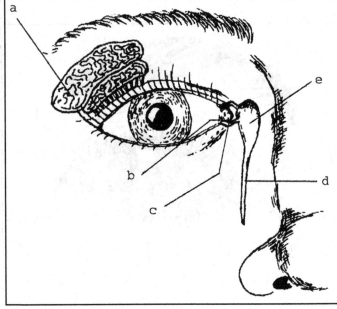

169. Label the following (Figure 12-5):

stroma   endothelium   Descemet's membrane

precorneal tear film   epithelium   Bowman's layer

Figure 12-5. Reprinted with permission of Nemeth SC, Shea CA. *Medical Sciences for the Ophthalmic Assistant.* SLACK Incorporated; 1988.

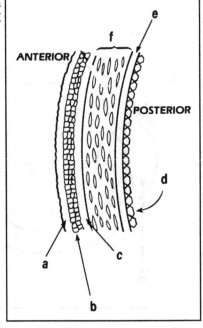

170. Label the following (Figure 12-6):

vitreous humor   lens

aqueous humor

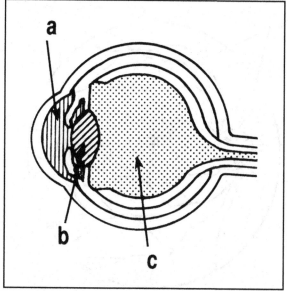

Figure 12-6. Reprinted with permission of Nemeth SC, Shea CA. *Medical Sciences for the Ophthalmic Assistant.* SLACK Incorporated; 1988.

171. Label the following (Figure 12-7):

lens   zonules   ciliary body

angle   cornea   iris

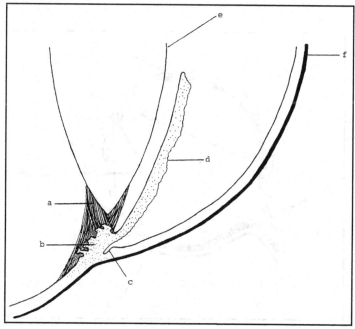

Figure 12-7. Drawing by Holly Hess Smith. Reprinted with permission of Gayton JL, Ledford JK. *The Crystal Clear Guide to Sight for Life.* Starburst Publishers; 1996.

172. Label the following (Figure 12-8):

optic nerve blood vessels macula

Figure 12-8. Drawing by Holly Hess Smith. Reprinted with permission of Gayton JL, Ledford JK. *The Crystal Clear Guide to Sight for Life.* Starburst Publishers; 1996.

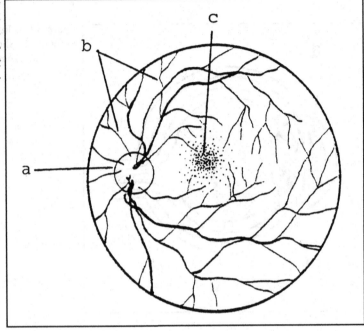

173. Label the following (Figure 12-9):

macula iris retina

cornea sclera optic nerve

lens

Figure 12-9. Drawing by Holly Hess Smith. Reprinted with permission of Gayton JL, Ledford JK. *The Crystal Clear Guide to Sight for Life.* Starburst Publishers; 1996.

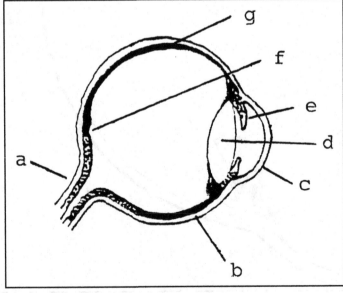

174. The primary goal of the eye's components is to:
a) interpret what is seen
b) focus incoming light onto the lens
c) focus incoming light onto the retina
d) maintain proper intraocular pressure

175. The term for the eye socket, which consists of parts of seven bones, is:
a) globe
b) orbit
c) bony chamber
d) orbital fissure

176. Most of the blood supply directly to the eye is supplied by the:
a) internal carotid artery
b) external carotid artery
c) ophthalmic artery
d) ophthalmic vein

177. How many extraocular muscles are attached to each eye?
a) 4
b) 5
c) 6
d) 7

178. The "plate" of connective tissue that serves as the underlying structure of the eyelids is the:
a) tarsus
b) Tenon's capsule
c) conjunctiva
d) meibomian glands

179. Asians and some children have a small vertical fold of skin nasally between the upper and lower lids. This is called a(n):
a) ptosis fold
b) epicanthal fold
c) ectropion
d) entropion

180. The main lacrimal (tear) gland is located:
a) under the brow
b) near the nose
c) in the lower lid
d) in the conjunctiva

181. Which of the following is *not* a component of the tear film layer?
a) mucin
b) water
c) oil
d) plasma

182. **Which is the correct route of tears as they are drained off the eye?**
    a) punctum, canaliculi, lacrimal sac, nasolacrimal duct
    b) nasolacrimal duct, canaliculi, lacrimal sac, punctum
    c) canaliculi, punctum, lacrimal sac, nasolacrimal duct
    d) punctum, canaliculi, nasolacrimal duct, lacrimal sac

183. **Which tear film layer acts to prevent or retard evaporation of tears from the eye?**
    a) lipid (oily) layer
    b) aqueous (watery) layer
    c) mucus layer
    d) epithelium

184. **The ocular media consists of:**
    a) the lens correction for ametropia
    b) contact lenses and intraocular lenses
    c) the eyelid, sclera, uvea, and optic nerve
    d) the tear film, cornea, aqueous, vitreous, and lens

185. **Which of the following is *not* a part of the optical media?**
    a) cornea
    b) aqueous/vitreous
    c) lens
    d) retina

186. **Which ocular structure refracts light the most?**
    a) tear film
    b) cornea
    c) aqueous
    d) lens

187. **The average adult corneal diameter, in millimeters, is:**
    a) 12 mm
    b) 10 mm
    c) 15 mm
    d) 8 mm

188. **Which corneal layer generally regenerates rapidly without scarring?**
    a) endothelium
    b) stroma
    c) Bowman's layer
    d) epithelium

189. **Which corneal layer acts to limit corneal hydration (edema)?**
    a) endothelium
    b) stroma
    c) Bowman's layer
    d) epithelium

190. How many muscles make up the iris?
 a) 1
 b) 2
 c) 3
 d) each strand is a muscle

191. Which of the following structures is responsible for aqueous production?
 a) ciliary muscle
 b) ciliary body
 c) trabecular meshwork
 d) islets of Langerhans

192. The hard, central core (nucleus) of the crystalline lens:
 a) is present in its adult form at birth
 b) is produced by the capsular envelope
 c) is formed from the inside out as fiber layers are produced at the center
 d) is formed as lens fiber layers are produced and compacted together

193. Which of the following is *not* true regarding the crystalline lens?
 a) It lies behind the pupil.
 b) It is suspended by zonules.
 c) It lies in the anterior chamber.
 d) It is encased in a capsular bag.

194. The physiological process by which one focuses on a near object is:
 a) phakomorphosis
 b) accommodation
 c) fixation
 d) stereopsis

195. Which of the following does *not* automatically occur when a patient focuses on a close-up object?
 a) narrowing of palpebral fissures
 b) pupils get smaller (miosis)
 c) eyes converge
 d) lens thickens (accommodates)

196. When a person looks at a near object:
 a) the ciliary muscle contracts, causing the zonules to relax, causing the lens to thicken
 b) the ciliary muscle relaxes, causing the zonules to relax, causing the lens to thicken
 c) the ciliary muscle contracts, causing the zonules to pull tight, causing the lens to thin
 d) the ciliary muscle relaxes, causing the zonules to pull tight, causing the lens to thicken

197. Which of the following is *not* a part of the uvea?
 a) choroid
 b) iris
 c) retina
 d) ciliary body

198. **The major function of the choroid is:**
    a) aqueous production
    b) accommodation
    c) blood supply to the retina
    d) blood supply to the cornea

199. **The retinal photoreceptor cells is/are known as:**
    a) pigment epithelium
    b) rods and cones
    c) rhodopsin
    d) carotene

200. **Which of the following is *not* true regarding cone cells?**
    a) They are concentrated in the foveal area.
    b) They outnumber the rods 20 to 1.
    c) They are responsible for color and central vision.
    d) They function best in daylight.

201. **Fibers from the retina travel through the optic chiasm in the following manner:**
    a) nasal fibers cross, temporal fibers do not cross
    b) temporal fibers cross, nasal fibers do not cross
    c) the upper half of all fibers cross, the lower half do not cross
    d) all fibers cross to the opposite side

202. **Because of the crossing of retinal fibers after leaving the optic nerve, an object in the patient's right field of view:**
    a) is perceived by the patient to be on the left
    b) is projected to the left optic tract
    c) is projected to the right optic tract
    d) is perceived by the patient to be closer than it actually is

203. **Your patient complains that he cannot see objects on his left with his left eye. Confrontation visual fields confirms this. You suspect a retinal detachment. What part of the retina would be affected if you are correct?**
    a) left eye, nasal side
    b) left eye, temporal side
    c) left eye, upper hemisphere
    d) right eye, temporal side

204. **The head of the optic nerve, visible with the ophthalmoscope, is called the:**
    a) optic radiation
    b) optic disc
    c) macula
    d) lamina cribrosa

Safety Glasses

205. The group that accredits standards in safety glasses and lenses is the:
a) American National Standards Institute (ANSI)
b) American Optical Association (AOA)
c) Council on Eye Safety (CES)
d) National Eye Institute (NEI)

206. The main features of safety frames include all of the following *except*:
a) they are impact-resistant
b) extended side protection required in some cases
c) do not conduct electricity
d) approved products are marked

207. Standard safety glasses are intended to be used:
a) only in industry
b) by adults only
c) on the job and on the street
d) when welding

208. Which of the following should always be prescribed safety lenses?
a) children and adults
b) postoperative cataract patients
c) health care workers
d) children and monocular patients

209. The key feature of safety lenses is that they:
a) are completely shatterproof
b) splinter under impact
c) are shatter-resistant
d) protect against radiation

210. The thinnest allowable width for a general wear, impact-resistant glass safety lens is:
a) 1.5 mm
b) 2.2 mm
c) 3.0 mm
d) 3.7 mm

211. The standard spectacle lens material used for safety in streetwear is:
a) impact-resistant glass
b) heat-treated glass
c) polycarbonate
d) aspheric

212. Occupational Safety and Health Administration (OSHA) standards require that a health care employer provide safety glasses and/or face shields for employees at risk for biological or chemical splashes. These safety glasses fall under the category of:
a) EOE regulations
b) personal protective equipment
c) incident reporting
d) unsafe work practices

213. **Welders must wear safety glasses or shields that will protect them from:**
    a) chemical splashes
    b) laser radiation
    c) infrared radiation burns
    d) ultraviolet radiation burns

Patient Instruction

Medication[6]

214. **To reduce systemic absorption of an eye drop, the patient should be instructed to:**
    a) use only half the prescribed dose and close his eyes
    b) avoid getting eye drops on his fingers
    c) put pressure over the punctum after instilling the drops
    d) blink rapidly after instilling the drops

215. **The patient should be told that the first step in applying any type of topical eye medication is to:**
    a) rinse the eyes with warm water
    b) perform lid hygiene
    c) wash the hands
    d) occlude the punctum

216. **Ophthalmic ointment is usually applied:**
    a) to the lower cul de sac
    b) to the cornea
    c) into the vitreous
    d) to the eyelashes

217. **When using eye drops, the patient should do all of the following *except*:**
    a) use 2 drops at a time to ensure effectiveness
    b) avoid touching the lids or eye with the bottle tip
    c) allow several minutes between instilling different types of drops
    d) avoid touching the bottle tip with the fingers

218. **If someone else is to instill eye drops for the patient, he can be told it is easiest to instill eye drops if the patient will:**
    a) close one eye
    b) open both eyes and look up
    c) hold her breath
    d) focus on the dropper tip

[6]My JCAHPO® VOW says that this category refers to teaching patients how to instill ocular medications and related issues. See also Chapter 9, *Pharmacology*, for specific patient instruction regarding ocular pharmaceuticals.

Tests[7]

219. A glare test might be indicated in a patient with:
   a) glaucoma
   b) macular degeneration
   c) hypertensive retinopathy
   d) posterior capsular cataracts

220. Your patient is a 10-year-old boy whose mother thinks he is having a problem with color vision. You evaluate him with the Ishihara pseudoisochromatic plates, which test for:
   a) red/green color vision defects
   b) blue/yellow color vision defects
   c) red/yellow color vision defects
   d) green/blue color vision defects

221. Your patient complains that he cannot see anything to his left. Which of the following will give the most detailed analysis of this problem?
   a) Amsler grid
   b) cover testing
   c) automated visual field
   d) visual acuity

222. Your patient sees 20/20, yet complains of "not being able to see." Which of the following tests might help in documenting the problem?
   a) pinhole test
   b) tonometry
   c) color vision test
   d) contrast sensitivity

223. A test done to estimate how much of a vision loss is due to cataracts and how much to retinal disease is:
   a) glare testing
   b) brightness acuity testing
   c) potential acuity testing
   d) OCT

224. Exophthalmometry reveals that your patient has bulging eyes. Which of the following is the eye care practitioner probably going to want tested?
   a) cholesterol levels
   b) heart function
   c) glucose levels
   d) thyroid function

[7]My JCAHPO® VOW says that this section refers to tests done "to determine the cause of a problem." There is some overlap between this section and others. For extraocular muscle and stereo testing, see Chapter 10, sections *Cover Tests* and *Stereoacuity*. For pupil testing, see Chapter 2. For tear testing, see Chapter 16, section titled *Tear Tests*.

225. **Your diabetic patient has decreased vision, but says he or she does not want to be dilated. You tell the patient that you will not do anything he or she does not want you to, but:**
    a) you cannot get an accurate IOP without it
    b) it is the best way for the doctor to get a good look at the back of the eye
    c) you can take nonmydriatic fundus photos instead
    d) the optic nerve is not visible without it

226. **Which of the following would be a way to explain a Schirmer's test to a patient?**
    a) "This will help us learn what is causing your floaters."
    b) "This will help us learn what is causing your eyes to feel gritty."
    c) "This will help us learn if your cataract is ready to be removed."
    d) "This will help us learn why you are having headaches."

227. **A "dye test" to evaluate the retina's blood vessels is:**
    a) retinal photography
    b) rose bengal angiography
    c) fluorescein slit-lamp test
    d) fluorescein angiography

228. **You are about to perform an A-scan on a patient with a suspected intraocular foreign body. You explain to the patient that:**
    a) the test involves use of laser technology
    b) the test uses a strong magnet to create an image
    c) the test uses ultrasound waves
    d) the test uses ultraviolet rays

229. **The doctor has asked you to measure a patient's central corneal thickness. You might explain this to the patient using any of the following *except*:**
    a) "Corneal thickness can be related to how we interpret your eye pressure readings."
    b) "This measurement uses ultrasound to measure your cornea."
    c) "This reading is just one aspect in determining if glaucoma is present."
    d) "This measurement is essential in fitting your contact lenses."

230. **The physician has ordered an OCT and left you in the room to explain the procedure to the patient. You tell her that the test:**
    a) uses ultrasound to image all the structures in the eye
    b) is used to further evaluate the patient's vision
    c) shows the layers of the retina
    d) determines aqueous outflow

231. **Your patient complains of a foreign body sensation. Which of the following would be most useful?**
    a) tonometry
    b) corneal topography
    c) keratometry
    d) topical fluorescein

232. **Which of the following helps determine the cause of an eye infection?**
a) biopsy
b) culture
c) rose bengal
d) complete blood count

233. **An established patient returns every 6 months or so complaining of decreasing vision. Refractometry has shown a gradual increase in astigmatism. The most helpful test to determine the cause of this would be a(n):**
a) keratometry
b) pachymetry
c) corneal topography
d) A-scan

234. **A patient returns for a 2-year exam, and her vision today with her glasses is 20/70. Two years ago, she was 20/25– with the same prescription. You perform a pinhole test, which improves her vision to 20/50+. This most likely indicates:**
a) the glasses were filled incorrectly
b) a new refraction should improve her back up to 20/25–
c) she has dry eye
d) there is some type of ocular pathology present

235. **Each of the following tests is standard in determining the cause of a red painful eye *except*:**
a) pachymetry
b) pupil check
c) slit-lamp exam
d) IOP check

236. **Your patient had 20/20 vision OD 9 months ago. Today, it is 20/60, without pinhole improvement. In the absence of obvious pathology, the eye care provider may want which of the following tests to help diagnose the problem?**
a) BAT
b) PAM
c) fluorescein angiogram
d) OCT of macula

237. **A patient complaining of floaters and flashes will need which of the following?**
a) B-scan ultrasound
b) dilated fundus exam
c) specular microscopy
d) macular photostress test

Procedures[8]

238. **A procedure done to help alleviate dry eye by keeping the tears on the eye is:**
   a) tarsorrhaphy
   b) epilation
   c) punctal occlusion
   d) tear inserts

239. **The eye care provider has determined that an infant's nasolacrimal duct is blocked. The procedure to rectify this problem is:**
   a) probe and irrigate
   b) Quickert-Dryden tube insertion
   c) dacryocystectomy
   d) punctal dilation

240. **Which of the following is used to remove an embedded metallic corneal foreign body?**
   a) spud or drill
   b) cotton-tipped applicator
   c) speculum
   d) anesthesiometer

241. **Botulinum toxin injection, or Botox (Allergan Inc, Irvine, CA), is used to relieve:**
   a) accommodative esotropia
   b) accommodative spasms
   c) blepharospasms
   d) migraine headaches

242. **Removal of an eyelash is called:**
   a) trichiasis
   b) epilation
   c) incision
   d) indentation

243. **A procedure done to resolve angle-closure glaucoma is:**
   a) goniotomy
   b) laser trabeculoplasty
   c) laser iridotomy
   d) glaucoma valve

244. **A procedure performed to clear a posterior capsule opacity is:**
   a) laser capsulotomy
   b) laser posteriotomy
   c) laser capsulorrhexis
   d) laser iridectomy

[8]According to my JCAHPO® VOW, procedures are "done to resolve problems detected on testing." This brings up a number of potential procedures. Refractometry could be considered a procedure, as it is done to resolve vision problems detected during visual acuity testing. Surgery (both minor and major, as well as laser) is definitely a procedure, but is covered in other places (see Chapters 11 and 20). First aid might also be thought of as a procedure; that is covered later in this chapter, in the section titled *Triage*.

245. Treatment of wet macular degeneration includes:
a) removal of diseased tissue
b) retinal tissue transplant
c) intravitreal injections
d) laser to open drainage sites

Treatments[9]

246. The post-surgical patient should be told to report the following symptoms, which may indicate wound infection:
a) itching, scaling, and redness
b) redness, swelling, and pain
c) tenderness and slight oozing
d) bruising, swelling, and itching

247. All of the following are true regarding care of skin sutures *except*:
a) do not get them wet
b) if a suture falls out, call the doctor's office
c) all sutures are absorbable and do not need to be removed
d) antibiotic ointment can be applied directly to the sutures

248. If the patient is to use warm compresses, she should be told to:
a) test the compress for excessive heat before applying
b) wet an electric pad to provide moist heat
c) use boiling water to make the cloth hot enough
d) use boiling water to sterilize the cloth

249. A hot compress is generally used to:
a) sterilize the area to prevent infection
b) increase patient comfort
c) increase the effectiveness of oral antibiotics
d) increase circulation to the area

250. An ice pack is generally used to:
a) increase circulation to the area
b) increase patient comfort
c) decrease bruising and swelling
d) decrease redness and discharge

251. The basic treatment for blepharitis is:
a) steroid ointment at night
b) antibiotic ointment and lid scrubs
c) antibiotic ointment
d) lid scrubs and steroid drops

[9]Treatments are meant to involve "ongoing care or aftercare." Thus, I have included aftercare for cataract surgery here. For patient instructions regarding glaucoma medications, see Chapter 9, section *Educate Patients on Medications*. For patient instructions regarding instillation of eye medications, see questions 214 to 218 in this chapter.

252. **A patient with which of the following might be taught how to perform lid scrubs?**
    a) blepharitis
    b) blepharoptosis
    c) blepharochalasis
    d) exophthalmos

253. **A patient with dry eye syndrome needs to be made aware that:**
    a) the condition will go away after a few days of treatment
    b) the condition will require indefinite treatment
    c) the condition is contagious
    d) the condition will get worse before it gets better

254. **A parent whose infant probably has a nasolacrimal duct obstruction should be told to:**
    a) apply the occluding patch as directed
    b) instill artificial tears every 2 hours
    c) massage the eyeball several times daily
    d) massage the nasolacrimal duct area several times a day

255. **Standard instructions for a patient with conjunctivitis include all of the following *except*:**
    a) if another family member develops symptoms, give him or her your eye drops
    b) do not share washcloths with anyone
    c) wash your hands before and after touching the eye
    d) do not share pillows with anyone

256. **A patient who has had a corneal foreign body removed in the office should be told to:**
    a) expect a foreign body sensation for the rest of the day
    b) use "numbing drops" as needed for pain
    c) expect the eye to feel better right away
    d) avoid heavy lifting

257. **After removal of a corneal foreign body, the patient should be warned that the eye may again have a foreign body sensation once the topical anesthetic wears off. This is because:**
    a) it is impossible to remove the entire foreign body
    b) rust forms from metallic foreign bodies
    c) there is an abrasion at the removal site
    d) there is decreased corneal sensation at the site

258. **A postoperative cataract patient is told to:**
    a) protect the eye from bright light
    b) sleep facedown
    c) avoid heavy lifting
    d) rub ointment vigorously into the eye

259. **The postoperative cataract surgery patient is generally sent home with:**
    a) an eye shield
    b) oral medications to lower intraocular pressure
    c) topical numbing drops
    d) a home IOP monitor

260. A postoperative cataract patient should be warned that:
a) the cataract can grow back
b) intraocular pressure may rise a year later
c) the intraocular lens implant can dislocate
d) the membrane behind the IOL can get cloudy

261. Following cataract surgery, the patient may notice:
a) a visual improvement in the fellow eye
b) vision has a bluish tinge
c) vertical diplopia
d) decreased depth perception

262. Following cataract surgery, the final refraction will usually take place:
a) 1 week after surgery
b) 4 to 6 weeks after surgery
c) once the intraocular pressure is normal
d) 6 months after surgery

263. The parent of a child who is being patched for amblyopia asks how the patch is going to help. You respond:
a) the patch prevents secondary infections
b) the weak eye is patched to relieve eye strain
c) the strong eye is patched to force the weaker eye to work harder
d) the patch prevents the eyes from crossing

264. A patient with which of the following might be taught how to do "pencil push-up" eye exercises?
a) amblyopia
b) convergence insufficiency
c) divergence insufficiency
d) exotropia

265. Your patient is given an Amsler grid for home use. She would be told all of the following *except*:
a) cover one eye at a time, checking each
b) post the grid on a wall, and stand 10 feet away
c) focus on the central dot
d) evaluate for missing or distorted areas

266. A patient using an Amsler grid at home should be told to contact the office if:
a) the lines appear to be straight
b) the lines appear to be wavy
c) there is any change in the way the grid looks
d) a dot appears in the middle of the grid

Eye Dressings

267. A properly applied pressure patch should:
   a) prevent the patient from moving his or her eye
   b) prevent the patient from opening his or her eye
   c) eliminate pain
   d) improve the patient's vision

268. To secure a pressure patch, it may be necessary to:
   a) shave the patient's eyebrows
   b) shave the patient's facial hair
   c) shave the patient's forehead
   d) shave the patient's eyelashes

269. When a pressure patch is properly applied, the tape:
   a) will prevent the patient from eating
   b) will prevent the patient from speaking
   c) will angle away from the edge of the mouth
   d) will go beyond the hairline of the forehead

270. If the tape of the pressure patch will not stick because the patient's skin is oily, the assistant may:
   a) use extra tape
   b) cleanse the skin with alcohol
   c) use an eye shield instead
   d) ask the physician for help

271. Use of a pressure patch in superficial corneal defects is generally indicated because:
   a) it helps create a smooth surface for healing
   b) it keeps light from entering the cornea
   c) the pressure makes healing faster
   d) the patch keeps the medicine on the eye

272. The patient should be told all of the following after application of a pressure patch *except*:
   a) to call the office if the eye opens under the patch
   b) to leave the patch on until told to remove it
   c) that the purpose of the patch is to promote healing
   d) to remove the patch if it is uncomfortably tight

273. An eye patch is commonly used after ocular surgery for all of the following *except*:
   a) to prevent infection and absorb discharge
   b) to protect the eye
   c) to stop bleeding and reduce swelling
   d) to improve visual acuity

274. The edges of an eye shield should:
   a) rest on the eyeball
   b) rest on the bones surrounding the eye
   c) fit over the nose
   d) permit no light to enter

275. **The purpose of the eye shield is:**
   a) to keep the eye shut
   b) to prevent light from entering the eye
   c) to protect the eye from physical injury
   d) to keep the eye from moving

Patient Flow

276. **A good rule of thumb when accompanying a patient with a physical disability is to:**
   a) try to anticipate his or her needs and give the appropriate help without being told
   b) offer no help even if he or she is struggling in order to support his or her independence
   c) ask if he or she wants or needs your assistance first
   d) automatically request that the patient ride in a wheelchair

277. **A patient can often be transferred from the wheelchair to the exam chair most easily by:**
   a) having the assistant physically lift him or her from one chair to the other
   b) removing the arms of both chairs so the patient can slide from one to the other
   c) transferring the patient first to a stretcher and from there to the exam chair
   d) using a step-stool

278. **To best assist a blind patient in the office, the assistant should:**
   a) use a wheelchair to move the patient
   b) offer the patient a cane
   c) offer his or her arm, and move slightly ahead of the patient
   d) gently guide the patient from behind

279. **When speaking to a blind patient, one should do all of the following *except*:**
   a) speak directly to the patient
   b) speak in a louder voice
   c) tell the patient when you leave and enter the room
   d) tell the patient what you are doing as the exam progresses

280. **Your patient has a guide dog. You should guide the patient by:**
   a) taking the dog's halter and guiding it to the exam room
   b) taking the patient's arm and directing him to the exam room
   c) requesting that the patient and dog follow you
   d) walking behind the dog and patient, telling them where to go

281. **Patient flow can be expedited by all of the following *except*:**
   a) chart preview
   b) scheduling fewer patients
   c) template-style exam forms
   d) protocol for handling phone calls

Triage[10]

282. The act of briefly assessing a patient's injury or illness in order to determine the urgency of treatment is:
    a) first aid
    b) patient flow
    c) triage
    d) first response

283. In the case that there is more than one patient needing attention, triage enables the screener to:
    a) determine the order in which the patients need care
    b) determine who is malingering and does not need care
    c) make sure the least serious condition is treated first
    d) make sure patients are seen in order of arrival

284. Which of the following is *not* one of the 3 highly emergent ocular situations that requires treatment within minutes?
    a) corneal transplant patient with symptoms of rejection
    b) sudden, painless loss of vision in one eye
    c) chemical burns
    d) penetrating injuries

285. Urgent ocular situations generally need to be seen:
    a) at the practice's convenience
    b) the same day
    c) within 24 to 48 hours
    d) within minutes

286. Which of the following is an example of an emergent condition?
    a) sudden onset of diplopia
    b) globe perforation
    c) chalazion
    d) obstructed nasolacrimal duct

287. Which of the following is an emergency?
    a) a 42-year-old patient who has just noticed an inability to read at near
    b) a 4-year-old with a crossed eye since birth
    c) a construction worker with a foreign body sensation
    d) a −1.00 myope who broke her glasses

288. Which of the following constitutes the *most* emergent complaint?
    a) gradual loss of vision in one eye
    b) flashes and floaters of 4 months' duration
    c) sudden, painless loss of vision in one eye
    d) painful red eye

---

[10] I have elected to include basic ocular first aid here, although it is not mentioned in the criteria.

289. **All of the following could be considered elective** *except*:
   a) diabetic eye exam
   b) refractive exam
   c) foreign body
   d) nonpainful lid lesions

290. **A patient phones in with a loss of vision. Which of the following is the most important set of questions from a triage point of view?**
   a) One eye or both? Was this sudden or gradual? Is there any pain?
   b) When was your last eye exam? Did they see anything they were concerned about?
   c) Is there any discharge? Does the eye feel gritty?
   d) Have you used any eye drops to try to relieve the symptoms? Did that help?

291. **Which of the following is most likely to have a disastrous visual outcome if not treated immediately?**
   a) conjunctivitis
   b) subconjunctival hemorrhage
   c) angle-closure glaucoma
   d) iritis

292. **A patient phones in complaining of a red eye. From a triage standpoint, which is the most important question?**
   a) When did this start?
   b) Is there any pain?
   c) Are you seeing double?
   d) Do you have glaucoma?

293. **All of the following can cause a painful red eye** *except*:
   a) angle-closure glaucoma
   b) conjunctivitis
   c) subconjunctival hemorrhage
   d) iritis

294. **Which of the following does** *not* **cause a red eye?**
   a) iritis
   b) conjunctivitis
   c) open-angle glaucoma
   d) angle-closure glaucoma

295. **Symptoms and signs for acute angle-closure glaucoma may include all of the following** *except*:
   a) severe pain
   b) decreased vision
   c) vomiting/nausea
   d) miotic pupil

296. **All of the following may trigger an angle-closure glaucoma attack** *except*:
   a) being dilated in the office
   b) being in a dark room
   c) sudden exposure to bright light
   d) sitting in a movie theater

297. **In angle-closure glaucoma:**
     a) the iris closes off the anterior chamber angle
     b) there is a sudden surge of aqueous production
     c) a miotic pupil prevents aqueous passage
     d) corneal edema closes off the anterior chamber angle

298. **Which of the following conditions gives a higher risk for developing an angle-closure glaucoma attack?**
     a) high hyperopia
     b) high myopia
     c) aphakia
     d) keratoconus

299. **The appearance of halos around lights during an attack of angle-closure glaucoma is due to:**
     a) lens edema
     b) corneal edema
     c) vitreous hemorrhage
     d) optic nerve damage

300. **Emergency treatment during an angle-closure glaucoma attack includes pressure-lowering medications and:**
     a) miotics
     b) mydriatics
     c) antibiotics
     d) corticosteroids

301. **In examining the pupil of a painful red eye, which would most likely be seen in iritis?**
     a) The affected eye would have a smaller pupil.
     b) The affected eye would have a larger pupil.
     c) The affected eye would have an oval-shaped pupil.
     d) Iritis does not affect the pupil size or shape.

302. **A 60-year-old patient calls with flashes and floaters in one eye, which started 2 days ago. You should:**
     a) schedule him or her for a routine eye exam in a month
     b) schedule him or her for a dilated exam in a week
     c) schedule him or her for an urgent visit right away
     d) reassure the patient that this is normal as one ages

303. **Which of the following symptoms could indicate a retinal detachment?**
     a) painful red eye
     b) curtain or veil over part of the vision
     c) halos around lights
     d) sticky discharge

304. **The classic symptoms for posterior vitreous detachment are:**
     a) sudden, painless loss of vision
     b) painful red eye
     c) flashes and floaters
     d) foreign body sensation

305. **Any eye injury is considered:**
   a) a reason to irrigate the eye
   b) a reason to apply a pressure patch
   c) vision-threatening until proven otherwise
   d) able to wait until the patient's turn in the exam room

306. **A patient comes to the office after getting chemicals in his eye. The first step is to:**
   a) assess vision
   b) apply a pressure patch
   c) instill topical anesthetic
   d) irrigate

307. **Which of the following causes the most severe chemical injury?**
   a) acetic acid
   b) hydrochloric acid
   c) nitric acid
   d) ammonia

308. **Before any treatment is started on a patient who presents with a foreign body in the eye, the most important question to ask is:**
   a) "Were you wearing safety glasses?"
   b) "Does the eye hurt?"
   c) "Does your vision seem to be affected?"
   d) "What were you doing when this happened?"

309. **Which of the following best indicates the severity of a deep, penetrating injury?**
   a) the patient's vision
   b) the ophthalmoscopic evaluation
   c) the external appearance of the eye
   d) the amount of pain the patient has

310. **If a patient has a perforated globe, the technician must:**
   a) apply a pressure patch
   b) irrigate the eye
   c) perform a tactile tension
   d) cover lightly and inform the physician

311. **Your patient complains of a foreign body sensation about an hour after grinding metal at work. The physician is in surgery and will not be available for over an hour. You should:**
   a) instill ointment for comfort
   b) dilate the pupil
   c) cover lightly
   d) give the patient oral pain medication

312. **It is best to remove a metallic corneal foreign body during the first 6 to 8 hours to prevent:**
   a) sympathetic ophthalmia
   b) formation of a rust ring
   c) epidemic conjunctivitis
   d) endophthalmitis

313. **Painful corneal burns due to ultraviolet light might occur (if one fails to protect the eyes) in all of the following situations *except*:**
    a) tanning booth
    b) direct viewing of a lunar eclipse
    c) welding
    d) snow skiing

314. **A patient has been hit in the eye with a tennis ball. Your best action is to:**
    a) ask him to come right in before the eye swells shut
    b) explain the symptoms of retinal detachment and have him call back if they appear
    c) make him an appointment for next week so the swelling has a chance to go down
    d) tell him to use an ice pack and call back if he has any problems

315. **All of the following can result from blunt trauma to the eye *except*:**
    a) blow out fracture
    b) traumatic hyphema
    c) retinal detachment
    d) trachoma

316. **A blow out fracture involves:**
    a) bones of the orbit and sinuses
    b) globe rupture
    c) airborne particles
    d) bones of the cheek and forehead

317. **A hemorrhage in the anterior chamber is:**
    a) a subconjunctival hemorrhage
    b) cells and flare
    c) a hyphema
    d) a vitreous hemorrhage

318. **Which of the following is the wrong thing to say to an injured patient?**
    a) "Dr. Pelham will do her best to help you."
    b) "I am sorry this happened to you."
    c) "I am sure you will be just fine."
    d) "Is there anyone I can call for you?"

Forms and Manuals

319. **The organization involved with ensuring employee health and safety is:**
    a) Joint Commission on Allied Health Personnel in Ophthalmology (JCAHPO®)
    b) Exempt Organization Entity (EOE)
    c) Occupational Safety and Health Administration (OSHA)
    d) Health Insurance Portability and Accountability Act (HIPAA)

320. **The "OSHA poster" must be displayed in the workplace and explains:**
    a) employee rights to a safe workplace and how to report problems
    b) hand washing requirements
    c) employee rights to a work environment free of harassment
    d) fire escape routes

321. **An employer's written plan regarding employee exposure to bloodborne pathogens is a(n):**
    a) Exposure Incident Report
    b) Report of Employee Hazards
    c) Exposure Control Plan
    d) Hepatitis B Vaccine Report

322. **You are concerned about the possible toxicity of the lens cleaner you use. Where can you look for information?**
    a) The office's Material Safety Data Sheet (MSDS) file.
    b) The office's Exposure Incident Report file.
    c) The office's exposure control plan.
    d) The office's employee handbook.

323. **An employer's written plan detailing expectations and procedures for the clinic would be the office's:**
    a) Exposure Control Plan
    b) Manual of Clinic Safety
    c) Standard Operating Procedures
    d) Job Descriptions

324. **A patient falls in your clinic. The practice will fill out a(n):**
    a) Safety Data Sheet
    b) Exposure Incident Report
    c) Incident Report
    d) Worker's Compensation Form

Legal Forms for Government Services

325. **An assessment that makes a statement about a patient's ability/inability to perform tasks that he or she needs and wants to do is an evaluation of:**
    a) impairment
    b) disability
    c) qualification
    d) vision loss

326. **A medical report of a patient's ophthalmic status (including vision assessment and documentation of ocular diseases/disorders) is an evaluation of that patient's:**
    a) quality of life
    b) disability
    c) impairment
    d) culpability

327. **The purpose of government-required forms regarding ocular health is generally to:**
    a) determine fault
    b) determine eligibility
    c) eliminate malingering
    d) justify legal prosecution

328. **Inaccuracy or errors made on a form for government benefits and services may:**
    a) deprive the patient of services he or she is actually qualified for
    b) accuse the patient of self-inflicted harm
    c) result in an OSHA citation to the practice
    d) result in a freeze on the practice's insurance reimbursements

329. **In order to qualify for many governmental benefits, acuity testing for the visually impaired commonly includes:**
    a) potential acuity testing
    b) uncorrected and best-corrected vision
    c) vision uncorrected and with current correction
    d) pinhole vision

330. **A person with 20/20 acuity in both eyes and normal visual fields:**
    a) would never qualify as having a visual disability
    b) is not eligible for any type of assistance
    c) may still be visually disabled
    d) does not have a visual impairment

331. **Your patient hands you a form to qualify him for a commercial driver's license (CDL). The main visual components in such an exam generally include:**
    a) IOP, confrontation fields, and central corneal thickness
    b) visual acuity, glare test, and stereo vision
    c) visual acuity, pupil evaluation, and dilated fundus exam
    d) visual acuity, visual fields, and color vision

332. **A patient usually presents with a form for a vision test related to obtaining a driver's license when:**
    a) getting a license for the first time
    b) getting a driving citation for the first time
    c) failing the acuity test at the license bureau
    d) failing the driving test at the license bureau

333. **As a result of vision testing, the eye care practitioner has written "daytime driving only" on the patient's drivers license form. This is an example of a(n):**
    a) restriction
    b) impairment
    c) allowance
    d) conviction

334. **Insurance that covers an employee who is injured on the job or develops a job-related illness is:**
    a) HIPAA
    b) Employee Incident Insurance
    c) Workers' Compensation
    d) Medicaid

335. **A Workers' Compensation form for a patient with a job-related eye injury will probably include:**
    a) nature and length of any disability
    b) statement regarding whether or not the worker was careless
    c) citations to the employer for unsafe environment
    d) citations to the employee for unsafe practices

336. **Which of the following might be covered under Workers' Compensation?**
    a) any eye injury
    b) an eye injury sustained while working on one's own car
    c) an eye injury sustained while on the job
    d) an eye injury sustained while working on a friend's house

337. **The United States government's health insurance plan for citizens over the age of 65 is:**
    a) Medicare
    b) Medicaid
    c) HIPAA
    d) Social Security

338. **A refraction is usually ruled by Medicare as:**
    a) an essential part of the routine eye exam
    b) a noncovered procedure
    c) covered at 50%
    d) covered if the physician can show need

339. **In order to be able to file Medicare for a patient, the patient must sign a(n):**
    a) informed consent
    b) assignment of benefits
    c) opt-out form
    d) financial statement

340. **Federal- and state-supported health insurance for those who cannot afford insurance is:**
    a) supplemental insurance
    b) Medicare
    c) Medicaid
    d) secondary insurance

341. **A federal law that includes a patient's right to protection of his or her personal health information is:**
    a) the Miranda Law
    b) OSHA
    c) HIPAA
    d) Amber Alert

342. **Patient forms pertaining to HIPAA would include:**
    a) release of information and privacy disclosure
    b) restriction of information and incident report
    c) assignment of benefits and financial statement
    d) health history and insurance information

Vital Signs

343. **The group of tests collectively known as "vital signs" include:**
    a) temperature, blood pressure, pulse, and respirations
    b) height, weight, and body mass index
    c) vision, pupils, and confrontation fields
    d) mental status, physical status, and psychological status

344. **Which of the following is considered the "normal" human body temperature?**
    a) 89.6° F
    b) 96.8° F
    c) 98.6° F
    d) 99.6° F

345. **If taking an oral temperature, accuracy depends upon:**
    a) when the patient last had something warm or cool in his or her mouth
    b) whether the patient is sitting or standing
    c) the patient having a normal pulse rate
    d) the time of day

346. **Before taking an oral temperature with a standard (nonelectronic) thermometer, one must first:**
    a) rinse the thermometer in hot water
    b) have the patient rinse her mouth
    c) tap the thermometer sharply on the table
    d) shake the mercury down into the bulb

347. **When checking temperature with a standard oral thermometer, the probe tip is placed:**
    a) between cheek and gum
    b) on top of the tongue
    c) under the tongue
    d) between the molars

348. **When using a standard oral thermometer, how long is the thermometer left in place before taking the reading?**
    a) 1 to 2 minutes
    b) 3 to 4 minutes
    c) 5 to 6 minutes
    d) until the probe "beeps"

349. **A temperature that is above normal generally indicates the presence of a(n):**
    a) infectious process somewhere in the body
    b) inaccurate method
    c) overheated patient
    d) swelling and pain

350. **When checking pulse, one should:**
    a) apply gentle pressure with the thumb
    b) apply the firmest pressure the patient can tolerate
    c) apply gentle pressure
    d) watch for the pulse-beat through the skin

351. **The usual place for checking pulse is:**
    a) in the arch of the foot
    b) in the soft tissue in front of the ear
    c) in the arm pit
    d) in the soft tissue of the wrist above the thumb

352. **Heart rate is generally recorded as:**
    a) systolic and diastolic
    b) beats per minute
    c) beats per second
    d) normal/abnormal

353. **Average heart rate in a human adult is:**
    a) 39 beats per minute
    b) 72 beats per minute
    c) 3 beats per second
    d) 100 beats per minute

354. **Pulse can additionally be evaluated by noting:**
    a) the ratio of breaths to pulse beats
    b) the amount of pressure applied until the pulse stops
    c) if the patient is in pain
    d) any irregularities in beat or strength

355. **The average adult human respiration rate is:**
    a) 1 breath per second
    b) 18 breaths per minute
    c) 30 breaths per minute
    d) 50 breaths per minute

356. **The best way to check respiration rate is to:**
    a) covertly evaluate it after the pulse has been checked
    b) place a hand on the patient's back and time the breaths
    c) ask the patient to breathe normally
    d) ask the patient to breathe once every 2.5 seconds

357. **Respiration can additionally be evaluated by noting:**
   a) if pinching the ankle causes an increase
   b) the ratio of pulse to breaths
   c) any unusual sounds or irregularities
   d) the patient's reaction to additional oxygen

358. **In a blood pressure of 120/80, the number 80 is:**
   a) the time length of the measurement
   b) the average of the measurement
   c) the diastolic pressure
   d) the systolic pressure

359. **The best time to take the patient's blood pressure is:**
   a) immediately after he or she enters the exam room
   b) right before dilation
   c) a few minutes after he or she has been seated
   d) when he or she is lying down

360. **Blood pressure (BP) is measured using a(n):**
   a) sphygmomanometer
   b) exophthalmometer
   c) electrocardiograph
   d) examiner's fingers

361. **The BP cuff is positioned:**
   a) above the knee
   b) around the wrist
   c) around the neck
   d) above the elbow

362. **When checking BP with a manual (nonelectronic) sphygmomanometer, the examiner holds the membrane of the stethoscope:**
   a) against the skin and inside the elbow
   b) against the neck at the carotids
   c) at the site of the radial pulse
   d) against the cuff

363. **The bulb of the sphygmomanometer is used to:**
   a) regulate the patient's heart rate
   b) keep the gauge visible
   c) pump air into the cuff
   d) measure pulse rate

364. **Air is released from the cuff by:**
   a) barely turning the screw on the bulb
   b) releasing pressure on the bulb
   c) asking the patient to exhale
   d) removing the cuff

365. **As the cuff initially deflates, the examiner must note the:**
    a) number of seconds before the heartbeat is heard
    b) gauge reading when the heartbeat is first heard
    c) gauge reading when the pulse stops
    d) reaction of the patient

366. **The BP cuff continues to deflate, and the heartbeat sound is lost. At this point, the examiner notes the:**
    a) time of the reading
    b) length of the reading
    c) gauge reading when the heartbeat is again heard
    d) gauge reading when the heartbeat fades

367. **In addition to the numeric measurement of BP, one also documents:**
    a) the length of the reading
    b) characteristics of the pulse
    c) which arm was used
    d) the patient's reaction

368. **Normal BPs fall into which range?**
    a) 110 to 140 systolic, 70 to 90 diastolic
    b) both systolic and diastolic over 100 but less than 150
    c) 120/80 to 150/100
    d) varies according to the patient's body mass index

369. **BP might be *especially* important in each of the following patients *except*:**
    a) the patient with a cataract
    b) the patient who is being prepped for a chalazion excision
    c) the patient who is using beta-blocker drops for glaucoma
    d) the patient who feels dizzy

370. **A BP of 120 to 139 systolic and 80 to 89 diastolic is considered:**
    a) normotensive
    b) hypotensive
    c) prehypertensive
    d) hypertensive

CPR[11]

371. **Which group is at most risk for developing cardiopulmonary arrest?**
    a) those with cardiovascular problems
    b) those with diabetes
    c) those with emphysema
    d) those with cancer

[11]While CPR training is no longer required by JCAHPO® for its certifications, it is advisable that people in the health care field be skilled in CPR.

372. If breathing and pulse are not present, brain death will usually occur:
   a) in 2 to 4 minutes
   b) in 4 to 6 minutes
   c) in 6 to 10 minutes
   d) in 10 to 14 minutes

373. The most common airway obstruction in an unconscious adult is:
   a) food
   b) the tongue
   c) displaced dentures
   d) ice

374. How many people survive cardiac arrest if someone performs chest compressions or CPR?
   a) 1 in 5
   b) 1 in 10
   c) 1 in 20
   d) 1 in 25

375. What is the first step in the rescue/CPR process?
   a) Activate 911 or an emergency response system.
   b) Assess responsiveness.
   c) Position patient.
   d) Check for pulse and breathing.

376. The correct rescuer position for performing chest compressions on an adult is:
   a) straddling the victim, hands interlaced, elbows straight
   b) at the victim's side, both hands on chest, elbows bent
   c) at the victim's head, heel of one hand on chest, elbow straight
   d) at the victim's side, hands interlaced, elbows straight

377. The correct depth for chest compressions in an adult is:
   a) 1 to 1.5 inches
   b) at least 2 inches
   c) 4 inches
   d) until the rib cage crackles

378. "Hands-only" CPR has been introduced to the public because:
   a) few people take CPR training
   b) previously only health care workers could perform CPR
   c) bystanders are reluctant to administer mouth-to-mouth breathing
   d) many areas are remote, and EMS is more than 15 minutes away

379. The rate of compressions in hands-only CPR is:
   a) 30 per minute
   b) one per second
   c) 100 per minute
   d) 120 per minute

380. **All of the following are true regarding automated external defibrillators** *except*:
   a) they can be used by any bystander
   b) they are appropriate to use on adults and children
   c) they provide a shock to restart the heart
   d) they are used until EMS arrives

Explanatory Answers

1.   c) An upper blepharoplasty ("lid lift") is the procedure used to treat dermatochalasis or redundant skin of the eyelids.
2.   b) Ptosis is a drooping upper lid.
3.   a) A procedure to remove a growth or other tissue is an excision. An incision is cutting into, but not necessarily removing, anything. A biopsy is when tissue is removed and sent to a lab for identification. A biopsy might be done once tissue is excised.
4.   c) A chalazion is often incised (cut into) and drained. Although not mentioned here, curettage may also be performed, where the exposed tissue is scraped.
5.   b) Surgery to improve appearance is cosmetic. Insurance is not likely to pay for it.
6.   a) In a biopsy, tissue is sent to a lab for identification. Usually, the concern is whether or not the tissue is malignant (cancerous).
7.   c) Removing tissue (such as skin) from one part of the body and transplanting it onto another area is a graft. (*Note:* When a *flap* is performed, the tissue to be transplanted is not totally removed, but left partially attached and rotated to cover the adjacent area needing repair.)
8.   d) An inward-turned eyelid is called an entropion; thus, the surgery is an entropion repair.
9.   c) An outward-turned eyelid is called an ectropion, so this surgery is an ectropion repair.
10. a) If a laceration involves the lower lid, next to the nose, the tear drainage system is involved. Permanent tearing may result if the drainage ducts are not properly aligned.
11. d) During fetal development, there is a membrane covering the nasolacrimal duct in the tear drainage system. This membrane usually disappears before birth, but sometimes remains. In this case, tears do not drain properly, and an infection can easily develop. The treatment is to open the membrane with a probe (thin wire) and then flush the drainage system with saline.
12. c) Punctal occlusion is sometimes used to prevent tears from draining off the eye's surface. Occlusion keeps the tears that are produced (not much, in a patient with dry eye) *on* the eye.
13. b) Another name for a corneal graft or transplant is a keratoplasty.
14. a) Radiation is not used with a corneal transplant.
15. c) A pterygium is a piece of fleshy tissue that grows from the conjunctiva onto the cornea. An "active" pterygium continues to grow and may need to be removed before it gets to the center and obscures vision.
16. a) In the case of recurrent corneal erosion, the eroded area is carefully scraped. The idea is to create a smooth surface so the cornea will be able to heal normally.
17. b) Logically, refractive errors are corrected using refractive surgery. Technically, any surgery that purposely alters the eye's refractive status could be considered refractive surgery, making cataract extraction with intraocular lens implant the most-performed refractive surgery.

18. a) RK and AK are performed with blades, not laser. Corneal implants are done by conventional surgery.

19. b) PRK involves removing the corneal epithelium (compared to creating a flap that is later replaced) and shaping the underlying corneal layer.

20. d) The excimer laser is used in refractive surgery. The YAG is a cutting laser, used for capsulotomy, adhesions, and iridotomy. The argon and krypton lasers are used in retinal vascular disease and in glaucoma procedures.

21. c) Topical anesthesia is used for refractive surgery.

22. b) In strabismus (esotropia, exotropia), the condition is often corrected by moving the location where the extraocular muscles attach to the eye and/or shortening a muscle. One muscle is recessed (its insertion moved farther back on the eyeball) and the other resected (part of it removed, making it shorter).

23. c) Anisometropia is a refractive problem where the refractive difference between the two eyes is 2.00 D or more. Strabismus surgery cannot change this; it must be resolved with optical correction. It is generally recommended that EOM surgery be done prior to a child's entering kindergarten so that the "crossed eyes" are no longer noticed (ie, for cosmetic reasons). The main hope, however, is that by aligning the eyes, they will quickly learn to "lock" together, resulting in stereo vision. This, in turn, can help prevent or resolve amblyopia.

24. c) By definition, a cataract is an opacity of the crystalline lens; it is not a growth.

25. a) Light entering an eye with a cataract is scattered and may result in halos around lights because the light is broken into its component colors.

26. a) As the lens opacity gets denser, the eye generally becomes more nearsighted or myopic. This can happen even in a farsighted/hyperopic eye and is known as a myopic shift. A person who needed glasses to read may now find he or she no longer needs them. This phenomenon is known as "second sight" or the "honeymoon" stage of cataracts.

27. a) See answer 25. The scattered light can cause objects to appear doubled, although "ghost image" is usually a better description.

28. d) Cataracts tend to cause a yellowing to a person's color vision. Often, after cataract surgery, a patient will notice that colors are more vivid.

29. b) A cataract may cause a general haze to the vision, as if looking through waxed paper.

30. b) It is current theory that every person will get cataracts if he or she lives long enough. It is just that mine may be ready to be removed when I am 57 (which I am not...yet!), and you may be 91 and not need yours removed yet.

31. c) Having open-angle glaucoma does not predispose one to cataracts.

32. a) A secondary cataract is caused by something else, such as trauma (including ultraviolet light), disease (eg, diabetes), or medication (eg, steroids).

33. d) Surgical extraction is the only current method of treating cataracts. Generally, a small opening is made in the eye just at the limbus. The cataract is broken into pieces using ultrasound, and the pieces are drawn out with suction. A clear plastic lens implant is then put in the place of the crystalline lens that was removed. Stitches are generally not needed.

34. b) Because laser is used to treat postoperative capsule opacity, people often think that the cataract is removed that way as well. Answer d is not recommended; you can educate the patient without implying that someone is ignorant! (By the way, the length of answer b should have clued you in that it was probably the correct answer!)

35. a) A PAM is used to estimate what vision will be once the cataract is removed. For other questions regarding the BAT, see Chapter 16, the section titled *Glare Testing*.

36. c) A patient who has macular degeneration may not notice much improvement after cataract surgery; the PAM may be able to help predict this. Explain it to the patient like this: If you have a great camera but the film is not good, you will not get a good picture regardless of the quality of the lens. The eye is like that. The lens is the implant, and the film is the retina. If the retina is diseased, having cataract surgery with a lens implant will not help much. (Exception: Sometimes, cataract surgery is performed for a patient with macular degeneration to improve his or her "getting around" vision, rather than the central vision.)

37. c) A dense cataract makes it difficult for the physician to see inside the eye to judge the health of the retina. A B-scan ultrasound might be done to make sure that the retina is not detached nor has any gross abnormality that might prevent vision improvement if the cataract was removed.

38. a) The A-scan ultrasound is used to measure the axial length of the eye prior to cataract surgery. It is one of several variables in determining the power of an IOL implant to be used once the cataract has been removed (see Chapter 16, the section titled *IOL Power Calculation*).

39. a) Cataract surgery invariably "bumps" the single-cell-layered corneal endothelium, which is already diseased in corneal dystrophy. Specular microscopy (also known as a cell count) may be done to evaluate the corneal endothelium prior to attempting cataract surgery to make sure it is healthy enough to withstand the operation.

40. d) Of the tests listed, the BAT gives the best evaluation of what a patient with cataracts actually sees now. The results can indicate a level of disability that is not evident on testing with the regular Snellen eye chart. Cataracts that are dense in the center can often cause vision to worsen in bright light because the pupil constricts. The BAT gives an actual measurement of how much worse the vision is in such bright conditions.

41. d) Years ago, a cataract was not removed until it was "ripe." But with modern technology, a cataract can be removed whenever the patient notices that his vision decrease is interfering with his activities of daily living.

42. a) Keratometry is used to measure the curvature of the cornea prior to cataract surgery. It is one of several variables used in determining the power of IOL implant to be used once the cataract has been removed. (See Chapter 6, *Keratometry*, as well as Chapter 16, the section titled *IOL Power Calculation*.)

43. d) The patient's intraocular pressure does not figure into the formula used to determine the power of an IOL implant.

44. c) Estrogen-based medications do not have any known effects on cataract surgery. Aspirin and blood thinners can cause operative and postoperative bleeding. Some treatments for erectile dysfunction have been known to cause the intraoperative complication of floppy iris syndrome.

45. c) Answer a might be tempting, but it sounds too much like a guarantee. Although unlikely, there could be some type of intraoperative complication where the surgeon will suture the wound.

46. a) The most commonly used type of anesthesia for cataract surgery is topical.

47. c) Phacoemulsification uses sound waves to break the cataract into small pieces, which are then removed by suction through a small tube.

48. c) Answers a and d are patently incorrect and sound like a (dangerous) guarantee that the patient will see perfectly without correction once the cataract has been removed. Answer b

is incorrect as well, because not everyone gets a "specialty" IOL (ie, multifocal or toric). Answer c is the only "safe" answer. (*Note:* While the use of "specialty" IOLs and monovision IOLs may obviate the need for glasses, that was not given as an option here.)

49. b) Patients are generally told not to bend over (ie, bending at the waist so that the head is dangling down). Inclining the head to read is okay, and it is fine to kneel to pick something up. Patients are also told not to lift anything heavy. Bathing is allowed, although the patient is cautioned not to get any water in the eye.

50. a) When a cataract is removed, the back part of the capsule that encloses the eye's natural lens is left in place to support the IOL. The capsule membrane is polished, but sometimes gets cloudy after surgery (a few months to a few years). The symptoms of a posterior subcapsular opacity are pretty much the same as those of a cataract: blurred/foggy vision, ghost images, and problems with glare.

51. b) Another name for a posterior capsule opacity is "secondary cataract," but this is a misnomer. Once removed, a cataract cannot grow back.

52. d) Posterior capsule opacity is treated with a YAG laser, which is used to make an opening in the center of the capsule. This clears the visual axis, improving acuity.

53. b) A "phakic IOL" is inserted into the eye without removing the natural crystalline lens. It is done for the purpose of correcting refractive errors.

54. d) The aim of all glaucoma treatment is to decrease intraocular pressure. This is generally done in one of two ways: increasing drainage/outflow or decreasing production/inflow of aqueous humor. Thus, glaucoma surgery might involve placing an implant devised to drain aqueous fluid out of the eye.

55. c) See answer 54.

56. d) The laser surgery for open-angle glaucoma is trabeculoplasty. The laser beam is aimed into the angle of the eye (between the cornea and iris root). The theory is that when the tissue heals, the scarring pulls the trabecular meshwork open, increasing aqueous outflow.

57. a) In glaucoma surgery using a valve, a "bubble" or bleb is created between the conjunctiva and sclera as a site for venting aqueous from the eye.

58. c) In angle-closure glaucoma, the iris butts up against the anterior lens surface and is then pushed into the angle of the eye, blocking the drainage of aqueous from the eye. A laser iridotomy is done to create an opening in the iris to allow the aqueous to drain even when the angle is blocked.

59. b) Removal of the vitreous is a vitrectomy (the suffix –*ectomy* refers to removal).

60. b) Laser photocoagulation is frequently used to seal, especially blood vessels. Answers a, c, and d are all retinal conditions that may respond well to photocoagulation. A hyphema is blood in the anterior chamber, which is not treated with laser.

61. c) A retinal detachment might be treated with laser (photocoagulation, to "fuse" tissue), a scleral buckle (a device that pushes the tissues together), or a "bubble" of gas or air (which puts internal pressure on the area of concern).

62. a) The medication given via intravitreal injection for macular degeneration is intended to interfere with neovascularization, or the growth of new, abnormal, fragile blood vessels.

63. d) An enucleation is the procedure for removal of the eyeball. Evisceration is removal of the contents of the globe but not the globe itself. Exenteration is removal of the globe and all associated muscles, fat, and tissue (including the eyelids). Ectropion is an out-turned eyelid.

64. b) After an eyeball is enucleated, an implant is placed into the eye socket to maintain the shape of the orbit. Without the implant, the orbit would tend to shrink, making it difficult to fit a prosthetic eye.

65. b) Diabetes results when the insulin-glucose (sugar) levels of the body are imbalanced. Answers a and d are symptoms of diabetes, but do not cause it.

66. a) A stable sugar level for about 6 weeks prior to refractometry is desirable for a good measurement. The refractometric measurement often varies as the sugar level fluctuates.

67. d) The word *proliferative* indicates that something is growing or spreading. Proliferative diabetic retinopathy occurs when new, abnormal blood vessels begin to spread into the retina of the diabetic. This is called neovascularization.

68. d) Diabetes itself is treated with answers b and c. Retinopathy is treated with laser.

69. c) High blood pressure (hypertension) affects mainly the retina.

70. a) Currently, the designation of hypertension starts when a person's blood pressure is consistently 140 to 159 systolic (or higher) and/or 90 to 99 diastolic (or higher). There is also a category known as "prehypertension," which ranges from 120 to 139 systolic and 80 to 89 diastolic. If the systolic is 180 or higher and/or the diastolic is higher than 110, emergency care is called for.[12]

71. d) As in diabetes, retinopathy caused by hypertension is treated with laser.

72. c) Cancer can spread to any organ or tissue, including the eye.

73. a) The condition of fatty deposits on the walls of the arteries is known as atherosclerosis. (Atherosclerosis is actually a form of arteriosclerosis, or hardening of the arteries.)

74. c) If a fatty plaque dislodges, travels through the bloodstream, and gets stuck in the central retinal artery, an occlusion can occur.

75. a) Any foreign material in the bloodstream has the potential for blocking blood vessels.

76. c) If the mother is infected with toxoplasmosis, herpes simplex, or gonorrhea (*Neisseria gonorrhoeae*), the infant is at risk. Toxoplasmosis would occur in utero, herpes simplex and *N. gonorrhoeae* during birth. Siderosis refers to iron deposits in the tissues, which is not something that would be transmitted from mother to child.

77. d) Herpes zoster is the virus that causes shingles.

78. d) Herpes zoster, or shingles, occurs in those who have been previously infected with the chicken pox (varicella).

79. a) The AIDS patient, with a lowered immunity, is subject to infection. One of the more common is herpes simplex.

80. c) Of course an AIDS patient *can* develop xanthelasma (yellowish lid lesions related to cholesterol), but in general this is not directly associated with AIDS. In addition to a, b, and d, recurrent conjunctivitis is also common.

81. b) Needle sticks remain the main source of transmission to medical personnel. The AIDS virus has been isolated from human tears, but there have been no known cases of transmission due to contact with contaminated tears.

82. b) Rheumatoid arthritis is commonly associated with dry eye, sometimes severe (keratitis sicca).

83. a) Exophthalmos, where the eye(s) bulge abnormally, is associated with thyroid eye disease. The instrument used to measure ocular protrusion is the exophthalmometer.

[12]These numbers come from the American Heart Association. Available at: www.heart.org/HEARTORG/Conditions/HighBloodPressure/AboutHighBloodPressure/Understanding-Blood-Pressure-Readings_UCM_301764_Article.jsp. Accessed 8/25/11.

84. b) Smoking pretty much affects the entire body. Externally, the smoke can contribute to dry eye. Smoking also increases the risk of retinal diseases, including diabetic and hypertensive retinopathy and macular degeneration. Tobacco amblyopia is visual decrease in an otherwise healthy eye, related to smoking.

85. d) Basal cell tumors are also known as basal cell carcinomas. This is a malignant tumor that should be removed and biopsied promptly.

86. b) A sagging, everted (out-turned) lid is known as ectropion.

87. a) An inverted lid is termed entropion.

88. b) An infected lash follicle produces a sty or hordeolum. (A chalazion is an infected meibomian gland.)

89. c) The condition of having inward-growing lashes—patients sometimes calls these "wild hairs"—is known as trichiasis.

90. c) An infected meibomian gland produces a chalazion.

91. a) Blepharitis is a common lid infection (*blephar-* referring to eyelids and *–itis* meaning an inflammation).

92. a) Ptosis refers to the drooping of an organ or structure. When speaking of the eye, the term refers to the drooping of the upper lid. *Blepharoptosis* would be even more descriptive and accurate.

93. d) The prefix *dermato-* indicates a condition involving the skin; the suffix *–chalasis* means relaxation. Thus, the combined term is dermatochalasis. (***Note:*** Some references make a distinction between blepharochalasis, which is a rarer problem involving intermittent swelling of the upper lids, and dermatochalasis, which is the common relaxing of the lid's skin.)

94. d) Dacryocystitis is the term for an infected tear sac. Canaliculitis is an infection of the canaliculus. Answers b and c are bogus.

95. c) A prolapse occurs when a structure slides out of place. The lacrimal gland can "fall" into the space between the globe and the conjunctiva, appearing as a yellowish, moveable mass under the conjunctiva on the superior area of the globe.

96. d) Extreme itching is more often associated with allergies and infections, not dry eye.

97. b) Schirmer's tear test measures the amount of tears produced in a 5-minute test period.[13]

98. a) Recurrent erosion syndrome is not related to a blocked nasolacrimal duct. Epiphora (tears streaming down the cheeks) and tearing in infants as well as chronic infections (occurring because microorganisms are not being flushed out of the system) are frequent hallmarks of this condition.

99. c) An SCH in and of itself is not serious. The patient can be reassured. The exception would be if the SCH was the result of trauma, in which case answer a would be appropriate. But do not read into the question!

100. d) A pinguecula appears as a yellow nodule, usually on the nasal side of the eyeball. A pterygium crosses onto the cornea, and the nodule associated with episcleritis generally is seen in a red eye. Xanthelasma appears on the lids.

101. d) Crusting is usually associated with bacterial conjunctivitis.

102. b) EKC is caused by a virus. The conjunctiva and usually the cornea are involved.

103. a) Giant papillary conjunctivitis is thought to be caused by constant irritation from contact lenses or other physical irritants such as a prosthesis or exposed suture.[14]

---

[13]See Chapter 16, section *Tear Tests*, subsection *Schirmer*.

[14]Available at: http://emedicine.medscape.com/article/1191641-overview. Accessed 4/1/11.

104. b) The sclera is the white of the eye, so the inflammation is known as scleritis. Episcleritis is an inflammation of the episclera and, in general, is not very painful (if at all). Uveitis is an inflammation of the uvea which includes the iris, ciliary body, and choroid; iritis is an inflammation of the iris.

105. a) Exophthalmos is the abnormal protrusion of an eye, also called proptosis. Buphthalmos is abnormal enlargement of the infant eye due to congenital glaucoma.

106. d) Arcus senilis is a creamy white deposit in the corneal tissue at the limbus. It is a cholesterol accumulation and may encircle the entire cornea or just part of it.

107. d) Neovascularization (in any part of the body) is the growth of new blood vessels. In the cornea, this is due to anoxia, or lack of oxygen. It is commonly associated with contact lens wear.

108. a) Trachoma is a contagious chlamydial (bacterial) infection that causes severe scarring, which often results in blindness.

109. b) The corneal dendrite typical of herpes simplex has a branched, tree-like appearance best seen with the cobalt blue light and fluorescein stain.

110. c) The hallmark of keratoconus is a bulging, cone-shaped cornea that thins at the center. This induces astigmatism. The condition can be progressive.

111. b) If only the corneal epithelium is involved, there will be no scarring. Corneal scarring generally occurs if the abrasion reaches the deeper stromal tissue.

112. d) A pterygium is a flesh-colored growth that extends from the conjunctiva and onto the cornea. If it grows far enough out onto the cornea, it will impair vision.

113. a) Recurrent erosion syndrome (RES) usually occurs in an eye that has had a previous corneal injury, maybe even years before. The weakened area adheres to the palpebral conjunctiva—which lines the inner lid—and is literally peeled off when the lid is opened, resulting in a new corneal abrasion with the typical foreign body sensation and light sensitivity.

114. d) Hyphema (-*hema* referring to blood) denotes the presence of blood in the AC. It is usually graded by the amount of the AC that is involved. A 50% hyphema would mean that half of the AC is filled with blood. A 100% hyphema is sometimes called an 8-ball hyphema, because the filled AC looks like a black 8-ball.

115. a) An hypopyon is the presence of white blood cells in the AC. It generally signals the presence of an infection. The other 3 answers are all bogus.

116. b) Prior to dilating patients, you should check the angles (the space in the AC where the cornea meets the iris). Dilating an eye with narrow angles could result in an angle-closure glaucoma attack.

117. c) Uveitis refers to inflammation of *any* part of the uvea: the iris, ciliary body, and choroid. Iritis indicates that the inflammation is limited to the iris. It is sometimes called anterior uveitis, which distinguishes it as being the "front" of the uvea (ie, not involving the choroid).

118. c) Open-angle glaucoma has no physical symptoms and tends to be hereditary. Halos around lights at night are sometimes associated with angle-closure glaucoma.

119. d) Most ophthalmologists agree that, in order for glaucoma to be diagnosed, there must be damage to the optic disc (head). Not mentioned here but also important is central corneal thickness. See also answer 127.

120. a) An infant's eye is more elastic than an adult's, so elevated intraocular pressure tends to distort and distend the globe. This causes buphthalmos, or "ox eye," in which the cornea takes up most of the palpebral fissure.

121. a) The symptoms of angle-closure glaucoma are redness, pain, blurred vision, and halos around lights.

122. d) The pupil in an angle-closure attack is mid-dilated. The pain can be severe to the point of nausea and vomiting.

123. d) Strabismus does not cause glaucoma.

124. a) There is no indication that a patient with rheumatoid arthritis is at a higher risk of developing glaucoma. Answers b through d do indicate an increased risk.

125. c) The fact that glaucoma screening generates public interest is not a plague, but a benefit. The other answers are problems inherent to screening programs.

126. c) Open-angle glaucoma is the most common type of glaucoma. Some sources identify more than 40 different types of glaucoma.

127. c) The classic hallmarks of glaucoma are increased IOP (tested with tonometry), loss of peripheral vision (evaluated with formal perimetry), and damage to the optic nerve head (as seen on ophthalmoscopy). Because a thin cornea is also associated with increased risk of glaucoma, a central—not peripheral—corneal thickness measurement is also taken.

128. d) Unfortunately, vision lost due to glaucoma is not recoverable even once the condition is controlled or treated.

129. b) Corneal edema has a prismatic effect, breaking light into its component colors, and thus creating halos around lights. Pressure build-up during an attack causes a breakdown in the pumping function of the corneal endothelium, and edema results.

130. b) Open-angle glaucoma cannot be cured; it can only be controlled. In this respect, it resembles diabetes and high blood pressure. Answers a, c, and d are true.

131. c) Because open-angle glaucoma has no physical symptoms, the patient is not driven to seek attention. The loss of peripheral vision occurs over a long period of time, often escaping the patient's notice. *Signs* are perceptible to the examiner, such as optic disc cupping or an elevated IOP reading.

132. d) As its name implies, the angle structure in open-angle glaucoma is open. Generally, it looks normal.

133. d) A patient with open-angle glaucoma needs an annual full exam including dilation, gonioscopy, and formal visual fields testing. Of course, he also needs periodic IOP checks during the year. The air-puff tonometer is not accurate enough to monitor glaucoma. Likewise, confrontation fields are not sensitive enough to monitor for field loss in glaucoma. Generally, it is safe to dilate a patient with open-angle glaucoma. Many practitioners also want an annual OCT.

134. a) In advanced open-angle glaucoma, the patient often retains a small temporal island of vision. Eventually, that is lost as well.

135. d) A patient with glaucoma who misses a pressure check undoubtedly should be contacted to reschedule. The importance of the exam and the gravity of the disease should be stated. Answer b is a breach of patient confidentiality.

136. c) The prefix *a-* means without, and *–phakia* refers to the lens. So, the condition of having no lens, generally due to surgical removal, is aphakia. In the term pseudophakia, *pseudo-* means false, referring to an intraocular lens implant (eg, a "false lens").

137. d) A luxated lens is dislocated; a subluxated lens is only partially dislocated. Lens dislocation may cause iridodonesis, where the iris seems to vibrate or shake because its support, the lens, has shifted or been lost.

138. c) Dizziness and nausea are not associated with uveitis. Redness is generally more marked at the limbus. Light sensitivity may be severe, and the pupil is generally smaller.

139. a) The longer eye of the myope predisposes him to retinal detachment.

140. c) Retinal detachment is generally painless.

141. a) PVD and retinal detachment can both be accompanied by floaters and flashes. However, PVD is more common.

142. d) Macular degeneration is an inclusive term meaning any degeneration of the macular tissue, the most common cause of which is aging. Years ago, it was called senile macular degeneration, but is now more often referred to as age-related macular degeneration (AMD).

143. b) Standard home care for patients with macular degeneration is Amsler grid (patient is shown how to use it and how often), UV protection (sunglasses and a hat with a brim), and vitamin therapy (often one of the "eye vitamins" now available on the market).

144. a) Treatment for macular degeneration (other than vitamin therapy) is for the wet form of the disease, where new abnormal blood vessels grow and leak fluid into the macular tissues.

145. d) A sudden, painless loss of vision (especially in just one eye) is the hallmark of a retinal artery occlusion. In this situation, the artery in the retina becomes blocked, cutting off the blood supply to the retina. Immediate treatment, within 30 minutes, is necessary.

146. a) Because the symptoms of a retinal vein occlusion are so similar to those of a retinal artery occlusion, the patient with sudden, painless loss of vision should always be triaged as if it were a retinal artery occlusion. If a vein is occluded, blood can still come into the eye via the arteries, but blood drainage from the retina is blocked or slowed. This happens most often in patients with high blood pressure. There may be a generalized blurring of vision or a field loss in an area related to the part of the retina that is affected.

147. d) Toxoplasmosis is passed in cat feces, thus the warnings for pregnant women to avoid cleaning the litter box and for children to play only in sand boxes that have been covered.

148. d) The spores of histoplasmosis infect a human via inhalation.

149. d) The classic optic nerve sign of open-angle glaucoma is optic nerve cupping, where the high IOP has killed axons, leaving empty space.

150. c) Endophthalmitis is a most serious infection of an eye following penetrating injury or surgery and can lead to loss of the eye.

151. c) Sympathetic ophthalmia is a rare but severe inflammation that develops in a noninjured eye in response to an injury in the other, generally weeks later.

152. b) The injured eye is enucleated in order to prevent or resolve inflammation from setting up in (and perhaps destroying) the uninjured eye.

153. c) Trachoma is a disease. The other answers all have a genetic basis.

154. Matching

cardiovascular	b, g, i, n, p
respiratory	c, h, k, q
endocrine	a, d, j, l
nervous	e, f, m, o, r

155. d) Oxygen is carried by the red blood cells, which contain hemoglobin.

156. b) Human circulation could be conceived to start and end at any number of points, because it is a cycle. The body's cells dump waste products into the capillaries, which lead to the veins, which lead to the heart. The heart pumps the blood to the lungs to get rid of carbon dioxide and to take on oxygen. The blood goes back to the heart where it is pumped through the arteries and then to the capillaries, where the cells have access to the now oxygen-rich blood.

157. b) As we breathe in, air enters the trachea ("windpipe") and goes to the lungs. In the lungs, the air enters the bronchus/bronchioles, alveoli, and then the capillaries. Humans do not have a gill arch!

158. c) During respiration, the blood gives up carbon dioxide, a waste product, and takes in oxygen.

159. b) Endocrine glands synthesize and release hormones.

160. c) Hormones are released into the bloodstream and are carried to the target organ.

161. d) Nerve cells release neurotransmitters, which are chemicals that transmit impulses from one nerve cell to another.

162. d) A reflex is the predictable, involuntary motor response to a stimulus.

163. a) The nervous system is structurally composed of the central and peripheral systems. (There are other divisions, but this is the structural division.)

164. c) Functionally, the nervous system is divided into the sensory and motor systems.

165. Labeling, Figure 12-1

anterior segment	a
posterior segment	b

166. Labeling, Figure 12-2

bulbar conjunctiva	c or f
eyelashes	l
lateral canthus	b
caruncle	h
eyebrow	k
pupil	e
plica (semilunaris)	i
eyelids	a
iris	d
palpebral fissure	j
sclera	f or c
medial canthus	g

167. Labeling, Figure 12-3

optic nerve	d
anterior chamber	a
vitreous	c
posterior chamber	b

168. Labeling, Figure 12-4

nasolacrimal duct	d
lacrimal gland	a
canaliculus	c
nasolacrimal sac	e
punctum	b

169. Labeling, Figure 12-5

stroma	f
precorneal tear film	a
endothelium	d
epithelium	b
Descemet's membrane	e
Bowman's layer	c

170. Labeling, Figure 12-6

vitreous humor	c
aqueous humor	a
lens	b

171. Labeling, Figure 12-7

lens	e
angle	c
zonules	a
cornea	f
ciliary body	b
iris	d

172. Labeling, Figure 12-8

optic nerve	a
macula	c
blood vessels	b

173. Labeling, Figure 12-9

macula	f
cornea	c
optic nerve	a
iris	e
sclera	b
lens	d
retina	g

174. c) Incoming light is ideally focused on the retina. (Interpretation occurs in the occipital cortex of the brain.)

175. b) The orbit (or bony orbit) is the socket in which the globe (eyeball) is situated.

176. c) The ophthalmic artery is the main blood source that enters the eye directly. (By the way, a vein conducts blood *out* of an organ.)

177. c) The movement of each eye is controlled by 6 extraocular muscles.

178. a) The tarsus, or tarsal plate, is a tough fibrous connective tissue that gives form to the eyelids.

179. b) The epicanthal fold is a small vertical fold of skin next to the nose. It is genetic in Asians and may appear in some children (who may later outgrow it).

180. a) The main tear gland is under the brow. There are accessory glands in the conjunctiva.

181. d) The tear film layer is made up of mucin, water, and oil.

182. a) Tears drain off the eye through the punctum into the canaliculi. From there, they go into the lacrimal sac and out the nasolacrimal duct.

183. a) The oily film that makes up the outer surface of the tear layer helps prevent evaporation of the underlying watery layer.

184. d) The ocular media are the transparent structures of the eye through which light passes. Some references might not include the tear film.

185. d) The retina is not considered a part of the optical media.

186. b) Light entering the eye is refracted three-fourths by the cornea and one-fourth by the remaining optical structures. The average crystalline lens has about 20 D of plus power. The cornea has 43.0 D.

187. a) The average adult cornea is 12 mm in diameter.

188. d) If only the epithelium is abraded, the cornea almost always heals without scarring.

189. a) The endothelial layer of the cornea acts as a "pump" to keep the cornea dehydrated and clear.

190. b) The two muscles of the iris are the dilator (which opens the pupil) and the sphincter (which closes the pupil).

191. b) Aqueous humor is formed by the ciliary body, which joins the iris and the sclera. The ciliary muscle controls the shape of the crystalline lens via accommodation. The islets of Langerhans are in the pancreas.

192. d) An infant's lens is soft throughout, like putty. The hard central core forms as layers laminate over time as we age.

193. c) The crystalline lens is in the posterior chamber, which lies behind the iris. (Do not confuse the posterior *chamber* with the posterior *segment*.) The zonules connect the lens—which is enclosed in a capsule—to the ciliary muscle.

194. b) Accommodation enables near vision by causing the pupils to constrict (miosis), the eyes to converge, and the ciliary muscle to contract. (See answer 196.)

195. a) A person might squint (narrow the palpebral fissures) when looking at a close object, but it is not an element of accommodation.

196. a) We need more "plus" power to view close-up objects. When the circular ciliary muscle contracts, the zonules are allowed to relax. This takes the tension off the lens, which also "relaxes" and thickens, making the lens "more plus."

197. c) The uvea is comprised of the choroid, iris, and ciliary body.

198. c) The choroid is the blood vessel-rich layer that underlies and nourishes the retina. The retinal pigment epithelium is the inner-most layer of the retina and overlies the choroid. Rhodopsin ("visual purple") is a visual pigment. Carotene is a pigment as well, but is not synthesized in the eye.

199. b) The light-receptor cells of the retina are the rods and cones.

200. b) The rods actually outnumber the cones by about 20:1.

201. a) As the nerve fibers exit the optic nerve and enter the chiasm, the nasal fibers cross from one side to the other. The temporal fibers stay on their original side.

202. b) An object to the patient's right would be perceived by the temporal retina of the left eye and the nasal retina of the right eye. Temporal retinal fibers stay on the side of origin; nasal retinal fibers cross to the other side. Hence, an object to the right would be projected to the left optic tract.

203. a) Objects on a patient's left are projected onto the nasal portion of the retina in the left eye.

204. b) The optic disc is the head of the optic nerve and is visible with the ophthalmoscope.

205. a) ANSI accredits the standards for a number of industries, products, and processes. The standards themselves must go through a specific accreditation process including, among other things, a consensus by experts in the field and input from the public sector.

206. c) Frames approved for safety glasses must be resistant to high impact and marked to identify them. If the temples are thin, extra side shields are required.[15]

207. c) Safety glasses are appropriate for use as street wear and on the job.

208. d) This is one case where the world "always" is acceptable! Children (who are more prone to impact) and monocular patients (who must protect his or her one good eye) should always have safety lenses.

209. c) No lens is completely shatterproof, but a safety lens resists shattering on impact.

[15]Available at: www.domesticpreparedness.com/userfiles/reports/MSA_ANSI-ISEA10.pdf. Accessed 08/25/11.

210. b) A glass safety lens for general use may be no thinner than 2.2 mm in any part of the lens. The standard for an industrial-use lens is 3 mm.

211. c) "Polycarb" is the safety lens usually prescribed for average streetwear in adults and children. Glass safety lenses are used primarily in industry.

212. b) The necessary personal protective equipment must be supplied by the employer and includes face shields, goggles, masks, gloves, and gowns.

213. d) The welding arc is ultraviolet radiation and can cause very painful corneal burns.

214. c) Placing a finger at the medial corner of the closed eye helps keep the drop on the eye and reduces drainage through the lacrimal system, and from there, to the body.

215. c) Hands should always be washed prior to touching the eye area.

216. a) To apply ophthalmic ointment, the lower lid is pulled down and ointment is placed in the "pocket" (cul de sac).

217. a) The eye will not usually hold more than one drop, so using two at a time is a waste.

218. b) If one eye closes, the other eye wants to close as well. Also, it is more difficult to close the eyes when looking up.

219. d) A patient with posterior capsular cataracts might have a problem with a decrease in vision when bright light causes the pupil to constrict. A glare test would assist in documenting this.

220. a) The Ishihara pseudoisochromatic plates evaluate for red/green color defects. This type of defect occurs almost exclusively in males.

221. c) A patient with a visual field loss would be most benefited by an automated visual field, which can help determine where in the visual pathway the problem is. An Amsler grid tests only the central 10 degrees to 20 degrees of vision, which is not enough in this case.

222. d) The standard "eye chart" is of high contrast, but the real world is full of shadows and low contrast. A contrast sensitivity test evaluates a person's ability to discern detail as the contrast becomes lower and lower.

223. c) The PAM gives a visual acuity that bypasses media opacities. For example, a patient with cataracts and macular degeneration has 20/100 acuity and a PAM of 20/40. One might expect that if there was no media opacity, the patient would have 20/40 vision, which is subnormal due to the macular degeneration.

224. d) Exophthalmos—or bulging of the eye, measured with an exophthalmometer—can be a sign of thyroid eye disease.

225. b) I often tell patients that dilation is like the difference between looking into a room through a window versus a keyhole. With dilation, we have opened the pupil in order to get a broader view of the eye's interior. I also frequently say that the dilated exam is the most important part of a diabetic eye exam.

226. b) Schirmer's is a test that evaluates tear output. Dry eye is a common cause of a gritty or sandy sensation. For more on tear testing, see Chapter 16, the section titled *Tear Tests*.

227. d) In fluorescein angiography, fluorescein dye is injected into a vein. Photographs (using a special filter) are taken as the dye enters the bloodstream of the eye, showing any areas of leaking and blockage.

228. c) The A-scan uses ultrasound. A retained intraocular foreign body will reflect the waves, revealing its presence as a "blip" on the scan.

229. d) Corneal thickness is not usually a factor in contact lens selection. The other statements are true.

230. c) The OCT uses low coherence light (not ultrasound) to image the layers of the retina. The results may indicate why a patient has subnormal vision, but that is not the best response of those given.

231. d) Instilling topical fluorescein dye and looking at the eye with a cobalt blue filter will cause any corneal abrasions to be visible when the dye pools in the defect.

232. b) A culture generally involves taking some material from the infected area (usually just rubbing the area with a cotton swab) and placing the sample on a culture plate to see what type of organism is causing the infection. Once this is determined, specific treatment can be given; certain bacteria respond better to certain types of antibiotics.

233. c) Corneal topography will generate a map of the corneal curvature and, if repeated over time, may reveal that this patient has keratoconus. The keratometer does not "read" a large enough area of the cornea to be the best answer in this scenario.

234. d) The pinhole only improves decreased vision caused by a refractive error, so a score of less than 20/20 pinhole vision generally indicates that some pathology is present, preventing the eye from having optimal vision.

235. a) The standard three causes of a red, painful eye are angle-closure glaucoma, iritis, and infection. In angle-closure glaucoma, the pupil is generally mid-dilated; in iritis, it is smaller than the fellow pupil; and in an infection, the pupil size is unaffected. Slit-lamp exam of the angles (for closure), anterior chamber (for inflammatory cells), the pattern of redness, the condition of the cornea, and any discharge also help differentiate between the three. IOP is elevated in angle closure, but normal in the other two.

236. d) The macular scan using the OCT may reveal underlying macular pathology that is not readily visible with the ophthalmoscope. While the fluorescein angiogram has its uses, it is not the best choice of the options given.

237. b)The dilated fundus exam (preceded, of course, by visual acuity, pupil check, IOP, and slit-lamp exam to check the angles) is standard procedure in the patient with floaters and flashes. Either of these can be caused by a benign vitreous detachment or the more ominous retinal detachment. There is no way to tell the difference without a fundus exam.

238. c) In punctal occlusion, the puncti—usually just the lower—are plugged with punctal plugs or sealed with laser or cautery. The idea is to keep whatever tears are made on the eye by blocking the drainage route.

239. a) To open a blocked nasolacrimal duct, a thin wire probe is inserted into the lower punctum and pushed through the obstructing membrane. The punctum is usually dilated first, but dilation alone will not open the duct.

240. a) A foreign body spud or a small drill may be used to remove a metallic foreign body that has lodged in the cornea. Any rust in the tissue around the foreign body must also be removed.

241. c) Botulinum toxin is used to relieve chronic lid twitching, or blepharospasm. It also is used in some cases of nonaccommodative strabismus.

242. b) Removal of an eyelash is called epilation. *Trichiasis* is the term for the condition where the lashes grow back toward the eye.

243. c) A laser iridotomy is a procedure in which a hole is punched into the iris so that aqueous can still exit the eye, even if the angle is occluded.

244. a) A cloudy posterior capsule is cleared in minutes using a laser to blast away the glazed-over center of the capsule, restoring vision. This is known as a capsulotomy.

245. c) Wet macular degeneration is treated by injecting anti-VEGF agents, or antivascular endothelial growth factor, which discourages the growth of new, abnormal blood vessels, into the vitreal cavity of the eye.

246. b) The symptoms of infection are redness, swelling, and pain. Itching and scaling are usually associated with allergy; mild tenderness and oozing are probably normal, as are bruising and swelling.

247. c) Not all sutures are absorbable; some need to be removed.

248. a) If the compress is too hot, the patient's skin may be burned. Answers b through d are dangerous or unnecessary.

249. d) Heat increases circulation in the area, promoting healing.

250. c) Cold is used to minimize or reduce bruising and swelling.

251. b) Lid scrubs and antibiotic ointment are commonly used to treat blepharitis. Steroids are usually avoided.

252. a) Blepharitis is treated, at least in part, by cleansing ("scrubbing") the lid margin daily to prevent build-up of oil and debris. This technique may also be termed "lid hygiene."

253. b) I often tell patients that dry eye is rather like high blood pressure. You cannot get rid of it, but you can control it. Dry eye is not, of course, contagious.

254. d) Some eye care practitioners advocate external nasolacrimal duct massage. The massage is started in the nasal canthus and worked downward toward the fold in the nose.

255. a) Treating a family member with another's medication is not wise. For one thing, there are many types of conjunctivitis, and treatment varies according to the cause.

256. a) Once a corneal foreign body is removed, an abrasion remains. The patient needs to be told this, and that the eye might still feel as though there is something in it. Such abrasions usually heal within 24 hours. Topical anesthetics ("numbing drops") are never prescribed for home use, as repeated instillation interferes with the healing process.

257. c) A corneal abrasion causes a foreign body sensation because every time the patient blinks, the lids rub over the raw spot. There is commonly an abrasion at the site where a foreign body was removed.

258. c) Following cataract surgery, the patient is told to avoid heavy lifting and straining, as this can cause a sudden rise in intraocular pressure.[16] Bright light may be uncomfortable, but it will not damage anything. The patient is generally told to sleep on the side opposite the operated eye, not facedown. Rubbing the eye is also to be avoided.

259. a) The operative eye is usually patched, and a shield is applied. IOP-lowering medications will be topical, not oral. Topical anesthetics ("numbing drops") are never prescribed for home use, as repeated instillation interferes with the healing process. And, did you know that there *is* such a thing as a home IOP monitor?[17] Postoperative cataract patients, however, are not sent home with these.

260. d) Many patients hear that cataracts "can grow back." By the time a post-cataract surgery patient is dismissed (generally at 4 to 6 weeks), she should understand that the membrane behind the implant can cloud over, causing the same symptoms as a cataract. The patient should then contact the office, as this problem is usually dealt with easily and in minutes by a YAG laser capsulotomy.

261. b) The cataract has the effect of causing vision to become dingy and yellowed. When the cataract is removed, objects are restored to their normal color. However, the patient often perceives this as being "bluer" than his or her preoperative vision.

[16]Available at: www.ncbi.nlm.nih.gov/pubmed/20333527. Accessed 7/17/11.

[17]Available at: http://emedicine.medscape.com/article/1978274-overview#aw2aab6b2. Accessed 7/17/11.

262. b) A final postoperative examination, including refractometry (and probably IOP and dilated exam), is generally done 4 to 6 weeks after surgery.

263. c) In patching (occlusion) therapy for amblyopia, the strong eye is patched to force the weaker eye to work harder. The hope is that the visual pathway will then develop normally, with an increase in visual acuity in the "lazy" amblyopic eye.

264. b) "Pencil push-ups" (convergence training) involves training the eyes to increase and hold convergence.

265. b) The Amsler grid is held at normal reading range, about 16 inches.

266. c) Did you get this one? Or did answer b fool you? Of course, the real COA® exam will not be intentionally tricky, but the point here is that the first time the patient looks at the grid, there may be wavy lines, distortions, and areas missing. The thing the patient is told to look for is any *changes* from the *initial* viewing. And yes, there *is* a dot in the middle of the grid!

267. b) The purpose of a pressure patch is to keep the eye closed.

268. b) You may have to shave some facial hair to get the tape to stick to the cheek. If the tape is not tight enough to keep the eye shut, pressure patching is useless.

269. c) Angle the tape away from the lips. There is no need to extend tape beyond the hairline; it will not stick.

270. b) Alcohol will cleanse away skin oil so the tape will stick.

271. a) Answers b through d sound good, but answer a is the best. If the cornea heals smoothly, there is less chance of developing recurrent erosion, where the eyelid pulls off the new cells.

272. d) If the pressure patch is put on correctly, it probably will be a little uncomfortable.

273. d) The role of the patch is to accomplish answers a through c.

274. b) The shield edges should rest on the orbital bones to prevent pressure on the globe.

275. c) The shield provides a rigid barrier to protect the eye.

276. c) Always ask a disabled person if he or she wants help.

277. b) Wheelchair transfers are easiest by removing the armrest of both chairs, enabling the patient to slide over. This avoids lifting.

278. c) Proper sighted-guide technique requires the guide to walk slightly ahead of the patient, with the patient's hand on your arm. Never push the patient. Some blind patients are not skilled with a cane. For some, the wheelchair option would be degrading.

279. b) A blind person is not deaf! The other answers are good rules of etiquette.

280. c) Never touch a guide dog! You need not touch the patient, either. Just tell him where you are going and lead the way.

281. b) It is not necessarily how many patients you see, but how you handle the ones you do see. Chart preview involves looking over a patient's record prior to his or her visit to be sure you are aware of the reason for the visit, any special patient concerns (eg, allergy to latex, claustrophobia), and any notes the physician left "for next time" (eg, dilation, pachymetry, A-scan). Template-style exam forms can expedite the exam and help ensure that you do not forget something. A phone call protocol should help minimize intra-exam interruptions as well.[18]

282. c) Triage is a cursory evaluation of a patient's needs and then categorizing them as emergent, urgent, or routine.

283. a) In the case of multiple patients, triage helps determine whose injuries or illness is most urgent. The more urgent the case, the sooner the patient is slated to be seen.

[18]Backer LA. Strategies for better patient flow and cycle time. *Fam Pract Manag.* 2002;9(6):45-50. Available at: www.aafp.org/fpm/2002/0600/p45.html. Accessed 10/16/2010.

284. a) Of the conditions listed, the corneal transplant rejection is the least emergent, although it probably warrants a same-day appointment. The situations in b, c, and d are highly emergent. Sudden, painless loss of vision in one eye (symptoms of central retinal artery occlusion) might be reversed with rapid treatment. Chemical burns should be irrigated immediately. Because a penetrating injury involves exposure of the ocular tissues to contamination, it is also a high-level emergency.

285. c) Urgent cases are seen within 24 to 48 hours.

286. b) See answer 284. Sudden onset of diplopia in an adult is usually considered urgent, not emergent.

287. c) The construction worker should be seen immediately. The 42-year-old probably has presbyopia, the 4-year-old has been waiting for 4 years, and the −1.00 myope can cope to some degree until being seen.

288. c) The most emergent of the conditions listed is the sudden, painless loss of vision in one eye. These can be the symptoms of central retinal artery occlusion, and there is a small window of opportunity during which treatment must start if there is to be any hope of regaining vision.

289. c) A foreign body is usually seen the same day (emergent/urgent). Conditions a, b, and d can be seen in a next available slot.

290. a) When a patient calls in with vision loss, you must first rule out the most emergent situation that can cause this: central retinal artery occlusion (CRAO). A symptom of CRAO is sudden, painless loss of vision in one eye.

291. c) Vision loss in angle-closure glaucoma can be permanent. Immediate treatment is imperative. Of course, iritis should be treated as soon as possible, but is not quite as crucial as a glaucoma attack.

292. b) Triage is the process of deciding how serious a condition is, and, thus, how soon it needs treatment. Generally speaking, a painful red eye is higher on the triage scale than a non-painful red eye. Double vision is not associated with redness. Usually, a person who knows he has glaucoma has the open-angle type.

293. c) A subconjunctival hemorrhage is red, but generally painless. Viral conjunctivitis can be particularly painful.

294. c) Open-angle glaucoma, in and of itself, does not cause an eye to be red. The other answers are classically accompanied by a red eye.

295. d) An attack of angle-closure glaucoma can include signs and symptoms as follows: redness, hazy cornea, mid-dilated pupil (not miotic), pain, vomiting, nausea, headache, eye ache, halos around lights, and decreased vision.

296. c) Answers a, b, and d all act to dilate the pupil, creating a potential for the iris to block the angle. A sudden bright light would cause the pupil to constrict, which is not associated with angle closure.

297. a) When angle-closure glaucoma occurs, the iris is pushing against the lens and angle. Aqueous production continues, but the fluid is not drained out, causing a rise in IOP. If the pupil were miotic, as suggested in answer c, the iris would be pulled *away* from the angle, increasing drainage.

298. a) The eye of a high hyperope is short, meaning there is not much room for the angle. This increases the chances of iris obstruction. It is also the reason that we check angle depth prior to dilation, to make sure the angle is not going to occlude during mydriasis or cycloplegia.

299. b) Corneal edema has a prismatic effect, breaking light into its component colors and thus creating halos around lights. Pressure build-up during an attack causes a breakdown in the pumping function of the corneal endothelium, and edema results.

300. a) The pupil in angle-closure glaucoma is mid-dilated. Miotics are used in an effort to constrict the pupil and pull the iris out of the angle. Mydriatics would keep the pupil dilated. Antibiotics would have no effect, nor would corticosteroids. Steroids can actually elevate the pressure when used for a period of time.

301. a) In iritis, the affected pupil is often smaller.

302. c) Flashes and floaters can be symptoms of a retinal detachment and should be seen on an urgent basis.

303. b) In addition to flashes and floaters, a retinal detachment can cause the appearance of a curtain or veil over part of the vision.

304. c) The classic symptoms of posterior vitreous detachment are floaters and flashes. These are also the symptoms of retinal detachment, however, and must be evaluated, usually the same day.

305. c) It is always better to overestimate the potential of an injury to threaten vision. Certain injuries should not be irrigated or pressure patched. A patient's ability to wait must be determined on a case-by-case basis. (The key to this question is the word *any*.)

306. d) The first step in a chemical splash to the eye is irrigation.

307. d) Ammonia is a base. Bases bind to lipids (fats) in the tissues and, thus, penetrate deeply. Acids cause surface burns, but do not adhere to the tissue or penetrate.

308. d) It is important to know how a foreign body got into the eye. If the foreign material was at a high velocity, the eye might have been penetrated.

309. b) A penetrating injury may have surprisingly little immediate effect on the patient's vision, the appearance of the eye, or the amount of pain. Looking inside the eye with the ophthalmoscope gives the best idea of the injury's severity.

310. d) If the globe is perforated, you do not want to put pressure on it or apply any drops, solutions, or ointments. Cover lightly with a sterile dressing and tell the doctor at once.

311. c) A foreign body under high velocity could have penetrated the eye (see answers 284 and 308 to 310). The physician is the one who would decide to give oral pain medication, not the assistant.

312. b) A rust ring forms around a metallic corneal foreign body in 6 to 8 hours. The rust stains the corneal tissue and must be removed with a drill or burr, or a foreign body spud.

313. b) A lunar eclipse does not emit significant ultraviolet light to damage the eye and may be viewed directly. A solar eclipse, however, should never be directly viewed.

314. a) A patient who has had a blow to the eye should be seen as soon as possible, before swelling makes it impossible to examine the globe. A dilated exam will be needed to determine if there is a detachment or any other retinal complications.

315. d) Trachoma is an infection, not an injury.

316. a) A blowout fracture involves the bones in the floor of the orbit, which actually separate the orbit from the sinuses.

317. c) A hyphema is blood in the AC.

318. c) Never tell a patient that everything will be all right. If the outcome is not satisfactory (a distinct possibility), the patient can claim that you guaranteed a successful outcome and sue your boss, and you, too.

319. c) OSHA is part of the United States Department of Labor. It was created in 1970 for the purpose of ensuring safety (including health safety) in the workplace.

320. a) OSHA is concerned with employee safety. The poster tells employees about their rights and how to report problems.

321. c) The Exposure Control Plan is part of OSHA's requirement for employee safety in the workplace where there is potential exposure to bloodborne pathogens.

322. a) MSDS sheets give information regarding a substance's ingredients, flash-point, storage requirements, handling requirements, and first aid for exposures. Your office should maintain a readily accessible file that contains MSDSs for materials used by employees in the performance of their jobs.

323. c) The practice's Standard Operating Procedures is a manual that usually includes job descriptions, provisions for training and evaluation of employees, office practices (vacation and sick-leave), code of conduct, and handling of personnel issues.

324. c) An Incident Report (ie, for non-employees) would be used to document any accidents on the property.

325. b) Statements regarding how a visual or other impairment has affected a person's quality of life evaluate the presence of a disability. The disability is "what's wrong," backed up by medical testing. The impairment is the effect that the disability has on the patient's life (eg, professionally, socially, and personally).

326. c) An assessment of a person's impairment includes medical data: the results of testing as well as a report of ocular disease.

327. b) See questions 325 and 326. The awarding of services and funds to disabled persons relies on determining eligibility.

328. a) Errors may mean that the patient is denied services for which he or she is eligible. Such a mistake can make a profound difference in a person's quality of life, or at the very least further delay such assistance.

329. b) Agencies generally want to know uncorrected and best-corrected acuity. (Vision with current correction might potentially be improved with a new refraction.)

330. c) Surprisingly enough, a person who has 20/20 vision and normal fields can still be disabled if one or both eyes is totally paralyzed (ophthalmoplegia) and/or there is severe diplopia. (*Note:* This explanation is simplified, but the point is to be aware that there is more to visual disability and impairment than acuity and fields.)

331. d) The minimum visual requirements for such a license would include visual acuity (usually uncorrected and best-corrected) visual fields, and color vision.

332. c) Visual acuity is generally tested at the licensing bureau. If the patient does not pass this test, then he is referred for a more formal eye exam.

333. a) Examples of such restrictions might include daytime driving only, must wear correction when driving, may not drive on interstates, or driving only within a specific radius from home.

334. c) Workers' Compensation is insurance paid by an employer to be used in the event that an employee is injured on the job or incurs a job-related illness.

335. a) As with any type of insurance claim, Workers' Compensation wants to know what type of disability the employee has suffered and how long that disability is likely to last, along with how soon (if ever) the employee can return to work, and whether or not rehabilitation will be required.

336. c) Workers' Compensation covers only on-the-job injuries.
337. a) Medicare is the federal insurance program that helps pay the cost of medical care for citizens 65 and older, as well as those with certain disabilities.
338. b) Medicare does not cover the cost of a refraction, nor does it usually cover certain special testing (eg, corneal topography or endothelial cell count), contact lenses, or fittings.
339. b) The Assignment of Benefits form allows the practice to file the patient's Medicare and other insurance and allows the practice to release pertinent medical information in pursuit of these payments.
340. c) Medicaid is supported by both state and federal funding (Medicare is federal only) and is designed to provide health insurance to the indigent of any age.
341. c) HIPAA was made law in 1996. One of its main features is the protection of personal health information. It also establishes regulations regarding electronic medical records.
342. a) A release of information form, as well as information regarding privacy, are standard office forms revolving around the HIPAA standards.
343. a) Vital signs include body temperature, blood pressure, pulse rate, and respiration rate.
344. c) Normal body temperature is 98.6° F, with some slight variation found between individuals.
345. a) It is recommended to wait 20 to 30 minutes before taking an oral temperature if the patient has had something warm or cold to drink or has been smoking.[19]
346. d) The mercury must be shaken down into the thermometer bulb before use.
347. c) An oral thermometer is placed under the tongue.
348. b) Leave the thermometer in the patient's mouth for 3 to 4 minutes before reading.
349. a) A fever *generally* indicates that an infection exists somewhere in the body.
350. c) Apply only gentle pressure, using the first two fingers. (The thumb has a pulse of its own, which might confuse things!) Heavy pressure might obstruct blood flow, so you will not feel a pulse.
351. d) The usual place to take a pulse is in the soft tissue of the wrist, above the thumb. There are pulses in other places, however, such as the neck, in the bend of the elbow, behind the knee, and next to the ankle.
352. b) Heart rate is measured as beats per minute.
353. b) The average human heart rate is 70 to 80 beats per minute.
354. d) In addition to the basic count of the heart rate, the pulse is also evaluated for patterns such as skipping or changes in speed and strength.
355. b) The average human respiration rate is 12 to 20. Eighteen is given as an average.[20]
356. a) Respirations are usually counted "on the sly"; after checking pulse, leave the fingers in place but count breaths instead of heart beats. If the patient knows you are counting breaths, it is difficult to breathe normally.
357. c) Are the breaths shallow or deep? Easy or labored? Quiet or is there some sort of noise such as wheezing or crackling? Is breathing even or irregular?
358. c) The lower of the 2 numbers in a BP reading is the diastolic pressure.

[19]Available at: http://firstaid.webmd.com/body-temperature?page=2. Accessed 7/16/11.

[20]DuBois L. *Clinical Skills for the Ophthalmic Examination: Basic Procedures*. 2nd ed. Thorofare, NJ: SLACK Incorporated; 2005.

359. c) Any exertion can alter the patient's "normal" BP reading, so wait several minutes before taking the reading. There is no need to have the patient lie down. After you have announced that you will be putting drops into his or her eyes is also not a good time to take the BP, as the patient's apprehension may cause a false elevation in the reading!

360. a) A sphygmomanometer is used to evaluate BP.

361. d) The cuff is placed on the patient's arm above the elbow. Shirt sleeves should be loosely pushed up above the BP cuff.

362. a) The stethoscope is held on the inside of the elbow, just below the cuff.

363. c) The bulb is used to pump air into the cuff. At some point, the heartbeat will be audible in the stethoscope. Continue to pump until the heartbeat disappears again.

364. a) Turn the screw on the bulb until the air just starts to escape, but not so fast that the cuff deflates rapidly.

365. b) You must listen for the heartbeat to start and note the reading on the gauge when this occurs.

366. d) The point where the heartbeat fades is when you note the second of the 2 readings that make up the BP measurement.

367. c) BP can actually vary from one arm to the other; patients can often tell you which arm is usually used.

368. a) Consistent readings somewhat lower than 120/80 are considered normal blood pressure.[21]

369. a) The patient scenarios in answers b, c, and d especially warrant a BP reading. If the cataract patient is about to have surgery, the BP would be needed then as well, but that was not part of the given answers.

370. c) Prehypertension is defined by the American Heart Association as consistent readings of 120 to 139 systolic and 80 to 89 diastolic.

371. a) People with heart problems are most at risk for cardiopulmonary arrest. (*Note:* The American Heart Association and the International Liaison Committee on Resuscitation periodically update and change the CPR guidelines. In 2000, it was decided that laypeople would no longer be taught to check for a pulse. Instead, after giving two rescue breaths, the layperson is to evaluate for "signs of circulation." These signs include movement, coughing, and breathing. The rationale behind this recommendation is that a victim in cardiac arrest will lose his or her pulse within 10 seconds of the attack. However, people who take CPR for health care personnel are still taught to check pulse. Other changes include activating 911 immediately [ie, after determining that the patient is unresponsive and prior to positioning and establishing an airway] if the victim is an adult. The exceptions are if the adult is a victim of drowning [submersion], trauma, or drug intoxication. In these cases, CPR is given for 1 full minute before 911 is activated. The child and infant victim are also given 1 minute of CPR before calling 911. The compression rate is 100 per minute for adult, child, and infant victims. Compression-to-breath ratio is 15:2 for adults, whether there is one rescuer or two. The ratio for children and infants is 5:1. CPR for health care personnel also includes instruction on using an automated electronic defibrillator [AED].)

372. b) Brain death occurs approximately 4 to 6 minutes after pulse and breathing cease.

---

[21]Classifications for hypertension are taken from the American Heart Association. Available at: www.heart.org/HEARTORG/Conditions/HighBloodPressure/AboutHighBloodPressure/Understanding-Blood-Pressure-Readings_UCM_301764_Article.jsp. Accessed 8/27/11.

373. b) The victim's own tongue is the most common obstruction to the airway. This occurs after the victim loses consciousness. (It is common for a person to choke on food, but not on his own tongue.)

374. b) Approximately 1 in 10 victims will survive cardiac arrest if chest compressions or CPR is performed.

375. b) The first step is always to assess responsiveness. The classic method is to gently shake or tap the victim's arm and shout "Are you okay? Are you okay?" (Consider the alternatives: 911 arrives, and the "victim" is only sleeping; you attempt to "position" a "victim," and he or she awakens, thinking he or she is being attacked!)

376. d) When performing compressions on an adult, the rescuer is kneeling at the victim's side, hands interlaced and placed on the victim's chest (two finger-widths above the xiphoid process), elbows straight. The rescuer's shoulders, elbows, and hands should be in line. Compressions originate from the shoulders and arms, not by bending the elbows or rocking the body.

377. b) In order for the compressions in an adult to be effective, they must be at least 2 inches deep.

378. c) In 2010, a report was released that found hands-only (or compression-only) CPR to be about as effective as CPR that includes emergency breathing on adults.[22] This is good news because bystanders are increasingly reluctant to perform mouth-to-mouth breathing on a person whose medical background (especially HIV status) is unknown. Rescue breathing is still indicated in children and infants.[23]

379. c) The compression rate in hands-only CPR is the same as in CPR that includes rescue breathing: 100 per minute. (Someone told me that if you pump to the tune of the song "Stayin' Alive" from the movie *Saturday Night Fever*, that you will be delivering 100 compressions per minute.)

380. a) While many automated external defibrillators actually tell you what to do step-by-step, they are to be used only by trained personnel. There are now pediatric-sized pads, and some automated external defibrillators have a switch to deliver a pediatric-appropriate shock.

[22]Svensson L, Bohm K, Castren M, et al. Compression-only CPR or standard CPR in out-of-hospital cardiac arrest. *N Engl J Med.* 2010;363:434-442. Available at: www.nejm.org/doi/pdf/10.1056/NEJMoa0908991. Accessed 6/25/11.

[23]Stein HA, Stein RM, Freeman MI. *The Ophthalmic Assistant.* 8th ed. Philadelphia, PA: Elsevier Mosby; 2006.

Chapter 13

Ophthalmic Imaging

Ledford JK.
*Certified Ophthalmic Assistant: Exam
Review Manual, Third Edition* (pp. 215-230).
© 2012 Taylor & Francis Group.

Slit-Lamp/Anterior Segment Photography

1. **Match the types of slit-lamp illumination to its definition:**

Term	Definition
diffuse	a) highlighting an area of interest by illuminating the structure behind it
direct	b) illumination source is shined at an oblique angle across the surface
indirect	of a structure
retroillumination	c) a softer lighting that evenly illuminates the entire subject without
tangential	highlighting any particular part

   d) illumination source is shined on another structure than the one of
   interest

   e) the illumination source is shined directly on the area of interest

2. **All of the following would be well documented using slit-lamp photography *except*:**
   a) pterygium
   b) hypertropia
   c) corneal scar
   d) iris lesion

3. **When performing slit-lamp photography, a photograph of the eye using low magnification and diffuse lighting is recommended to:**
   a) judge the patient's tolerance to the flash
   b) judge the corneal reflection
   c) provide identification
   d) provide orientation

4. **By convention as well as for ease of use, the illuminator in slit-lamp photography is usually positioned:**
   a) nasally
   b) temporally
   c) temporally for OD and nasally for OS
   d) nasally for OD and temporally for OS

5. **You are taking a slit-lamp photo of an iris lesion that may be melanoma. The illumination technique of choice is:**
   a) diffuse
   b) direct
   c) indirect
   d) retroillumination

6. **You are taking a slit-lamp photo of a cortical cataract. The illumination technique of choice is:**
   a) diffuse
   b) direct
   c) indirect
   d) retroillumination

7. **The technique for taking photographs of the angle structures of the anterior eye is:**
   a) goniography
   b) trabeculography
   c) iridography
   d) pupillography

8. **The method used to take photographs of the endothelial layer of the cornea is:**
   a) specular photomicrography
   b) fluorescein angiography
   c) corneal topography
   d) retroluminar reflectography

Fundus Photography[1]

9. **Before taking the fundus photograph, it is important to do all of the following *except*:**
   a) check the patient's record to confirm the requested photographs
   b) enter patient information into a log manual or camera imprint system
   c) study any previous fundus photos that the patient has had
   d) make sure that the patient has had a visual field test

10. **The most important thing to do before using any fundus camera each day should be:**
    a) confirm the diopter compensator is at the "+" setting
    b) ensure all patients are dilated with homatropine
    c) check to see that the eye piece is correctly set
    d) clean the camera lens whether or not it is dirty

11. **Setting the fundus camera eye piece should be done:**
    a) with one eye shut, in dim light or darkness
    b) with both eyes open, in dim light or darkness
    c) with both eyes open in a normally lit room
    d) with one eye shut in a normally lit room

12. **When setting the ocular of the fundus camera system, one must:**
    a) remove one's own correction
    b) turn the ocular to the maximum plus position, then rotate down
    c) turn the ocular to the maximum plus position, then rotate up
    d) turn the ocular to the maximum minus position, then rotate up

13. **If you continue to turn the fundus camera ocular past the first point of clarity:**
    a) the reticle will become sharper yet
    b) you can compensate for the patient's refractive error
    c) you may induce your own accommodation
    d) the resulting photograph will be sharper

[1]Many fundus cameras no longer have an eye piece, but rather a viewing screen. Questions 10 through 13 are included here for the sake of completeness, as a number of offices still employ analog (non-digital) cameras.

14. **Proper pupil dilation to facilitate fundus photography requires:**
    a) any dilation is acceptable
    b) dilation is not necessary
    c) a minimum pupil size of 4 to 5 mm
    d) a minimum pupil size of 8 mm

15. **Inadequate dilation results in photographs with:**
    a) half of the frame unexposed
    b) a general blur
    c) a gray, fuzzy quadrant
    d) a grainy appearance

16. **In fundus photography, high corneal astigmatism can be compensated for by:**
    a) use of the correction device in the fundus camera
    b) placing the dioptric correction dial on "+" for plus cylinder
    c) placing the dioptric correction dial on "−" for minus cylinder
    d) having the patient wear a toric contact lens during photography

17. **In order to image eyes with high refractive errors, it is best to:**
    a) place a contact lens on the patient's eye to compensate
    b) reset the eye piece reticle to compensate
    c) set the diopter compensation device built into the camera
    d) remember that eyes with high refractive errors cannot be photographed

18. **To take a photo of the external eye with the fundus camera (eg, to document corneal edema that interferes with a clear view of the fundus):**
    a) change the diopter setting to "−"
    b) change the diopter setting to "+"
    c) have the patient sit back from the camera
    d) a slit-lamp camera must be used

19. **Gross focusing with the fundus camera is generally accomplished by:**
    a) turning the eye piece until the subject is clear
    b) moving the joystick
    c) having the patient lean forward or back
    d) changing the magnification setting

20. **Focusing the fundus camera can be simplified by:**
    a) starting with the camera all the way back, then moving it forward
    b) starting with the camera all the way forward, then moving it back
    c) focusing the donut on the patient's closed lid before composing the photograph
    d) positioning the fixation light directly in front of the camera lens

21. **To allow scanning of the patient's retina without moving the base of the camera mount:**
    a) move the fixation light and ask the patient to follow it
    b) use the joystick
    c) adjust the chin cup
    d) swing the camera on its pivot

22. **When correctly positioned, the orange-yellow background of the fundus should be:**
     a) at an even color saturation across the viewing field
     b) darker in the periphery of the viewing field
     c) lighter in the periphery of the viewing field
     d) unevenly saturated across the viewing field

23. **Once the fundal image is correctly positioned and focused:**
     a) fire the camera
     b) ask the patient to blink, then fire the camera
     c) have the patient sit back and rest a moment
     d) take repeated photographs quickly, warning the patient not to blink

24. **You are attempting to take fundus photographs and see a blue-gray halo around the subject. To correct this, you should:**
     a) move the camera closer
     b) move the camera further back
     c) reduce illumination
     d) increase illumination

25. **You are attempting to take fundus photographs and notice a whitish haze in the center of the subject. This may mean that:**
     a) the patient is highly myopic
     b) the patient is highly hyperopic
     c) the patient has his or her eye closed
     d) the camera has drifted to one side

26. **You are centering on the macula when a light yellow crescent appears in the upper left of the viewing field. This is caused by:**
     a) the illumination being set too high
     b) a reflection off of a cataract
     c) the pathology in the fundus
     d) a reflection off of the edge of the pupil

27. **In the scenario above, you should:**
     a) reduce illumination
     b) move the camera slightly down and to the right
     c) move the camera slightly up and to the left
     d) use the dioptric compensation device

28. **Periodic photographs to monitor the progress of a disease might be needed in all of the following *except*:**
     a) hypertensive retinopathy
     b) aphakia
     c) diabetic retinopathy
     d) glaucoma

29. **The primary area of interest in the fundus photo of a glaucoma patient is:**
     a) the optic disc
     b) the macula
     c) the retinal vessels
     d) the choroid

30. **Fundus photos of a patient with macular degeneration would focus on the:**
    a) optic disc
    b) retinal periphery
    c) fovea
    d) superior field

31. **In a standard diabetic survey, a series of photos are taken that include:**
    a) five overlapping fields of view
    b) four fields of view to document every quadrant
    c) seven overlapping fields of view
    d) two photos: one centered on the disc and one centered on the macula

32. **The technique that uses fundus photography to evaluate retinal blood flow is:**
    a) specular microscopy
    b) cyanine green evaluation
    c) fluorescein angiography
    d) optical coherence tomography (OCT)

33. **In fundus photography, the red-free filter is used to evaluate:**
    a) nerve fibers
    b) for intraocular copper
    c) blood vessels
    d) pseudomembranes

34. **If the patient is to have fundus photos of both eyes:**
    a) go from the right eye to the left eye without stopping to avoid patient fatigue
    b) wait 30 minutes between photographing the right and left eyes
    c) allow the patient to rest in between eyes until the fixation light can be seen
    d) use stronger dilating drops on the second eye

35. **Poor detail on a fundus photograph can be caused by all of the following *except*:**
    a) improper focusing
    b) hazy media
    c) retinal pathology
    d) failing to set the eye piece accurately

External Photography

36. **The camera most often used in external ophthalmic photography is a(n):**
    a) instant still camera
    b) video camera
    c) twin-lens reflex 35 mm camera
    d) single-lens reflex 35 mm camera

37.   **A key feature of a camera to be used in ophthalmology for external photography is that it can:**
       a) be focused at about 4 inches from the subject
       b) provide enough magnification to image a single eye
       c) accept a micro lens
       d) be coupled to a slit lamp

38.   **Regarding lighting for external ophthalmic photography:**
       a) a ring light is preferred
       b) professional portrait lighting is preferred
       c) an adjustable "point source" flash is preferred
       d) no special lighting is needed

39.   **All of the following are important when illuminating the subject for external photography *except*:**
       a) avoid shadows falling on the area of interest
       b) provide an even illumination across the area of interest
       c) direct the illumination from the nasal aspect
       d) avoid large flash reflection from the cornea

40.   **External photographs taken prior to strabismus surgery will include (at a minimum):**
       a) upgaze, downgaze, and primary positions
       b) a head shot, primary position, and angle of deviation
       c) nine positions of gaze plus a head shot
       d) right gaze, left gaze, primary position, plus a head shot

41.   **The patient has given verbal agreement to be a model in "before and after" photographs of a blepharoplasty. In order to legally display the full head shots, you will need:**
       a) a standardized background
       b) to just eliminate the patient's name from the display
       c) enlargements of the photos
       d) the patient's written consent

42.   **External photographs of a patient might be required for insurance purposes in which of the following types of ocular surgery?**
       a) emergency repair of lid laceration
       b) upper blepharoplasty
       c) lacrimal intubation
       d) cataract extraction

Diagnostic/Standardized A-Scan[2]

43.   **Ultrasound is a valuable diagnostic tool because it:**
       a) is safe because there is no radiation exposure
       b) can be performed in the office
       c) can be repeated frequently to follow the patient's condition
       d) all of the above

[2]My JCAHPO® VOW says this is "understanding and use of the probe and readings." For axial length A-scan, see Chapter 16.

44. **Ultrasound employs the use of:**
    a) light rays
    b) sound waves
    c) laser rays
    d) electromagnetic waves

45. **The term *A-scan* refers to a:**
    a) one-dimensional amplitude scan
    b) two-dimensional brightness scan
    c) three-dimensional scan
    d) none of the above

46. **The "A" in A-scan stands for:**
    a) axial
    b) amplitude
    c) anti-orbital
    d) audio

47. **The term *biometry* could refer to measuring the:**
    a) axial length of the eye
    b) thickness of an extraocular muscle
    c) height of a tumor
    d) all of the above

48. **In standardized or diagnostic A-scan, the purpose of the scan is generally to:**
    a) calculate intraocular lens power
    b) calculate anterior chamber depth
    c) evaluate abnormalities
    d) evaluate the aqueous

49. **In standardized/diagnostic A-scans, the probe tip is placed:**
    a) perpendicular to the visual axis
    b) relative to the area of interest
    c) so sound waves will fall on the macula
    d) so sound waves will fall on the optic nerve

50. **Gain is:**
    a) whether or not an accurate reading has been obtained
    b) the strength of the sound waves emitted by the probe
    c) the false lengthening of an A-scan because of the tear film bridge
    d) the sensitivity, or electronic amplification, of the sound wave signal

51. **Extra echoes between the anterior and posterior lens spikes indicate:**
    a) a poor A-scan that should be repeated
    b) a malfunctioning probe
    c) a dense cataract
    d) none of the above

52. **Label the parts of an A-scan echo (Figure 13-1):**

peak	width	baseline	descending limb or falling edge

ascending limb or leading edge

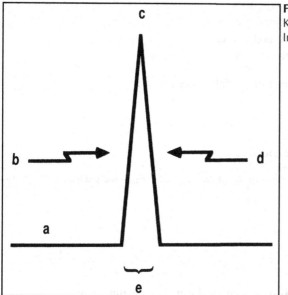

Figure 13-1. Reprinted with permission of Kendall CJ. *Ophthalmic Echography.* SLACK Incorporated; 1990.

53. **Which biometric measurements may be performed with the standardized A-scan?**
a) axial eye length
b) optic nerve thickness
c) tumor height
d) all of the above

54. **Unwanted echoes that do not represent ocular structures are known as:**
a) pseudo-echoes
b) artifacts
c) reverberations
d) echoes of confusion

55. **Label the following structures on the A-scan pictured below (Figure 13-2):**

posterior lens	orbital fat	cornea
retina	anterior lens	sclera

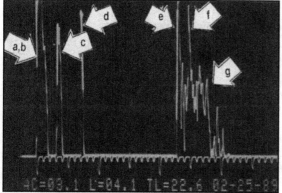

Figure 13-2. Reprinted with permission of Kendall CJ. *Ophthalmic Echography.* SLACK Incorporated; 1990.

Corneal Topography[3]

56. **All of the following are true regarding computerized corneal topography *except*:**
    a) it evaluates four points of the corneal apex
    b) it measures the curvature of the anterior cornea
    c) it displays the results with a color-coded "map"
    d) it analyzes light reflected from the cornea

57. **Corneal topography is useful in each of the following *except*:**
    a) fitting rigid contact lenses
    b) monitoring keratoconus
    c) monitoring endothelial drop-out
    d) preoperative refractive surgery evaluation

58. **"Cold" colors (blues and greens) on a corneal topography map indicate which of the following?**
    a) a flatter area
    b) a steeper area
    c) an area of irregularity
    d) the apex of a cone

59. **The common pattern of astigmatism on a corneal topography map is a:**
    a) ring
    b) tear-drop shape
    c) bow-tie shape
    d) pie wedge shape

60. **Potential candidates for refractive surgery who currently wear contact lenses:**
    a) may have to leave the lenses out and have repeat corneal topography
    b) do not need repeat topography if they are wearing soft lenses
    c) should have corneal topography performed while wearing the contact lenses
    d) should use rewetting drops frequently prior to topography

61. **The corneal topography map most commonly used is the:**
    a) Placido ring map
    b) keratometry map
    c) refractive map
    d) axial map

62. **Corneal topography is useful in each of the following *except*:**
    a) evaluation of corneal sensitivity
    b) evaluation of corneal warpage
    c) evaluation of high astigmatism
    d) determination of the incision site for cataract surgery

[3]Also known as *photokeratoscopy* or *videokeratography*.

63. **Which of the following would you expect to see on the corneal topography of a patient who has had laser refractive surgery for myopia?**
a) new bow-tie pattern
b) bluer center
c) bluer periphery
d) red/orange center

64. **Which of the following would provide the most useful information in order to evaluate a patient with keratoconus?**
a) keratometry
b) retinoscopy
c) corneal topography
d) corneal pachymetry

65. **A postoperative refractive surgery patient is complaining of glare and ghosting. Which of the following would provide the most helpful analysis?**
a) slit-lamp evaluation
b) endothelial cell count
c) corneal anesthesiometry
d) corneal topography

66. **All of the following can result in inadequate corneal topography _except_:**
a) pupil centered in the rings
b) poor fixation
c) eye not opened wide enough
d) long eyelashes

Scanning Laser Tests for Glaucoma/Retina[4]

67. **Match the following (some answers will be used more than once):**

Technology	Feature
Heidelberg Retinal Tomography (HRT)	a) confocal laser
Glaucoma Diagnosis (GDx)	b) can be adapted for corneal imaging
Optical Coherence Tomography (OCT)	c) uses polarized laser light
	d) uses "near infrared" light

68. **The purpose of using scanning laser devices to image and evaluate the retina is to:**
a) generate normative data
b) detect subtle changes in the retinal structure
c) detect subtle visual field defects
d) perform a cell count

69. **The topographical map acquired by scanning laser tests is generated by:**
a) a fundus image
b) scans at various tissue depths
c) comparing the scan to industry standards
d) comparing the scan to normative data

[4]Given that HRT, GDx, and OCT are very similar, I have not separated them except for the first question.

70. **Scanning laser tests (HRT, GDx, OCT) generate results that are:**
    a) color-coded to indicate thickness of tissues
    b) color-coded to show index of curvature
    c) shown in grayscale
    d) comparable to fluorescein angiography

71. **Which of the following would *not* generally be evaluated using scanning laser tests?**
    a) optic nerve cupping
    b) macular swelling
    c) vitreous detachment
    d) a glaucoma suspect

72. **When using scanning laser as an aid in diagnosing glaucoma, the area of interest is the:**
    a) fovea
    b) retinal nerve fiber layer
    c) optic radiations
    d) retinal pigment epithelium

73. **Scanning laser testing software evaluates the probability that:**
    a) the reading is accurate
    b) further changes will occur
    c) evaluated tissues are normal
    d) changes are caused by operator error

Explanatory Answers

1. Matching:
diffuse	c)
direct	e)
indirect	d)
retroillumination	a)
tangential	b)

2. b) Answers a, c, and d are all entities of the anterior segment that would be ideal to document via slit-lamp photography. If one wished to document hypertropia, an external photograph showing both eyes in relation to each other would be needed.

3. d) Before photographing pathology, take a photo of the entire eye using diffused lighting. (The diffuser is a foggy-looking filter that flips up over the slit-lamp's illumination source.) This helps orient the viewer when photos are examined later, as well as provides documentation of the eye's general appearance. Keep in mind, it is very difficult to identify a patient from a shot of a single eye!

4. b) Illumination for slit-lamp photos is usually directed from the temporal side. This convention helps orient the viewer, for one thing. For another, it avoids the physical limitations of the patient's nose when positioning the illuminator.

5. b) Direct illumination is used for opaque entities. (A subject that is more see-through would be better photographed using indirect illumination.)

6.   d) Using retroillumination, the light reflection from the retina (giving a bright orange/red background) will show any lens opacities in silhouette.

7.   a) A goniolens is used to view the angle structures of the eye at the slit lamp; it is placed directly on the anesthetized cornea. Photographs can then be taken of the angle structures.

8.   a) Specular photomicrography is a special technique used to capture images of the cornea's single-layer endothelium. The endothelium does not regenerate and is key in maintaining the cornea's clarity. The cells can get bumped and damaged during any kind of intraocular surgery, so evaluating the endothelium's health prior to surgery can be very important (especially if the patient has some type of corneal degeneration/dystrophy). The cells in the photo are examined for health as well as number (thus the term *cell count*).

9.   d) A visual field test is not a prerequisite for having fundus photos.

10.   c) Check the eye piece! (That is the first rule when using any piece of focusable eye equipment.) If the lens is not dirty, do not touch it. Homatropine is not necessary for dilation; usually, weaker drops are used. The dioptric compensator should be set on a patient-by-patient basis.

11.   b) The eye piece should be set in dim light (or in the dark) with both eyes open. On the fundus camera, this means that one eye is looking through the eye piece and the other eye is not. This is difficult to do, perhaps, but is the best method.

12.   b) The fundus camera ocular is set like any other eye piece. Turn it all the way to maximum plus. Looking through the eye piece, turn slowly toward the minus. Stop when the image is clear. Do not pass the clear spot in search of more clarity. It is not necessary to remove your correction. But, if you wear your glasses sometimes, and other times do not, you will have to reset the ocular.

13.   c) Going past the first point of image clarity adds minus to the ocular, which forces your eye to add plus (accommodate) to compensate. The resulting photographs will not be clear. You are not compensating for the patient's refractive error, but your own. During photography, if the image seems to go in and out of focus, yet the camera and patient are stationary, this probably is due to the accommodation of the photographer. Have the patient sit back, and check the focus of your ocular(s) again.

14.   c) Four to 5-mm dilation would be the minimum size for fundus photos (8 mm would be best, of course, but it is not the minimum). (*Note:* There are now "nonmydriatic" fundus cameras available that require 3.3 mm as the minimum size.)

15.   b) In addition to causing pupil cuts (not listed), inadequate dilation can cause a general blur on the photographs.

16.   a) Some fundus cameras have an astigmatic correction device that is used much like the dioptric compensation setting. The dioptric compensation device is for spherical refractive errors, not cylindrical.

17.   c) If the patient is highly hyperopic or myopic beyond the normal focusing ability of the camera, the diopter compensation device is used.

18.   b) If you set the dioptric compensation device to "+," it is possible to take a photo of the external eye using the fundus camera.

19.   b) Gross focusing can be accomplished by moving the joystick. On some fundus cameras, fine focusing is accomplished by turning a focusing knob on the camera. The subject is never focused by turning the oculars or by asking the patient to move. Changing the magnification setting will make the image larger, but not more focused.

20. c) Have the patient close both eyes while you align and focus the "donut" on the closed lid. This will put you very close to being in focus when the patient opens his or her eye. It is also more comfortable for the patient and allows you to avoid fumbling around with the camera, looking for the eye. If the fixation light is in front of the camera, it will get in the way of the photograph.

21. d) To scan the patient's retina, swing the camera on its pivot. If you move the joystick, you are moving the camera base. If the patient follows the fixation light or moves his or her chin, you are going to lose your field of view.

22. a) The orange-yellow background color of the fundus should be even across the viewing field.

23. b) Ask the patient to blink just before you fire the camera. This clears the tear film and increases the chances of the lids being open widely when you snap the picture.

24. a) A blue-gray halo around the subject indicates that you are too far back. Move the camera closer. If you are too close, you will see a whitish haze in the center of the subject.

25. d) See answer 24. The whitish central haze means you are too close.

26. d) The little yellow crescent is caused by a "pupil cut."

27. b) To compensate for a pupil cut, move the camera directly opposite from the crescent.

28. b) Fundus photography is used in all of the listed situations except aphakia. Aphakia is a condition, not a disease, and does not require photographic monitoring.

29. a) The optic disc is the primary object of interest in monitoring glaucoma patients.

30. c) The fovea is the center of the macula. (This was essentially an ocular anatomy question.)

31. c) The diabetic survey includes pictures of seven overlapping fields.

32. c) In fluorescein angiography, fluorescein dye is injected into a vein, and fundus photographs are taken in rapid succession as the dye fills the blood vessels.

33. c) The red-free filter (which is green) makes the blood vessels appear black, increasing contrast for evaluation.

34. c) Allow the patient to rest briefly between photos of both eyes. This allows him or her to recover from being "dazzled" before being required to see the fixation light.

35. c) Retinal pathology does not cause blurred photos in and of itself.

36. d) The single lens reflex (SLR) 35 mm camera remains the camera of choice for external ophthalmic photography. It can easily be equipped with accessory lenses to accommodate different focusing needs.

37. b) External ophthalmic photography is often taken on a 1:1 ratio, where the photograph is life-sized. A *macro* (not micro) lens is often used to enhance image quality when taking close-up photos.

38. c) The point source flash reduces the amount of reflection from the cornea. The flash is often mounted to the camera with a moveable bracket so the flash can be rotated into the most advantageous position for the area being imaged. If taking an external image of corneal pathology, the reflection from a ring light might totally obliterate the area of interest.

39. c) If the flash/illumination is coming from the nasal aspect, the nose and brows may cast a shadow across the area of interest.

40. c) External photography generally includes one head shot for orientation and documentation. A strabismus series would then involve shots showing just the two eyes in the nine positions of gaze. (External photos for ptosis or plastics would include a head shot, then both eyes in primary position, upgaze, and downgaze.)

41. d) If the patient can be identified from the picture, a written consent is needed before displaying or publishing the photo. Verbal consent is not enough. If only the eyes appear in the photo (ie, the patient cannot be identified), the consent is not needed.

42. b) Insurance companies will evaluate the photographs for evidence that the drooping upper lids are interfering with the patient's peripheral vision. They will probably also want to see two sets of visual fields: one with the lids in their natural, lower position and another with the lids taped up, simulating the patient's peripheral vision once the surgery is done.

43. d) Ultrasound uses sound waves, not radiation. The measurement is easily done in the office, and repeat readings can be taken to follow the patient's progress.

44. b) Sound waves are used in ultrasound.

45. a) The A-scan has a one-dimensional amplitude.

46. b) "A" stands for amplitude. (Anti-orbital is a bogus term.)

47. d) Biometry refers to the measurement of a living tissue, be it the length, thickness, or height. When talking about A-scans, it *usually* means axial length, so do not feel bad if you chose answer a!

48. c) Standardized/diagnostic A-scan is usually used in conjunction with B-scan. The purpose is to measure abnormal structures as well as evaluate for tissue type. (Certain tissue types have unique reflective spikes.)

49. b) Unlike axial length A-scans, in diagnostic A-scans, the probe is placed wherever appropriate in order to image the area of interest.

50. d) Gain is the sensitivity, or electronic amplification, of the sound wave signal.

51. c) A dense cataract can cause extra echoes between the anterior and posterior lens echoes.

52. Labeling, Figure 13-1:

peak	c)
width	e)
ascending limb or leading edge	b)
baseline	a)
descending limb or falling edge	d)

53. d) The A-scan is a versatile instrument that can be used to measure any of the items listed.

54. b) An artifact is an unwanted echo that is not due to any structure in the eye. Artifacts may be caused by air bubbles in the probe, pneumatic retinopexy (retinal detachment treatment that involves injecting air into the eye), and echoes bouncing off intraocular foreign bodies (including intraocular lenses).

55. Labeling, Figure 13-2

posterior lens	d)
orbital fat	g)
cornea a),	b)
retina	e)
anterior lens	c)
sclera	f)

56. a) Corneal topography evaluates some 6000 points across the entire corneal surface. Keratometry, on the other hand, measures only four points in the 3-mm central optic zone.

57. c) Corneal topography evaluates the cornea's external curvature, not the specific nature of the cornea's innermost endothelial layer. This would be evaluated using specular microscopy. The other uses are valid.

58. a) The "cooler" colors indicate flatter areas. By contrast, the "warmer" colors (red/orange) represent steeper areas. It is important to note that green may also be used to denote "normal." Some displays can be "normalized," which means that the green would represent the areas of "average" curvature specifically for that patient's eye.

59. c) The classic representation of astigmatism looks like a bow-tie of similarly hued colors different than the rest of the image.

60. a) The contact lens patient who wants refractive surgery may have to discontinue lens wear for days or weeks prior to surgery. Repeat corneal topography will be done at intervals until the scan shows that the patient's corneal curvature has stabilized and that corneal warpage is not present. This applies even to those who wear soft contact lenses.

61. d) The axial map is the most commonly used.

62. a) Corneal sensitivity is evaluated with an aesthesiometer, not topography.

63. b) The cornea's center is flattened in myopia, so one would expect to see a center with cooler colors. (Warm colors [red/orange] in the center would indicate steeper curvature, as in hyperopic correction.)

64. c) Corneal topography creates a map of the cornea's surface. The keratometer measures only a tiny portion of the cornea. Retinoscopy of a patient with keratoconus can be confusing and difficult. Pachymetry is useful (eg, to evaluate corneal thinning), but this is not the best answer.

65. d) Corneal topography can show the location of the ablation zone. If the pupil does not fall within the central portion of the zone, visual disturbances can occur.

66. a) The ideal alignment is achieved when the pupil is centered in the rings.

67. Matching:

HRT	a, b
GDx	a, c
OCT	b, d

68. b) The purpose behind the scanning abilities of the HRT, GDx, and OCT is to detect and monitor changes in the retinal structure, generally before other testing (eg, visual fields) can detect such changes. These devices have emerged as key in determining whether or not a patient has glaucoma and whether or not treatment needs to be initiated or changed.

69. b) The scanning laser devices generate topographical information by scanning tissues at different depths, much like an MRI or CT scan. While the scan may be compared to normative data, this does not generate the map itself.

70. a) The display/printout results of scanning laser devices are color-coded to indicate tissue thickness.

71. c) Scanning laser technology is ideal for evaluating the optic nerve, macula, and nerve fiber layer (for glaucoma). Vitreous detachment would not generally warrant such scanning.

72. b) In glaucoma, atrophy (degeneration) of the nerve fiber layer is a key in diagnosis. (Damage to the nerve fibers generally occurs in a characteristic pattern, yielding the classic visual field defects seen in glaucoma.) The fovea is the center of the macula; the optic radiations are beyond the globe itself and run to the occipital cortex; the retinal pigment epithelium is another layer of the retina between the rod and cone cells and the choroid.

73. c) Scanning laser testing software gives a probability that the evaluated tissue is normal by comparing the patient's reading with normative data. Thus, the care provider might tell a patient, "The chances that this finding is normal is only 5%."

Chapter 14

Refractometry

Ledford JK.
Certified Ophthalmic Assistant: Exam
Review Manual, Third Edition (pp. 231-250).
© 2012 Taylor & Francis Group.

Refractive Errors[1]

1. **Label the following (Figure 14-1):**

   compound hyperopic astigmatism
   emmetropia
   mixed astigmatism
   simple hyperopic astigmatism

   compound myopic astigmatism
   hyperopia
   myopia
   simple myopic astigmatism

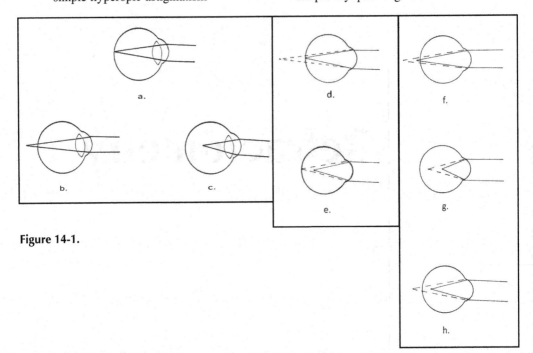

Figure 14-1.

2. **Which of the following prescriptions denotes emmetropia?**
   a) +2.00 sphere
   b) –2.00 sphere
   c) Plano + 2.00 × 180
   d) Plano sphere

3. **In hyperopia:**
   a) the object image focuses on the retina
   b) the object image focuses on the cornea
   c) the object image focuses in the vitreous
   d) the object image focuses beyond the macula

4. **Myopia can be caused by:**
   a) irregular curvature of the cornea
   b) removal of the crystalline lens
   c) an eyeball that is "too long"
   d) a stretched-out retina

[1]While not listed as a criteria item per se, knowledge of refractive errors is expected of the COA®
candidate.

5. **A refractive error of +2.00 + 2.00 × 180 would be classified as:**
   a) mixed astigmatism
   b) compound hyperopic astigmatism
   c) compound myopic astigmatism
   d) simple hyperopic astigmatism

6. **The condition of having no lens is referred to as:**
   a) astigmatism
   b) ametropia
   c) aphakia
   d) pseudophakia

7. **Farsightedness may be caused by all of the following *except*:**
   a) heredity
   b) removal of the crystalline lens
   c) orbital tumor
   d) migraine headaches

8. **If your patient complains of blurred vision at near, the most likely cause is:**
   a) hyperopia
   b) presbyopia
   c) astigmatism
   d) need more information

9. **The classic symptom of myopia is:**
   a) blurred vision at near
   b) blurred vision at distance
   c) blurred vision at near and distance
   d) headaches

10. **All of the following are characteristic of nearsightedness *except*:**
   a) it tends to be hereditary
   b) it tends to accelerate during adolescence
   c) the patient is more prone to retinal detachment
   d) presbyopia is delayed

11. **Astigmatism occurs when:**
   a) the cornea is irregularly curved
   b) the cornea is curved equally in all directions
   c) an individual reaches his or her 40s
   d) the retina is irregularly curved

12. **A 12-year-old patient complains of problems seeing the board at school. Most likely the patient is:**
   a) myopic
   b) presbyopic
   c) malingering
   d) hyperopic

13. **A 45-year-old male who has never worn glasses complains of decreased near vision. Most likely he is:**
    a) myopic
    b) presbyopic
    c) astigmatic
    d) aphakic

14. **Presbyopia is caused by:**
    a) removal of the crystalline lens
    b) loss of muscle tone in the ciliary muscle
    c) degeneration of the zonules
    d) loss of elasticity of the crystalline lens

15. **A classic complaint of the presbyopic patient is:**
    a) "I cannot see where I'm going in a dark movie theater."
    b) "My arms are too short."
    c) "My eyes itch and burn."
    d) "My eyes draw and pull."

16. **Using a plus lens or an add corrects presbyopia because:**
    a) it restores plus power lost by the crystalline lens
    b) it restores minus power lost by the crystalline lens
    c) it neutralizes the patient's hyperopia
    d) it neutralizes the patient's astigmatism

17. **A presbyopic myope with distance correction may find that his or her near vision improves if the patient:**
    a) closes one eye
    b) wears contact lenses
    c) holds the reading material closer
    d) takes off his or her glasses

18. **A presbyopic patient who is prescribed his or her first pair of single-vision reading glasses should be told:**
    a) that distant objects will appear blurred through the glasses
    b) that near objects will appear blurred through the glasses
    c) that the glasses can be worn for all activities
    d) to wear the glasses at all times to get used to them

19. **Your patient is delighted because suddenly, at age 65, she can now read without her bifocals. The most likely cause of this symptom is:**
    a) cataract
    b) hyperopia
    c) presbyopia
    d) ocular hypertension

20. **A 75-year-old patient states that he wears contact lenses because he had cataract surgery without implants. You need to remove the contacts for part of the exam, but the patient objects. Why?**
a) He is virtually blind without them.
b) He can read without the contacts, but cannot drive.
c) He can drive without the contacts, but cannot read.
d) His eyes are more comfortable with the lenses in.

21. **A 2-year-old male wearing -15.00 lenses screams if you take his glasses off. Why?**
a) He has gotten used to feeling them on his face.
b) He is totally blind without them.
c) He cannot see more than several inches beyond his face without them.
d) He is probably punished at home if he takes the glasses off.

22. **A new patient calls, complaining of poor vision with some glasses made elsewhere. She wants to start over with your doctor. You should:**
a) refuse to see her because she should really go back to her original physician
b) make the appointment, and ask her to bring the problem glasses plus her previous glasses
c) tell her to return to her optician
d) make the appointment, and ask her to bring only her previous glasses

Automated Refractometry

23. **The automated refractor is an example of:**
a) subjective testing
b) objective testing
c) self-testing
d) vision testing

24. **An automated refractor reading is especially helpful when the patient:**
a) is new and has no glasses
b) has a previous refraction on record
c) has cataracts
d) has a written glasses prescription with him or her

25. **An autorefraction reading would be helpful in all of the following cases *except*:**
a) prescribing glasses (without subjective testing)
b) following cataract surgery
c) evaluating an aphasic patient
d) evaluating the refractive error of a child

26. **The key instruction to the patient during automated refractometry (AR) is:**
a) "Don't blink."
b) "Tell me if the image blurs."
c) "Look straight ahead."
d) "Hold your breath."

27. Some autorefractors allow the assistant to manipulate the reading in order to provide the clearest image possible. This pushes the AR into the realm of:
    a) subjective testing
    b) retinoscopy
    c) prescribing
    d) duochrome testing

28. Patient prep for an AR could include all of the following *except*:
    a) explaining the procedure
    b) sanitizing areas of patient contact
    c) adjusting the table height for comfort
    d) instilling topical anesthetic

29. Performing an AR after the patient is dilated:
    a) provides no useful information
    b) will be inaccurate
    c) is needed when prescribing bifocals
    d) may reveal additional hyperopia

30. An AR measurement may be used:
    a) to plug into an intraocular lens formula
    b) to confirm change between current glasses and refraction
    c) as a glasses prescription
    d) to guide laser-assisted in situ keratomileusis (LASIK) surgery

31. All of the following could result in erroneous AR measurements *except*:
    a) posterior subcapsular cataract
    b) central corneal scar
    c) glaucoma
    d) miosis

32. The target in most autorefractors simulates distance viewing in order to avoid:
    a) accommodation
    b) unequal pupil size
    c) induced prism
    d) visual fatigue

33. An appropriate use of an AR measurement would be:
    a) to select final contact lens power
    b) use in intraocular lens (IOL) calculation
    c) starting point for retinoscopy
    d) starting point for subjective refractometry

34. Error in AR measurement can result from:
    a) inaccurate pupillary distance
    b) having the instrument in a lighted hallway
    c) using the incorrect cylinder format
    d) induced prism

35. **An AR might include all of the following additional features** *except*:
    a) visual acuity
    b) glare testing
    c) keratometer
    d) cover testing

Manifest Refractometry

36. **Which of the following is** *true* **regarding the difference between "refraction" and "refractometry"?**
    a) Objective measurement is used in refractometry.
    b) Only refractions are written in the patient's chart.
    c) Clinical judgment is used in a refraction.
    d) Only a licensed practitioner can perform refractometry.

37. **Which of the following will give the technician the most useful information regarding the patient's refractive status?**
    a) the history
    b) the muscle balance check
    c) the slit-lamp exam
    d) the fundus exam

38. **All of the following patients could reasonably be expected to have alterations to his or her refractive status** *except*:
    a) a diabetic
    b) a pregnant woman
    c) a patient with cataracts
    d) a patient taking allergy shots

39. **In order to avoid compromising the distance measurement, refractometry should be performed prior to:**
    a) tonometry
    b) retinoscopy
    c) pupil exam
    d) muscle balance testing

40. **A slit-lamp exam is useful before refractometry in order to:**
    a) determine if astigmatism is present
    b) measure the intraocular pressure (IOP)
    c) check the clarity of the media
    d) determine if refractometry is needed

41. **Label the parts of the refractor (Figure 14-2):**

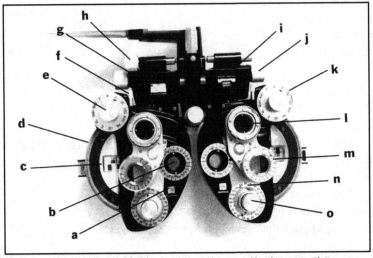

Figure 14-2. Reprinted with permission of Jim Ledford, PA-C, PhD.

pupillary distance (PD) adjusting knob

cylinder power

cylinder power dial

prism

PD scale

sphere dial

aperture convergence lever

cross-cylinder

sphere power

3-diopter sphere dial

level

aperture

cylinder axis dial

aperture knob

leveling screw

42. **Before beginning the refractometric measurement on an adult, it is important to:**
    a) explain the procedure
    b) have an autorefractor reading
    c) make sure he or she can read 20/20
    d) instill artificial tears to clear the tear film

43. **All of the following are appropriate adjustments to the refractor (phoroptor) before starting the distance measurement *except*:**
    a) set to the patient's PD
    b) set to an appropriate vertex distance
    c) converge the apertures
    d) make sure the instrument is level

44. **All of the following are true regarding fogging *except*:**
    a) it may be used to avoid giving too much plus at near
    b) it may be used to help prevent giving too much minus
    c) it can be used as an alternative to occlusion
    d) it can be used to relax accommodation

45. **Fogging is accomplished by:**
    a) placing a polarized lens in front of the eye to blur the vision
    b) placing the Bagolini lens in front of the eye to blur the vision
    c) placing enough plus power in front of the eye to blur the vision
    d) placing a Maddox rod in front of the eye to blur the vision

46. **In general, the first step in refractometry is to:**
    a) correct as much of the refractive error as possible with cylinder
    b) correct as much of the refractive error as possible with sphere
    c) find the cylinder power using the cross-cylinder
    d) find the cylinder axis using the astigmatic dial

47. **When offering the patient changes in spheres, a good general rule is to:**
    a) refine the axis before the power
    b) offer more plus first
    c) offer more minus first
    d) always use minus cylinder

48. **You have no prior record on your young patient, and he has never worn glasses. His vision is 20/80 uncorrected. A correction of –1.50 sphere brings his vision up to 20/30; –2.00 and –2.50 sphere gives no improvement in vision. Your next step should be:**
    a) record the final measurement as –1.50 sphere
    b) see if –1.75 or –2.25 sphere will help
    c) use the duochrome test
    d) check for astigmatism

49. **If your patient has more than 6.00 D of astigmatism:**
    a) you cannot use the refractor
    b) the cross-cylinder will not work
    c) the fogging technique must be used
    d) an auxiliary cylinder lens must be used

50. **The astigmatic dial[2] is useful for:**
    a) finding the exact cylinder power
    b) refining astigmatic correction
    c) finding the exact cylinder direction
    d) estimating the cylinder axis

51. **The astigmatic dial looks like:**
    a) a telephone dial
    b) a clock face
    c) a circular grid
    d) a circle with horizontal lines

---

[2]The new JCAHPO® criteria for refractometry says simply "Manifest Refractometry" without any further details. I have elected to include questions on the astigmatic dial.

52. **When using plus cylinder, if the patient says that all the lines on the astigmatic dial seem to be equally clear:**
    a) the test is over; proceed directly to cross-cylinder refinement
    b) turn the cylinder axis knob 45 degrees, and ask again if any lines are darker
    c) add +0.50 sphere, and ask again if any lines are darker
    d) open the aperture, and try the test with both eyes together

53. **In plus cylinder, if the patient says that the lines on the astigmatic dial running from 12 to 6 are clearer, you will set your axis cylinder at:**
    a) 90 degrees
    b) 180 degrees
    c) 0 degrees
    d) 45 degrees

54. **In minus cylinder, if the patient says that the lines on the astigmatic dial running from 12 to 6 are clearer, you will set your axis cylinder at:**
    a) 45 degrees
    b) 90 degrees
    c) 135 degrees
    d) 180 degrees

55. **When using the astigmatic dial, once you have set your axis, you should:**
    a) add cylinder until all lines are equally clear
    b) add sphere until all lines are equally clear
    c) use the cross-cylinder until all lines are equally clear
    d) remove the dial and refine with the cross-cylinder

56. **You are measuring a patient from scratch (no retinoscopy, lensometry, or prior records). Your best spherical correction is +2.00 sphere for 20/60 vision. You use the astigmatic dial and find that the lines are equally black with cylinder −1.50 × 180. What is your next step?**
    a) Change the sphere setting to +2.75.
    b) Change the sphere setting to +1.25.
    c) Refine the cylinder axis.
    d) Record the measurement.

57. **The cross-cylinder is used:**
    a) to refine cylinder axis and power
    b) to refine sphere axis and power
    c) to refine sphere and cylinder power
    d) to refine sphere and cylinder axis

58. **Before cross-cylinder testing, it is important to:**
    a) be close to the sphere power endpoint
    b) refine sphere power to the endpoint
    c) measure for bifocal add
    d) balance the two eyes

59. **On cross-cylinder testing:**
    a) the power of the sphere should always be measured first, then its axis
    b) the axis of the sphere should be measured first, then its power
    c) the power of the cylinder should be measured first, then its axis
    d) the axis of the cylinder should always be measured first, then its power

60. **When refining the axis using minus cylinder, you should follow which dot on the cross-cylinder?**
    a) red
    b) white
    c) blue
    d) there are no dots on the cross-cylinder

61. **You are using plus cylinder and are refining cylinder power. The present cylinder power is +0.50. The patient says that the letters are more clear when the white dot is showing on the cross-cylinder. What should you do now?**
    a) rotate the axis toward the white dot
    b) change the cylinder power to zero
    c) change the cylinder power to +1.00
    d) stop because you are at the endpoint

62. **You are using minus cylinder and are refining cylinder power. The present cylinder power is –1.00. The patient says that the letters are clearer when the white dot is showing on the cross-cylinder. What should you do now?**
    a) switch to plus cylinder
    b) change the cylinder power to –1.50
    c) change the cylinder power to –0.50
    d) change the sphere power by +0.50

63. **The generally accepted endpoint for the cross-cylinder test (for either axis or power refinement) is:**
    a) when the first choice is better than the second choice
    b) when the second choice is better than the first choice
    c) when the two choices appear equal
    d) when the patient states his or her vision is most comfortable

64. **Your patient reads 20/20 with the following setting: –2.00 + 1.25 × 065. To refine the sphere, you first change the sphere setting to –1.75. The patient says the 20/20 line is now a bit blurred. You show her –2.00 again, and she says it is clearer. Now, you change the sphere to –2.25. The patient says the letters are smaller but clearer. She cannot read 20/15 at any setting. What is your next step?**
    a) see if –2.50 helps
    b) record the final measurement as –2.25 + 1.25 × 065
    c) record the final measurement as –2.00 + 1.25 × 065
    d) record the final measurement as –1.75 + 1.25 × 065

65. **The duochrome technique[3] of refining sphere depends on:**
    a) the fact that green rays are refracted more than red rays
    b) red rays will appear orange, and green rays will appear blue
    c) the patient having normal color vision
    d) contrast sensitivity to red light as opposed to green light

66. **The duochrome test is useful to:**
    a) determine a patient's color vision
    b) help prevent giving too much plus
    c) help prevent giving too much minus
    d) refine cylinder correction

67. **Before beginning the duochrome test, do all of the following *except*:**
    a) occlude one eye
    b) get a final distance correction
    c) place a red filter in front of the eye
    d) fog with +0.50 sphere

68. **If the patient says that the letters in the red panel are sharper, you should:**
    a) record this as your endpoint
    b) add more cylinder
    c) add more plus power to the sphere
    d) add more minus power to the sphere

69. **The endpoint for the duochrome test generally is accepted to be when the letters:**
    a) in the red panel are clearer
    b) in the green panel are faded out
    c) are equally clear in both panels
    d) are no longer visible in both panels

70. **How is the duochrome test done if a patient is red-green color blind?**
    a) The duochrome test cannot be used.
    b) Place a Maddox rod in front of the right eye.
    c) Place a Bagolini lens in front of the right eye.
    d) Refer to left and right sides instead of red and green.

71. **If the patient is accommodating during refractometry, this may result in:**
    a) a prescription that has excess plus
    b) a prescription that has excess minus
    c) a prescription without necessary cylinder correction
    d) a prescription that will cause the eyes to relax too much

72. **All of the following may be used to reduce or eliminate accommodation *except*:**
    a) duochrome test
    b) bringing the distant eye chart closer
    c) fogging
    d) topical cycloplegics

[3]The new JCAHPO® criteria for refractometry says simply "Manifest Refractometry" without any further details. I have elected to include questions on duochrome testing.

73. **A patient whose prescription is inaccurate due to accommodation will have to:**
    a) relax accommodation in order to see clearly when wearing the correction
    b) have prism in the lenses to reduce diplopia
    c) accommodate in order to see clearly when wearing the correction
    d) have a bifocal for near vision

74. **If a patient is known to be myopic:**
    a) one need not worry about accommodation
    b) one must still reduce or eliminate accommodation
    c) the eye has no ability to accommodate
    d) avoiding too much minus is not critical

75. **The ideal distant refractometric measurement:**
    a) leaves vision slightly blurred on the plus side to avoid overminusing
    b) is slightly overminused in order to stimulate accommodation
    c) causes as much accommodation as possible
    d) gives the clearest vision possible and relaxes accommodation

76. **Balancing[4] is performed:**
    a) with the right eye occluded
    b) with the left eye occluded
    c) with both eyes open
    d) while standing on one foot

77. **The purpose of balancing is:**
    a) to ensure that the vision is the same in each eye
    b) to make sure that the eyes are accommodating equally
    c) to ensure that the measurement in each eye is as nearly the same as possible
    d) to make sure that the eyes are not crossing

78. **Your healthy patient has clear media, although you have not looked at the retina. Your best refractometric measurement yields only 20/40 vision. What should you do next?**
    a) Record the measurement as final.
    b) Label that eye as amblyopic.
    c) Get a pinhole vision.
    d) Perform a stereo test.

Reading Add

79. **To test for the reading add, the standard near card is placed:**
    a) at the distance preferred by the patient
    b) at 10 inches
    c) at 14 inches
    d) at 20 inches

[4]The new JCAHPO® criteria for refractometry says simply "Manifest Refractometry" without any further details. I have elected to include questions on balancing.

80. **The general rule for determining the reading add is to:**
    a) give the least amount of plus possible
    b) give the maximum amount of plus
    c) go by the standard age chart
    d) never give more than +3.00

Special Cases

81. **Using a trial frame might be preferable over using the refractor (phoroptor) when:**
    a) the patient has facial deformities
    b) the patient already wears glasses
    c) performing retinoscopy first
    d) the patient has a head tremor

82. **When measuring the refractive error of a patient with low vision, it is helpful to:**
    a) speak a little more loudly and slowly
    b) urge him or her to choose quickly between lens options
    c) use larger steps (ie, 0.50 or larger) for refinement
    d) use smaller steps of 0.25 to increase accuracy

83. **The best instrument to use when measuring the refractive error of a low vision patient is:**
    a) trial lenses and trial frame
    b) phoroptor
    c) automated refractometer
    d) prisms to create separate images for each eye

84. **The patient with nystagmus should be refracted using:**
    a) no special adaptations
    b) the astigmatic dial
    c) +3.00 lens instead of an occluder
    d) −3.00 lens instead of an occluder

Explanatory Answers

1. Labeling:

compound hyperopic astigmatism	f)
emmetropia	a)
mixed astigmatism	h)
simple hyperopic astigmatism	d)
compound myopic astigmatism	g)
hyperopia	b)
myopia	c)
simple myopic astigmatism	e)

2. d) Emmetropia is the absence of refractive error, hence no correction (plano sphere) is required.

3.   d) The hyperopic eye does not have enough plus power to focus the image on the retina. Instead, the image falls beyond the retina/macula. (Technically, of course, this is not possible, except in a "virtual" sense.)

4.   c) The myopic eye is usually longer than average, causing the image to fall in front of the retina.

5.   b) Hyperopia combined with plus cylinder astigmatism is termed *compound hyperopic astigmatism.*

6.   c) The prefix *a-* means without. The term *-phakia* refers to the lens. So, *aphakia* means without a lens.

7.   d) Migraine headaches do not cause any type of refractive error. An orbital tumor can cause farsightedness if it has pushed the retina forward.

8.   d) The answer depends on the age of the patient and her previous refractive status. There is not enough information here to make a good choice.

9.   b) Myopia is "nearsightedness"; the patient's vision is at near (ie, blurred at a distance).

10.   d) Myopia does not delay presbyopia; the myopic eye ages at the normal rate. (It is true, however, that a mildly myopic patient might not notice the effects of presbyopia until later than average.) The myopic eye tends to be longer than normal. This may result in the retina's being stretched, predisposing one to retinal detachment (as in answer c).

11.   a) Irregular curvature of the cornea is the textbook definition of astigmatism.

12.   a) A young patient who is having trouble seeing at a distance is most likely myopic. Presbyopia begins around age 40. Hyperopia blurs the near vision. Malingering means to lie, and we have to assume most patients (regardless of age) are telling the truth!

13.   b) Presbyopia begins around age 40 and onward, whether the patient has worn glasses before or not. Myopia blurs vision at a distance. Astigmatism would likely have been detected by age 45. Aphakia is the condition of having no crystalline lens in the eye, and the patient is legally blind without correction (eg, intraocular lens, contact lens).

14.   d) As we age, the lens forms layers that compact, forming a hard nucleus. Thus, the lens loses its elasticity. It is true that the ciliary muscle tone decreases, but this is not the major factor in presbyopia.

15.   b) The loss of near vision is often compensated for by holding reading material at arm's length. Thus, the patient complains that his or her arms are too short.

16.   a) It takes more plus to see up close. When the presbyopic eye has lost the ability to add enough plus, the plus is restored by using glasses with plus lenses.

17.   d) A myope is corrected with minus power. Thus, taking off his glasses adds plus power to the eye, bringing near objects into better focus.

18.   a) The focal distance of a pair of reading glasses is usually 14 to 16 inches. Anything further away than that will be blurry. The patient should be warned about this.

19.   a) The onset of cataracts causes a myopic shift in the refractive error, often restoring reading vision lost by presbyopia.

20.   a) A patient with no crystalline lens is legally blind without contacts or glasses. Driving home without them would be impossible. Even walking around the office would be difficult and possibly embarrassing.

21.   c) A –15.00 myope is not totally blind without glasses, but is certainly legally blind. A 2-year-old cannot articulate his frustration at not being able to see—he can only cry.

22.   b) You might suggest that she see the original doctor or optician, but do not refuse to see her. If she brings both pairs of glasses, you can analyze them and hopefully find the problem.

23. b) The autorefractor takes the reading with no response from the patient, treating the patient as an "object." This is an easy way to remember the difference between *obj*ective and *sub*jective.

24. a) In cases b and d, there is information from which a refractometric measurement could be started. A patient with cataracts may not get an accurate AR measurement because of the opacities, plus the information given in the question does not state whether or not the patient has been seen before. An AR on the new patient (ie, with no refractive record in your practice) who has no glasses (ie, from which to read a prescription) would be the most useful of the bunch.

25. a) It is not usually accepted practice to prescribe an AR as glasses; subjective refinement via refractometry is required. An AR would be useful in all of the other cases. Aphasia means "without speech."

26. c) Alignment is key for a good AR reading. Most autorefractors are so fast that blinking will not interfere with the reading. Besides, a good tear film means a clearer path of light during the analysis. If the patient talks during the reading, alignment will be disturbed. Holding the breath makes no difference.

27. a) Subjective testing of any kind involves asking for a response from the patient. Still, the reading would not be prescribed directly under most circumstances; refinement using lenses would still be done. Most autorefractors use the principles of retinoscopy: evaluating how light reflects from the eye in order to suggest a possible refraction.

28. d) Topical anesthetic is not required for an AR.

29. d) If a patient accommodates (ie, focuses at near) during an AR, then the reading may be less hyperopic than the patient actually is. When accommodating, the eye adds "more plus" to itself, which the AR responds to by adding more minus.

30. b) In cases where there is either little or no difference between the refraction and the patient's current glasses, or there is a good bit of difference but little vision improvement, an AR gives another piece of information that may help confirm that the manual refraction (MR) is accurate. An example might be where the MR shows an axis change of 30 degrees compared to the patient's glasses but improves vision only a little.

31. c) Glaucoma itself would make little difference in an AR measurement. Any media opacity (eg, posterior capsular cataract, central corneal scar) can diffract incoming light and render the measurement unusable. Miosis (small pupil) can also make it difficult to get an accurate reading.

32. a) See answer 29. However, the fact that the patient knows that the target is not actually far away can, itself, induce accommodation.

33. d) The AR is generally entered into the phoroptor and then refined. Selecting a final contact lens power and gathering data for IOL calculation are matters of evaluating the patient's vision using subjective methods. Generally, the AR takes the place of retinoscopy.

34. b) Dim lighting is recommended, as peripheral lighting may inhibit the instrument from aligning properly. PD does not factor into the measurement; in fact, many autorefractors measure and provide this information.

35. d) Cover testing is an evaluation of the extraocular muscles, not of the eye's refractive system. An AR with a built-in eye chart is great because it helps verify the accuracy of the reading. Many models also have glare and keratometry capabilities, increasing the instrument's usefulness.

36. c) *Refractometry* is the measurement of a patient's refractive error (by objective and/or subjective means) and usually is recorded in the patient's chart. *Refraction* includes the clinical judgment necessary to arrive at the prescription based on the refractometric measurement. Ophthalmic medical personnel are allowed to perform refractometry. Refractions are only performed by those licensed to do so (ie, an optometrist or an ophthalmologist).

37. a) The history will tell you much that can affect the measurement: the presence of any systemic or ocular disease that may affect vision, any medications that can affect vision, past vision history, past problems with glasses, or visual symptoms. The option of doing a slit-lamp exam prior to refractometry is preferable, but not as necessary as knowing the patient's history.

38. d) As a general rule, taking allergy shots does not affect the measurement. Answers a, b, and c can change the measurement.

39. a) Refractometry should be done prior to tonometry or any other procedure that applanates the cornea (A-scan, B-scan, pachymetry, cell count, etc). With any of these tests, there is the possibility of some corneal abrasion and/or edema, which can affect the patient's vision and thus the measurement. Retinoscopy is done prior to refractometry in order to provide a starting point. The pupil test might dazzle the patient for a minute, but you can proceed once he or she recovers.

40. c) The slit-lamp exam will indicate the clarity of the tear film, cornea, aqueous, lens, and vitreous (collectively called the *optical media*), giving you an idea of the prognosis of the measurement. Unless the patient has marked keratoconus, astigmatism will not be seen with the slit lamp. Applanation tonometry can compromise corneal clarity. The necessity for refractometry is determined by factors other than the slit-lamp exam.

41. Labeling:

PD adjusting knob	j)
cylinder power	a)
cylinder power dial	o)
prism	m)
PD scale	g)
sphere dial	d)
aperture convergence level	f)
cross-cylinder	l)
sphere power	c)
3-diopter sphere dial	k)
level	i)
aperture	b)
cylinder axis dial	n)
aperture knob	e)
leveling screw	h)

42. a) Patient education is one of the keys to successful measurements. An autorefractor reading might be nice, but is not necessary. Obviously, not everyone can read 20/20 (or they would not need us). If the tear film is inadequate, eye drops may be needed, but they are not required on every patient.

43. c) Always set the PD, vertex distance, and level before measuring. The apertures are converged to test the reading (near) vision, not the distance.

44. a) Fogging is used to reduce accommodation during refractometry, which helps prevent giving too much minus. It also can be used instead of occlusion, but is not used to avoid giving too much plus at near.

45. c) To fog, add enough plus sphere to blur the vision. (There is no set amount, but I prefer +3.00.)

46. b) The measurement starts by working with spheres. You want to correct as much of the refractive error as possible with sphere.

47. b) Always offer more plus first, whether you are going from +2.00 to +2.50, or from –6.25 to –5.75. More minus frequently looks better to an eye that is accommodating. Sphere has no axis.

48. d) If sphere alone does not correct a patient to 20/20, it is not time to stop! Start looking for astigmatism. If –2.00 and –2.50 sphere did not improve, it is a waste of time to try –1.75 and –2.25. The duochrome test is performed after best visual acuity has been obtained using spheres and, if necessary, cylinder.

49. d) Cylinder power in most refractors goes up to 6.00 D, but there is an auxiliary cylinder lens that you can snap into the aperture to add more. The cross-cylinder is not dependent on a certain amount of astigmatism.

50. d) The astigmatic dial is useful in estimating the cylinder axis. You still must refine with the cross-cylinder.

51. b) The astigmatic dial looks like a clock face.

52. c) If you are using plus cylinder and the lines on the dial appear equally black, add a little sphere (ie, move in a more plus direction) and ask again. In minus cylinder, give –0.50. Either way, you are moving the image off the retina enough to see if there is another meridian of focus.

53. a) For plus cylinder, set the cylinder axis parallel to, or in line with, the darkest lines as the patient sees them.

54. d) In minus cylinder, set the cylinder axis perpendicular to, or 90 degrees away from, the darkest lines as the patient sees them.

55. a) After setting your axis, slowly give the patient cylinder power until the lines appear to be equally clear.

56. a) For every 0.50 D of minus cylinder, you should now add 0.25 D of sphere in the plus direction. This is to maintain equivalence. In plus cylinder, for every 0.50 D of cylinder, you should subtract 0.25 D of sphere.

57. a) Use the cross-cylinder to refine cylinder axis and power. (Spheres do not have an axis.)

58. a) If the spherical component of your measurement is too far off, your cylinder will not be correct. You will be trying to neutralize with cylinder what would be better corrected with sphere.

59. d) Always measure the cylinder axis first. (This is one of the few exceptions to my warning about the word *always*.) If the axis is not refined first, you cannot get the accurate power.

60. a) If you are using minus cylinder and are refining axis, follow the red dot. There are no blue dots. Conversely, if you are using plus cylinder, then follow the white dot.

61. c) When refining power, the red dot means subtract, which is the same as "giving minus," and the white dot means add, which is the same as "giving plus," regardless of whether you are working in plus or minus cylinder. If you are at cylinder power +0.50 and the patient likes the white dot choice better, you are going to move to +1.00 cylinder power. (In reality, you could alternately choose to go to +0.75, adding just +0.25, but that was not offered as an answer in this question.)

62. c) See answer 61. The white dot means give plus, so you should move from –1.00 to –0.50.

63. c) The cross-cylinder actually straddles a setting, so on one choice, the patient sees the setting with a little "plus" and on the other choice with a little "minus." When straddling the correct reading, each choice is equidistant from that setting, and the choices will look about the same.

64. c) Remember that a minus lens minifies. (You also could say that, compared to a +6.00, a +2.00 minifies.) The patient's impression that the letters have gotten smaller is generally an indication of too much minus. But, it is best to check vision with yet smaller letters to see if there is an improvement. Therefore, you return to the previous setting of $-2.00 + 1.25 \times 065$ as your end-point.

65. a) Green rays are refracted more than red rays, so red hits the retina first. Adding minus moves the red rays behind the retina (virtually speaking) and pushes the green onto the retina. There is a difference of 0.50 to 0.75 D between the red and green wavelengths. Normal color vision is not required (see answer 70). *Note:* The duochrome test may also be called the bichrome test.

66. c) The duochrome test is used to prevent giving the patient too much minus sphere. It is not a color vision test, nor is it used to refine cylinder. The only time you have to worry about giving a patient too much *plus* is when measuring the reading add.

67. c) The red filter is not used in the duochrome test. Fogging the eye with +0.50 makes the letters in the red darker, so you can move toward the green by –0.25 steps.

68. d) If the letters in the red are sharper and more distinct, remove 0.25 D of sphere (ie, reduce plus or increase minus). Go in small steps so you do not miss the endpoint and overminus.

69. c) The endpoint is when the letters on both sides are equally clear. Some practitioners recommend that you leave the patient "one click into the green," but that was not given here as a choice.

70. d) Even a red-green color blind patient who cannot distinguish between vivid hues can be tested using the duochrome if you refer to the left and right halves of the screen instead of the colors. No special lenses or tricks need to be used.

71. b) If the patient accommodates, he or she has added plus power to the eye. This is neutralized with minus sphere, or the removal of plus sphere, during the measurement. If prescribed by the practitioner, this spectacle lens will not have enough plus, and the eye will have to strain when wearing it, causing even more accommodation to be required for clear vision.

72. b) Methods to control or reduce accommodation include the duochrome test, fogging, and topical cycloplegics. Bringing the distant chart closer will stimulate accommodation.

73. c) See answer 71.

74. b) It is a common misconception that if the patient is known to be myopic, you need not worry about accommodation. This is not true. You might easily refract a young myope who only needs –2.00 sphere as a –4.00 or more.

75. d) As a general rule, the ideal situation for distance is for accommodation to be relaxed and vision to be as clear as possible.

76. c) Both apertures are open during balancing. (Standing on one foot?! I thought it was time for a little levity; optics can get pretty heavy!)

77. b) The goal in balancing is to make sure that the eyes are accommodating equally. Ideally, of course, this means that neither eye is accommodating at all for distance vision.

78. c) Anytime a healthy-looking eye does not refract to 20/20, do a pinhole vision. If the pinhole improves the vision, you should be able to improve acuity with the correct lenses. If the pinhole does not improve the vision, your refractometric measurement is probably the best you can do, and the doctor will look for pathology.

79. a) The technician should measure the distance preferred by the patient, place the near test card at that distance, and move in the direction of plus, giving the least amount of add that will enable the patient to read clearly and comfortably at that distance. It is then important to document the distance at which the add was measured.

80. a) In general, be cautious with giving plus. The goal is to leave half of the patient's accommodation (if there is any) in reserve. If you give the maximum plus that the patient will tolerate, you totally eliminate natural accommodation at near. The age chart may be a guide, but each patient should be measured. Some patients will need more than +3.00. The word "never" should have indicated that answer d was not correct.

81. d) A patient with head tremors will be easier to work with using the trial frame. It would be difficult to keep such a patient aligned with the refractor. A patient with facial deformities may not be able to wear or tolerate a trial frame. Retinoscopy is more conveniently done using the refractor.

82. c) Use larger steps for low-vision patients to provide more contrast between the compared lenses. No need to speak louder; they can hear. Go more slowly, rather than quickly. Small steps are harder for them to see and judge.

83. a) Because low-vision patients often need lenses of high power, thus making vertex distance a very important issue, the trial frame is the instrument of choice. In addition, objective methods do not work well in low-vision patients with media problems. The trial frame also makes it easier to offer the patient larger increments when changing lenses. Low-vision patients may not appreciate a 0.50 D change and may require higher increments to appreciate the difference. By the same token, a 0.50 D cross-cylinder may not provide enough contrast, either. Use one that provides at least 1.00 D. Also, if the patient has a central scotoma, the small apertures in the phoroptor do not provide enough field of vision. For the same reason, full aperture trial lenses are best as well. Finally, the trial frame allows the patient to adopt any head posture that seems to clear the vision a bit.

84. c) Occluding one eye may make the nystagmus worse. Fog the untested eye with +3.00 of plus; using minus would probably stimulate accommodation. Just do not forget to switch when you go to measure the other eye and to remove the +3.00 when doing that final vision check and documenting your results.

Chapter 15

Spectacle Skills

Ledford JK.
*Certified Ophthalmic Assistant: Exam
Review Manual, Third Edition* (pp. 251-254).
© 2012 Taylor & Francis Group.

Transpose Cylinder Readings[1]

1. A patient who had an eye exam last week comes into the office upset. He shows you two prescriptions for glasses: the one your doctor issued last week and another from an out-of-town doctor dated 2 months ago. "One of these has got to be wrong," he says. "Look how different they are!"

    Prescription #1:
    OD: –2.50 – 1.75 × 087
    OS: –1.75 – 2.25 × 112

    Prescription #2:
    OD: –4.25 + 1.75 × 177
    OS: –4.00 + 2.25 × 022

    Your response to the patient would be to explain:
    a) refraction is subjective and he probably gave different responses the last time
    b) the other office's prescription is incorrect
    c) the prescriptions are merely written in different formats
    d) the need for another appointment to recheck the measurement

2. Transposition applies to which of the following lenses?
    a) spherical
    b) spherocylindrical
    c) prismatic
    d) bifocal/trifocal add

3. Transposition applies to which of the following refractive errors?
    a) mixed astigmatism
    b) simple myopia
    c) simple hyperopia
    d) mixed emmetropia

4. Transposition is used to:
    a) convert prism so it is equal between the two eyes
    b) give the best correction possible without using cylinder
    c) calculate the power of an intraocular lens implant
    d) convert plus cylinder to minus cylinder

5. Transposition is accomplished by:
    a) adding axis and cylinder, keeping the sphere the same
    b) adding sphere and cylinder, changing the cylinder sign, and keeping the axis the same
    c) adding sphere and cylinder, and changing the axis 90 degrees
    d) adding sphere and cylinder, changing the cylinder sign, and changing the axis 90 degrees

6. Care must be taken to figure the transposition correctly, because an error:
    a) may result in induced prism
    b) may result in an incorrect prescription
    c) may make it impossible to fit the lenses into the frame
    d) may make the lenses thicker than they should be

[1]The only item under Spectacle Skills in the new JCAHPO® COA® guidelines is transposition.

7.   **Transpose +2.00 – 1.00 × 075:**
     a) +1.00 + 1.00 × 075
     b) –2.00 + 1.00 × 165
     c) +1.00 + 1.00 × 165
     d) –2.00 + 1.00 × 165

8.   **Transpose –3.00 + 2.00 × 090:**
     a) + 3.00 – 2.00 × 180
     b) –1.00 – 2.00 × 090
     c) –1.00 – 2.00 × 180
     d) +1.00 – 2.00 × 180

9.   **Transpose –1.25 – 6.25 × 173:**
     a) –7.50 + 6.25 × 083
     b) –4.00 + 6.25 × 083
     c) –1.25 – 7.50 × 063
     d) -7.50 + 6.25 × 063

10. **Transpose Plano +3.75 × 027:**
     a) –3.75 – 3.75 × 117
     b) +3. 75 – 3.75 × 117
     c) –3.75 – 3.75 × 177
     d) +3.75 sphere

11. **Transpose +1.25 + 1.25 × 154:**
     a) +2.50 – 1.25 × 064
     b) Plano – 1.25 × 064
     c) Plano – 1.25 × 109
     d) +1.25 – 2.50 × 109

12. **Transpose –0.75 + 4.25 × 001**
     a) +0.75 – 4.25 × 091
     b) +0.75 – 3.50 × 091
     c) –0.75 – 4.25 × 089
     d) +3.50 – 4.25 × 091

Explanatory Answers

1.   c) The prescriptions have merely been transposed. Be sure to keep your explanation in terms that the patient can understand. You probably need not demonstrate the process, but could just tell the patient that the two offices just use different lens formats.

2.   b) A spherocylindrical lens combines a sphere and cylinder to correct for astigmatism. A spherical lens does not need to be transposed. Prism or the segments of multifocal lenses are likewise unaffected by transposition.

3.   a) Patients with astigmatism (of any type: myopic, hyperopic, or mixed) have cylinder in their prescription. Simple myopia and hyperopia are spherical errors, without any astigmatic/cylindrical correction. There is no such thing as mixed emmetropia; emmetropia itself is the lack of a refractive error.

4.   d) Transposition is the mathematical formula used to change plus to minus cylinder format and vice versa. (By the way, answer b actually involves using spherical equivalent, another optical formula, but in this case the incorrect one.)

5.   d) Transposition involves adding the sphere and cylinder powers algebraically, changing the cylinder power sign, and rotating the axis by 90. If the original axis is *less* than 90, it can be rotated by *adding* 90 as in the following examples: original axis is 045, add $45 + 90 = 135$; original axis is 002, add $2 + 90 = 092$. If the original axis is *more* than 90, it can be rotated by *subtracting* 90 as in the following examples: original axis is 092, subtract $92 - 90 = 002$; original axis is 169, subtract $169 - 90 = 079$.

6.   b) If you goof, the patient will get the wrong prescription.

7.   c) Algebraically add sphere and cylinder: $+2.00 + (-1.00) = +1.00$, sphere. Change cylinder sign: $+1.00$. Rotate axis by 090: $90 + 75 = 165$. Answer: $+1.00 + 1.00 \times 165$.

8.   c) Algebraically add sphere and cylinder: $-3.00 + 2.00 = -1.00$, sphere. Change cylinder sign: -2.00. Rotate axis by 090: $90 + 90 = 180$. Answer: $-1.00 - 2.00 \times 180$.

9.   a) Algebraically add sphere and cylinder: $-1.25 + (-6.25) = -7.50$. Change cylinder sign: $+6.25$. Rotate axis by 090: $173 - 90 = 083$. Answer: $-7.50 + 6.25 \times 083$.

10.   b) Algebraically add sphere and cylinder: 0 [Plano] $+ 3.75 = +3.75$. Change cylinder sign: -3.75. Rotate axis by 090: $27 + 090 = 117$. Answer: $+3.75 - 3.75 \times 117$.

11.   a) Algebraically add sphere and cylinder: $+1.25 + 1.25 = +2.50$. Change cylinder sign: -1.25. Rotate axis by 090: $154 - 90 = 064$. Answer: $+2.50 - 1.25 \times 064$.

12.   d) Algebraically add sphere and cylinder: $-0.75 + 4.25 = +3.50$. Change cylinder sign: -4.25. Rotate axis by 090: $1 + 90 = 091$. Answer: $+3.50 - 4.25 \times 091$.

Chapter 16

Supplemental Skills

Ledford JK.
*Certified Ophthalmic Assistant: Exam
Review Manual, Third Edition* (pp. 255-270).
© 2012 Taylor & Francis Group.

Intraocular Lens Power Calculation[1]

1. **When calculating intraocular lens (IOL) powers, one must enter:**
   a) visible corneal diameter
   b) desired postoperative refraction
   c) pupil size
   d) current refractive error

2. **You are inputting data for IOL calculations and notice that the K readings are 44.5/42.75. This type of reading:**
   a) should prompt you to repeat the measurement
   b) alerts you that lenticular astigmatism may exist
   c) alerts you that axillary astigmatism may exist
   d) is acceptable

3. **Almost all of the formulas for calculating IOL power:**
   a) are based on achieving emmetropia after surgery
   b) are based on measuring the aphakic eye
   c) are based on the same general equation
   d) are based on using an anterior chamber lens

4. **The manufacturer of a given IOL often supplies a specific number that must be entered into the IOL calculations when the lens is to be used. This number is referred to as a(n):**
   a) A-constant
   b) fudge factor
   c) personal identification number
   d) optical constant

5. **Which of the following poses problems in obtaining accurate measurements for IOL calculations?**
   a) patients with aphakia
   b) patients who have had corneal refractive surgery
   c) patients with posterior subcapsular cataracts
   d) patients with dense brown cataracts

6. **When calculating IOL power, each of the following are necessary *except*:**
   a) white-to-white corneal diameter
   b) axial length
   c) a calculation formula
   d) K readings

[1]See also *Laser Interferometry* (IOLMaster) at the end of this chapter.

Anterior Chamber Depth

7. **When using a penlight to estimate the depth of the anterior chamber, the following technique is best:**
    a) shine the light flatly from the side, in the plane of the iris
    b) shine the light from the front, and see whether there is a narrow angle
    c) shine the light from the front so that the light enters the pupil
    d) shine the light so that posterior synechiae can be seen

8. **When using a penlight to estimate anterior chamber depth, an open angle would appear:**
    a) to have a shadow on the nasal part of the iris
    b) to have a shadow around the pupil
    c) to have a shadow superiorly
    d) to have little or no shadow

9. **Estimating the anterior chamber depth with a penlight works because:**
    a) a narrow angle and bowed iris cast a shadow on the iris
    b) a narrow angle and bowed iris cause a change in the iris color
    c) an open angle and deep chamber cast a shadow on the iris
    d) the pupillary response of a narrow angle is decreased

10. **It is important to estimate the anterior chamber depth prior to dilation because:**
    a) open angles may precipitate an angle-closure glaucoma attack
    b) narrow angles may precipitate an angle-closure glaucoma attack
    c) narrow angles do not dilate as well and therefore require stronger dilating drugs
    d) open angles dilate quickly and therefore require weaker dilating drugs

11. **In slit-lamp assessment of the corneal periphery, the dark interval should be a minimum of approximately how much of the total corneal width for the angle to be considered open and safe for dilation?**
    a) one-half
    b) three-fourths
    c) one-fourth
    d) one-third

12. **When evaluating anterior chamber depth with the slit lamp, the illumination technique used is:**
    a) cobalt blue filter
    b) narrow beam
    c) wide beam
    d) pinpoint beam

Pachymetry

13. **Measuring corneal thickness via nonoptical pachymetry involves the use of:**
    a) specular microscopy
    b) ultrasound
    c) the slit-lamp microscope
    d) a contact mirrored lens

14. **One of the keys in accurate pachymetry is:**
    a) aiming the probe at the optic nerve
    b) aiming the probe at the macula
    c) maintaining contact with the coupling gel
    d) holding the probe perpendicular to the corneal surface

15. **Pachymetry readings are routinely taken prior to:**
    a) cataract surgery
    b) retinal surgery
    c) refractive surgery
    d) plastic surgery

16. **When performing pachymetry prior to refractive surgery, it is generally best to begin:**
    a) with the corneal periphery at 12:00
    b) with the central cornea
    c) with the mid-periphery at 12:00
    d) a scleral reading for calibration

17. **The type of pachymetry used to evaluate a glaucoma suspect is:**
    a) optical coherence tomography
    b) central corneal curvature
    c) peripheral corneal thickness
    d) central corneal thickness

18. **The average central thickness of the human cornea is:**
    a) 43 D
    b) 50 mm
    c) 545 µm
    d) 655 µm

Calibrate Biometry Instruments

19. **The IOLMaster must be calibrated daily using a:**
    a) calibration weight
    b) set of metal spheres of known curvature
    c) "test eye"
    d) calibration bar

20. **If a biometry instrument fails to calibrate properly, one should:**
    a) adjust the measurements appropriately
    b) remove the instrument from use
    c) make a note in the patient's record along with the measurement
    d) apply the manufacturer's "fudge factor" to the formula

Tear Tests

Schirmer's

21. **The Schirmer's test might be indicated in all of the following *except*:**
    a) dry eye
    b) contact lens pre-evaluation
    c) epiphora
    d) dacryocystitis

22. **The difference between Schirmer's test I and II is:**
    a) the length of the test
    b) the type of strips used
    c) the use of an anesthetic
    d) there is no difference

23. **Schirmer's test I is used to measure:**
    a) reflux tears
    b) reflex tears
    c) normal tearing
    d) epiphora

24. **Schirmer's test II is used to measure:**
    a) reflux tears
    b) reflex tears
    c) normal tearing
    d) drainage rate

25. **Measuring time for the Schirmer's test is:**
    a) 1 minute
    b) 2 minutes
    c) 5 minutes
    d) 10 minutes

26. **All of the following are true regarding the Schirmer's test *except*:**
    a) it requires expensive equipment
    b) it is brief
    c) it is portable
    d) it can be done at bedside

27. **A normally functioning lacrimal gland will produce how much wetting on a Schirmer's test strip after 5 minutes?**
    a) 1 mm
    b) 2.5 mm
    c) 6 mm
    d) 10 mm

Tear Break-Up Time

28. **All of the following are used in evaluating tear break-up time (TBUT) *except*:**
    a) slit-lamp microscope
    b) tear filter papers
    c) fluorescein dye
    d) cobalt blue light

29. **Just prior to the beginning of the TBUT test, the patient is instructed to:**
    a) take a deep breath and hold it
    b) squeeze the eyes shut tightly
    c) look up
    d) blink

30. **When performing the TBUT test, the observer is looking for:**
    a) the appearance of dry spots
    b) pooling of the fluorescein dye
    c) reflex tearing
    d) drainage of tears off the eye

31. **A TBUT of which of the following would indicate tear film dysfunction?**
    a) 10 seconds
    b) 20 seconds
    c) 30 seconds
    d) 40 seconds

Rose Bengal

32. **Rose bengal is:**
    a) a treatment for dry eye
    b) used in checking intraocular pressure
    c) used to dilate the pupil
    d) a staining agent

33. **A patient with which of the following potential diagnoses would be tested with rose bengal?**
    a) glaucoma
    b) corneal foreign body
    c) severe dry eye
    d) contact lens fitting

34. **Each of the following might be evaluated using rose bengal *except*:**
    a) corneal endothelial drop-out
    b) corneal abrasion
    c) corneal herpes simplex
    d) keratitis

35. **Each of the following is true regarding rose bengal *except*:**
    a) stinging may be severe
    b) it requires the use of the cobalt blue filter
    c) it stains tissue a reddish-pink color
    d) it is available in drop and strip form

Glare Testing

36. **Glare testing is used to identify:**
    a) irregular curvature of the crystalline lens
    b) decrease in vision due to glare conditions
    c) decrease in contrast sensitivity
    d) macular stress adaptation

37. **In which of the following would glare testing be most appropriate?**
    a) pterygium
    b) keratoconus
    c) posterior subcapsular cataract
    d) IOL calculations

38. **When performing a brightness acuity glare test, it is best to do which of the following?**
    a) Allow the patient to adjust to the light level before reading the letters.
    b) Do glare testing through the phoroptor.
    c) Time how long it takes for the patient to read the letters.
    d) Calibrate the instrument.

Color Vision Testing

39. **Which eye structure is responsible for color vision?**
    a) choroid
    b) rods
    c) cones
    d) optic nerve

40. **The photosensitive pigments of the eye are sensitive to:**
    a) red, green, and blue
    b) red, blue, and yellow
    c) red, green, and yellow
    d) green, blue, and yellow

41. **Color vision testing is used to detect all of the following *except*:**
    a) presence of normal color vision
    b) type and severity of color defect
    c) those who may not qualify for certain jobs
    d) differentiate between congenital or acquired color blindness

42. **The Ishihara color plates are useful:**
    a) for screening purposes, such as job applications
    b) for detailed information on a patient's color defect
    c) as a basis for referral to a neuro-ophthalmologist
    d) only for those who already know they have a defect

43. **To test a patient with the color pseudoisochromatic plates:**
    a) the plates should be held at 10 inches
    b) the patient should be tested without correction
    c) the patient should be tested with near correction, if worn
    d) the patient must have at least 20/30 vision at near

44. **Illumination for the color plates test:**
    a) varies according to the type of test administered
    b) should come from an easel lamp in a dark room
    c) should be natural daylight
    d) should be one-fifth of the room light

45. **Before proceeding with the actual color plate test:**
    a) the patient is shown a sample that is discernable to normal and abnormal alike
    b) the patient is shown a sample that is discernable only to those with a color deficit
    c) the lights should be dimmed
    d) the patient should be dilated

46. **A color plate that shows no obvious number to normal and abnormal alike is useful because:**
    a) it identifies those with vision too poor to do the regular test
    b) a malingerer may invent a number, thus identifying him- or herself
    c) it causes the patient to be more alert
    d) it creates doubt, so that the patient is unaware of his or her score

47. **How long should the patient be given to recognize the figure in a color plate?**
    a) 2 to 3 seconds
    b) 10 to 15 seconds
    c) 30 to 40 seconds
    d) as long as he or she needs

48. **Young children can be tested using the color plates:**
    a) only if they know numbers
    b) only if they know colors
    c) by having them trace the number/figure
    d) by having them describe the number/figure

49. **When using color plates, a score indicates abnormal color vision:**
    a) when the patient misses 5% of the plates
    b) when the patient misses 10% of the plates
    c) when the patient misses 20% of the plates
    d) varies according to the type of test

50. **Hereditary color defects most often fall into which category?**
    a) red-green
    b) blue-yellow
    c) monochromic
    d) multichromic

51. **Hereditary color vision defects affect:**
    a) males and females equally
    b) more males than females
    c) males only
    d) females only

52. **Hereditary color vision defects usually affect:**
    a) both eyes equally
    b) one eye more than the other
    c) one eye only
    d) the dominant eye

53. **Which of the following should be color-vision tested one eye at a time?**
    a) suspected blue-yellow defect
    b) suspected red-green defect
    c) suspected congenital color defect
    d) suspected acquired color defect

54. **Acquired color vision defects:**
    a) can often be cured by wearing a green contact lens on one eye
    b) can often be cured if the causative factor is eliminated
    c) can often be cured by retinal surgery
    d) can often be cured by injections of photosensitive pigment

55. **If the patient is suspected of having an acquired color vision defect, all of the following apply *except*:**
    a) each eye can have a different degree of deficit
    b) the defect tends to remain stable over time
    c) he or she will tend to make color errors scattered all across the color wheel
    d) they can resolve

56. **When should a child have his or her color vision checked?**
    a) Only if there is a family history of color blindness.
    b) Prior to age 4.
    c) Before starting school.
    d) By age 10.

57. **Color vision defects in children are frequently detected among those with:**
    a) reading disabilities
    b) retinoblastoma
    c) sickle cell disease
    d) attention deficit disorder

Contact A-Scan[2]

58. **The axial length of an average adult eye is:**
    a) 21 to 22 mm
    b) 23 to 24 mm
    c) 26 to 27 mm
    d) 29 to 30 mm

59. **The axial length of the eye is important in the calculation of:**
    a) contact lens parameters
    b) corneal graft power
    c) IOL power
    d) keratometric parameters

60. **In evaluating an axial length scan, the retinal echo must be:**
    a) to the right of the scleral and orbital echoes
    b) the shortest of the scan
    c) in the center of the scan
    d) to the left of the scleral and orbital echoes

61. **In an axial length A-scan, if there is only one tall echo from the back of the eye with no other echoes behind it, this indicates:**
    a) the presence of a tumor and that an x-ray should be done
    b) that the sound beam is directed to the macula and the measurement is correct
    c) that the sound beam is directed to the optic disc and the measurement is incorrect
    d) that the sound beam is directed at the macula and the measurement is incorrect

62. **A measurement error of 1 mm in an axial eye length could result in an unwanted postoperative refractive error of as much as:**
    a) 0.1 D
    b) 1.0 D
    c) 0.3 D
    d) 3.0 D

63. **When comparing the axial lengths of a patient's left and right eye, how much of a difference between the eyes should signal you to repeat the measurement of both eyes?**
    a) 1.0 mm
    b) 0.5 mm
    c) 0.3 mm
    d) 0.1 mm

[2]This category specifically designates contact A-scan versus immersion and IOLMaster methods. For diagnostic A-scan questions, see Chapter 13.

64. **An A-scan can be artificially shortened due to:**
    a) pressing on the globe too hard with the probe
    b) not using enough topical anesthetic
    c) measuring through a dilated pupil
    d) high hyperopia and astigmatism

65. **Which of the following A-scans would you use (Figure 16-1)?**

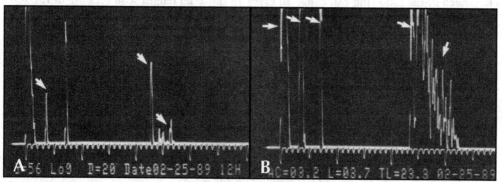

Figure 16-1. Reprinted with permission of Kendall CJ. *Ophthalmic Echography.* Thorofare, NJ: SLACK Incorporated; 1990.

Laser Interferometry (IOLMaster)

66. **Laser interferometry uses which type of laser light?**
    a) microwave
    b) ultrasonic
    c) infrared
    d) polarized

67. **The IOLMaster eliminates which of the following sources of error?**
    a) shortened axial length due to compression
    b) distorted corneal curvature due to improper alignment
    c) inaccurate corneal diameter measurements due to parallax error
    d) mathematical formula selection errors

68. **When positioning the IOLMaster for the axial length reading:**
    a) only the center of the visual axis may be used
    b) only a totally clear cornea is readable
    c) focus can be moved off-axis to obtain a clear reading
    d) the probe tip must be perpendicular to the corneal surface

69. **The IOLMaster evaluates each of the following *except*:**
    a) horizontal corneal diameter
    b) corneal curvature
    c) refractive error
    d) anterior chamber depth

70. **For safety reasons, the limit for the number of readings that may be taken per eye per day with the IOLMaster is:**
    a) 5
    b) 10
    c) 15
    d) 20

71. **Each of the following can cause an error in the axial length scan reading of the IOL-Master *except*:**
    a) patient wearing contact lenses
    b) patient wearing spectacles
    c) patient not fixating
    d) patient with retinal detachment

72. **The ideal IOLMaster axial length graph is:**
    a) a tall, central spike with only one peak and smaller spikes on either side
    b) a tall, central spike with two peaks and smaller spikes on the left
    c) a tall spike with only one peak and smaller spikes to the left
    d) a small, central spike and taller spikes on either side

73. **With the IOLMaster, the ideal signal-to-noise ratio is:**
    a) 0 or less
    b) 0.5
    c) 1.5
    d) 2.0 or more

Explanatory Answers

1. b) The desired postoperative refraction must be entered into the equation in order for the proper IOL to be selected. In some cases, it may be best for a plano postoperative refraction. However, some patients may prefer to be left a little nearsighted in order to read without correction following surgery. Other possibilities exist as well.

2. d) In the absence of other problems (such as vastly dissimilar K readings between the two eyes), this reading is within the normal range. You were not given enough information to indicate whether or not lenticular astigmatism was present.

3. c) Nearly all of the IOL calculation formulas are based on the same type of equation in which the axial length of the eye, the depth of the anterior chamber, tissue velocity, and the refractive powers of the cornea and IOL are factors.

4. a) The A-constant is a number provided by the IOL manufacturer that is specific to that type of IOL. The number is entered into the IOL calculation formula.

5. b) It can be very difficult to obtain accurate corneal power readings (by Ks, IOLMaster, or corneal topography) on patients who have previously had corneal refractive surgery.

6. a) The white-to-white corneal diameter measurement is used in the event an anterior chamber lens is needed. The other answers, in addition to desired postoperative refraction, are all needed input for IOL calculation. There are various formulas that can be used; which one is used depends on several factors, including surgeon preference.

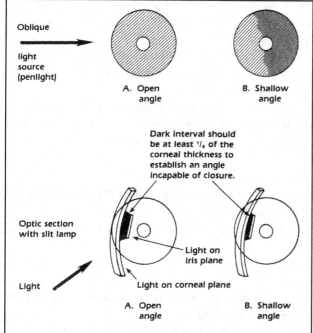

Figure 16-2. Techniques for assessing the angle opening. Top: Penlight method. Bottom: Slit lamp method. (Reprinted with permission of Nemeth SC, Shea CA. *Medical Sciences for the Ophthalmic Assistant.* Thorofare, NJ: SLACK Incorporated; 1988.)

7. a) The light should be directed from the side when using a penlight to estimate chamber depth, to see if the iris casts a shadow across the anterior chamber past the pupil (Figure 16-2).

8. d) Because the iris is lying flat, little or no shadow would be cast across the angle (see Figure 16-2).

9. a) If the angle is narrow or the iris is bunched up, a shadow is cast across the angle (see Figure 16-2).

10. b) Dilating a narrow angle can lead to an angle-closure glaucoma attack. Irreversible vision loss can result.

11. c) If you are using the slit lamp to evaluate the chamber depth, an open angle would have a dark interval one-fourth (or more) of the total corneal width (see Figure 16-2).

12. b) A narrow beam (the narrowest available) directed at the limbus from about 60 degrees is used to evaluate chamber depth. This method puts a sharply focused beam of light on the cornea and an unfocused beam on the iris. The dark band in between these two is the object of your interest, because it represents the depth of the anterior chamber (ie, the space between the cornea and iris). Compare the width of the shadow to the width of the corneal band (see Figure 16-2). If the shadow is one-fourth to one-half as wide as the corneal band, then the angle is open (or the chamber is deep). If the shadow is less than one-fourth that of the corneal band, then the angle is narrow (or the chamber is shallow). If the shadow is missing, then the cornea and iris are so close together that the angle is closed or nearly closed (or the chamber is flat).

13. b) Pachymetry is usually performed with an ultrasonic measurement. (There is an optical pachymeter that uses the slit lamp, but in general the ultrasonic unit is easier to use and more portable.)

14.   d) The probe must be held perpendicular to the portion of the corneal surface being measured. When measuring central cornea, this is not too difficult. The hard part is measuring the periphery, where the cornea is more curved.

15.   c) The thickness of the cornea is vital information in refractive surgery, where instruments are used to alter the shape of the cornea in order to change the patient's refractive error. An error could result in a perforation or inaccurate correction.

16.   b) The central cornea should be the easiest to measure, because it is easier to maintain proper alignment in this position. It is also the thinnest part of the cornea, providing a number with which to compare subsequent readings. Therefore, it is best to start the measurements with the central cornea.

17.   d) Research has shown that a person with a thinner cornea is more likely to develop glaucoma than someone with a thick cornea. Therefore, measuring the central corneal thickness has become standard of care in evaluating glaucoma.

18.   c) The average corneal thickness is about 545 μm. (Answer d, 655 μm, is the average corneal thickness at the limbus.)

19.   c) Each instrument is supplied with a "test eye" that is used daily for calibration prior to measuring any patients.

20.   b) Anytime that a biometry instrument fails the calibration test, it should be removed from service. Call the manufacturer for further instructions.

21.   d) Dacryocystitis is an infection of the tear sac and does not affect tear production.

22.   c) Schirmer's test I does not use topical anesthetic; Schirmer's test II does.

23.   b) Because no anesthetic is used, the Schirmer's test I measures tears that form as a response to irritation. These are called *reflex tears*.

24.   c) The use of anesthetic in Schirmer's test II eliminates the tearing due to irritation by the test strip. Thus, normal tearing is measured.

25.   c) Both Schirmer's tests have a 5-minute test time.

26.   a) Test strips are the only expense of the Schirmer's test (plus topical anesthetic, if used), and they are relatively inexpensive (as far as medical supplies go).

27.   d) A Schirmer's test of 10 mm or more is considered normal.

28.   b) TBUT does not use tear filter papers. Do not be confused by fluorescein-impregnated strips!

29.   d) Just before you begin timing the TBUT test, have the patient blink. This spreads the fluorescein dye over the cornea. Timing is begun just after the blink, and the patient is asked not to blink again until told to do so.

30.   a) Time is counted until the fluorescein shows that the tear film is breaking down, evidenced by the appearance of dry spots where the dye seems to "open up."

31.   a) The TBUT is considered abnormal if less than 10 to 15 seconds. (References vary between 10 and 15 seconds, but all agree that 10 seconds or less is abnormal.)

32.   d) Rose bengal (it is actually a derivative of fluorescein) is a staining agent used to identify dead or degenerated epithelial cells.

33.   c) Severe dry eye (keratoconjunctivitis sicca, often associated with autoimmune diseases such as rheumatoid arthritis) is the classic diagnosis for which rose bengal testing is performed. The dye causes dead or degenerated epithelial cells as well as mucus to stain red.

34.   a) The point of this question is to emphasize that rose bengal is used to evaluate conditions involving epithelial (not endothelial) cells, including cornea and conjunctiva. Most practitioners will use standard fluorescein dye for these indications, however.

35.   b) Rose bengal does not require use of the cobalt blue or any other filter. The other state-
       ments are true.
36.   b) The glare test helps measure the patient's acuity in the presence of marked glare. In
       certain situations (notably media opacities, such as posterior subcapsular cataracts, corneal
       scarring, posterior capsule opacity, etc), glare will cause a drop in vision by causing the
       patient's pupil to constrict. This forces the patient to try to look directly through the opac-
       ity.
37.   c) Glare testing in the presence of posterior subcapsular cataracts is especially dramatic
       because the glare causes the pupil to constrict (see answer 36).
38.   a) Allow the patient a few seconds to adjust to the level of light before asking him or her to
       read the chart.[3] If the patient has had a change in his or her refractive error, trial frames and
       lenses should be used as the phoroptor blocks some of the light from the brightness acuity
       tester (BAT). The BAT is factory calibrated. The *macular photostress test* is where a bright
       light is shown into the patient's eye for 10 seconds (the BAT may be used, although this is
       not considered a glare test), then time is counted until the patient can read letters two lines
       larger than his or her original acuity. Normal recovery is 0 to 30 seconds, but can be much
       longer in patients with macular problems.
39.   c) The cone cells are responsible for color vision. The rods function in dim lighting and
       give only shades of gray. The optic nerve is a conductor, but does not collect light itself,
       nor does the choroid.
40.   a) The eye's pigments are sensitive to red, green, and blue. Do not be confused by the so-
       called primary colors listed in answer b.
41.   d) A color vision test in and of itself cannot differentiate between congenital or acquired
       color defects. Certain professions may reject applicants who do not have normal color
       vision. (Of note, some tests merely give a yes/no and type of defect present, while others
       identify the severity of the deficit.)
42.   a) The standard pseudoisochromatic color plates are to be used as a screening device. For
       more detailed color-vision information, other tests are needed (such as arrangement tests).
43.   c) The patient should wear habitual near correction when being tested with the color plates.
       The plates should be held at 14 to 16 inches.
44.   a) Read the instructions for your particular set of color plates to get illumination require-
       ments.
45.   a) The color plate test starts with a figure that everyone can see, regardless of whether a
       color deficit exists or not.
46.   b) A patient may try to fool you by inventing a number for the "blank" plate.
47.   a) The patient should be given 2 to 3 seconds to identify the number in the color plates.
48.   c) Ask young children to trace the pattern formed by the different-colored dots with a cotton
       swab (to avoid marring the test plates).
49.   d) The number a patient can miss before being considered abnormal also varies from one
       test to another. Consult the instructions.
50.   a) Most hereditary defects are red-green.
51.   b) The incidence of hereditary color vision defects is 8% in males and 0.5% females, but
       either gender may be affected.
52.   a) Both eyes are usually affected equally in hereditary color vision problems, so the screen-
       ing color test can be done with both eyes together.
53.   d) If one suspects an acquired color defect, the eyes should be tested separately.

[3]Available at: www.agingeye.net/cataract/BATMANUAL.pdf. Accessed 12/10/11.

54. b) If the cause of an acquired color deficit is removed, color vision may return to normal.

55. b) An acquired defect (as opposed to a congenital defect) tends to gradually worsen unless the cause is treated. Because an acquired defect may affect the eyes differently, each eye should be tested separately. (Congenital defects can be tested with both eyes together.) Instead of making matching errors in a specific color range, as with a congenital defect, those with acquired defects tend to make matching errors scattered all across the color wheel. (There are, of course, exceptions.)

56. c) Before starting school is a good time to test a child's color vision. Answer a is wrong because of the word "only."

57. a) Children with reading disabilities often have color vision deficits as well.

58. b) The average adult eye is 23 to 24 mm.

59. c) Axial length is essential in the calculation of IOL powers. Contact lens parameters are external. Axial length does not figure into keratometric readings. Transplanted corneal grafts do not have calculated power.

60. d) The retinal echo is to the left of the scleral and orbital echoes (because the sclera and orbit are behind the retina).

61. c) If the A-scan beam is falling on the optic disc, only one echo will appear from the back of the eye. Because the reading should be taken from the macula, this would be an inaccurate measurement.

62. d) An error of 1 mm on the A-scan measurement can be translated to an undesired postoperative refractive error of about 3.0 D.

63. c) A difference in axial length between the two eyes of *less* than 0.3 mm is considered a normal variation. A difference of 0.3 mm or more is just cause for repeat measurements.

64. a) Pushing on the globe artificially shortens the eye. A high hyperope usually has a shorter eye, but it is naturally shorter, not artificially so.

65. b) In Figure 16-1B, all echoes are clearly defined, tall, and steeply rising. Figure 16-1A shows insufficient anterior lens, retinal, scleral, and orbital fat echoes.

66. c) Laser interferometry uses infrared laser light.

67. a) The IOLMaster measures axial length without contacting the cornea, so there is no artificial shortening of the measurement due to pressing on the globe with an ultrasonic probe.

68. c) Unlike conventional ultrasonic measurements, the IOLMaster reading is not dependent on measuring from the visual axis. Sometimes, maneuvering the focus a little bit around the visual axis will give a more ideal display. This way, the scan can be obtained even in the presence of small media opacities. There is no physical contact between the instrument and the patient's eye.

69. c) The IOLMaster does not perform automated refractometry readings.

70. d) No more than 20 measurements should be taken on an eye in a single day. (In fact, the instrument has a built-in safety feature that prevents this.)

71. b) In cases of high refractive errors (more than 6 D), the measurement may be taken with the patient wearing his or her spectacles. (This is only done so that the patient can see the fixation light/device.)

72. a) The ideal axial length scan on the IOLMaster is a tall, central spike that has only one peak. (It is important to zoom in on this spike to make sure that there are not multiple peaks; otherwise, you may miss this.) There should be smaller spikes on either side.[4]

73. d) A signal-to-noise ratio of 2.0 or more is desirable. But the axial length display must also be considered in identifying useable measurements.

[4]Available at: www.meditec.zeiss.com/C1256CAB00599F5D?Open. Accessed 8/25/11.

Chapter 17

Tonometry

Ledford JK.
*Certified Ophthalmic Assistant: Exam
Review Manual, Third Edition* (pp. 271-284).
© 2012 Taylor & Francis Group.

Goldmann Applanation Tonometer

Clean[1]

1.   **When cleaning the applanation tonometer, one must be careful not to:**
     a) remove the biprism
     b) bend the pressure-sensitive arm
     c) turn the adjustment knob
     d) cause scleral rigidity

2.   **The applanation tonometer unit itself may be cleaned by:**
     a) immersing in 3% hydrogen peroxide
     b) spraying and wiping with electronics cleaner
     c) gently wiping with damp cloth and mild soap
     d) spraying with disinfectant

3.   **The tonometer tip should be cleaned:**
     a) prior to being sterilized
     b) prior to being autoclaved
     c) prior to being boiled
     d) prior to being disinfected

Disinfect[2]

4.   **The tonometer tip should be disinfected:**
     a) morning and night
     b) first thing each day
     c) every 10 minutes
     d) between each patient

5.   **To best disinfect the tonometer tip, one should:**
     a) wipe it with a moist tissue
     b) swipe it with an alcohol wipe
     c) put it in a 10-minute soak in 3% hydrogen peroxide
     d) place it in the autoclave for 15 minutes

6.   **With regular use, soaking the tonometer tip in alcohol:**
     a) will not affect it
     b) will cause the numbers to fade
     c) will cause etching on the face
     d) will cause the plastic to soften

7.   **Failure to properly rinse the tonometer tip after disinfecting and prior to using it could result in:**
     a) corneal chemical burn
     b) inaccurate readings
     c) etching of the tip's surface
     d) clouding of the mires

[1]My JCAHPO® VOW says that this category refers to overall maintenance.
[2]My JCAHPO® VOW says that this category refers to cleaning (ie, degerming) between patients.

Calibrate

8. **Check calibration on the Goldmann applanation tonometer by:**
    a) placing the tip on a test block
    b) measuring an eye of known pressure
    c) use of a calibration bar
    d) returning it to the manufacturer

9. **When calibrating the Goldmann applanation tonometer at the 2 setting, the tonometer head should move:**
    a) no more than ±0.50 from the tested position
    b) 1.0 from the tested position
    c) freely in every position
    d) not at all

10. **The test positions for calibration of the Goldmann applanation tonometer are:**
    a) 0, 22, and 45 mm Hg
    b) 0, 20, and 60 mm Hg
    c) 10, 20, and 50 mm Hg
    d) 0, using a test block

11. **If you are calibrating an applanation tonometer for the 20 mm Hg setting, the drum will read:**
    a) 1
    b) 2
    c) 4
    d) 5

12. **If the applanation tonometer falls outside of the calibration allowance:**
    a) add or subtract from the final reading to offset the problem
    b) bend the tonometer arm until calibration is accurate
    c) turn the screw in the tonometer arm until calibration is accurate
    d) return the tonometer to the manufacturer for calibration

Measuring[3]

13. **The applanation tonometer measures intraocular pressure (IOP) by:**
    a) measuring the amount of pressure needed to indent the cornea
    b) measuring the amount of time needed to flatten the cornea
    c) measuring the IOP directly
    d) measuring the amount of pressure needed to flatten the cornea

14. **IOP as measured by applanation is recorded as:**
    a) mm Hg
    b) gm/mm^2
    c) a scale from 0 to 18
    d) lb/in^2

[3]While measuring is not, itself, listed as a criteria item, my JCAHPO® VOW states that COA® candidates are expected to know how to measure IOP with an applanation tonometer.

15. **Once the cornea is applanated, the force of the applanation tonometer is increased or decreased:**
    a) until the outer edges of the mires touch
    b) until the edges of the mires overlap
    c) until the inner edges of the mires touch
    d) until the upper mire is larger

16. **Wide mires in applanation tonometry will result in:**
    a) accurate readings
    b) falsely low readings
    c) falsely high readings
    d) increased patient comfort

17. **Thin mires in applanation tonometry will result in:**
    a) accurate readings
    b) falsely low readings
    c) falsely high readings
    d) decreased patient comfort

18. **All of the following can cause applanation tonometry errors *except*:**
    a) too much or too little fluorescein
    b) lack of contact with the eyelid
    c) misalignment of mires
    d) dirty tonometer face

19. **All of the following can result in inaccurate applanation readings, with no compensation method available, *except*:**
    a) astigmatism
    b) pterygium
    c) corneal scars
    d) corneal graft

20. **The applanation tonometer is preferred in cases of low scleral rigidity because:**
    a) it does not displace an appreciable amount of aqueous and, therefore, does not cause distention of the ocular structures
    b) it does not flatten the cornea and, therefore, does not cause distention of the ocular structures
    c) it is performed with the patient in a seated position and, therefore, gravity can equalize distention of the ocular structures
    d) topical anesthetic is used and, therefore, does not cause distention of the ocular structures

21. **The biprism design of the applanation tonometer:**
    a) makes it easier to align than an indentation tonometer
    b) makes it more accurate than indentation tonometry
    c) offsets scleral rigidity factors
    d) makes it more comfortable than indentation tonometry

22. **Each of the following is an advantage of applanation tonometry** *except*:

a) it gives an excellent binocular view of the mires

b) it is the most accurate method of checking IOP

c) the tonometer tip is easily cleaned and disinfected

d) it is accurate even in the presence of low scleral rigidity

23. **Disadvantages of applanation tonometry include all of the following** *except*:

a) it is expensive

b) slit-lamp models are not portable

c) it can be difficult to learn to use

d) one must use a chart to convert the reading

24. **Match the following with the drawings using each answer only once. (All drawings reprinted with permission of Herrin MP.** *Ophthalmic Examination and Basic Skills.* **Thorofare, NJ: SLACK Incorporated; 1990.)**

proper position for measurement	too close
reading is too low	too far back
reading is too high	too much fluorescein
vertical position is off	not enough fluorescein

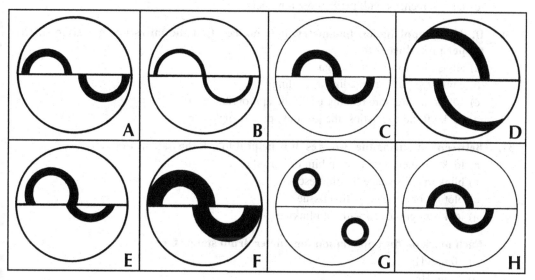

25. **You have just realized that you instilled regular fluorescein into an eye with a soft contact. What do you do next?**

a) perform the applanation over the lens

b) remove the lens, and rinse it immediately

c) irrigate the eye with the lens in it

d) slide the lens to the side, and take the measurement

26. **For proper applanation, the slit-lamp light should be set up as follows:**

a) at a 60 degree angle, with the cobalt blue filter, and with the light source completely open

b) at a 45 degree angle, with the red-free filter, and with the light source completely open

c) at a 90 degree angle, with the cobalt blue filter, and a narrow beam

d) at a 60 degree angle, with the cobalt blue filter, and a pinpoint light beam

27. **During applanation tonometry, the patient is instructed to:**
    a) close the eye not being tested, hold his or her breath, and look up
    b) open both eyes, breathe normally, and look to the right
    c) open both eyes, breathe normally, and look straight ahead
    d) open both eyes, hold his or her breath, and look straight ahead

28. **Each of the following can be key in accurate applanation tonometry *except*:**
    a) the patient should loosen a tight collar
    b) the patient should clamp his or her teeth
    c) the patient should not strain to reach the slit lamp
    d) the patient should relax the shoulders and neck

29. **Your patient is a 45-year-old executive. You have just taken his applanation tonometry reading, and it is 28. There is no history of glaucoma in the family. His readings for the past 10 years at annual exams in your office have been 20. You lean back, scratch your head, then ask the patient to:**
    a) come back for a reading in the afternoon
    b) drink a lot of water to see if this will affect the pressure reading
    c) loosen his tie and collar, then repeat the measurement
    d) let you recheck with the Schiøtz tonometer

30. **If, during applanation tonometry, it is noticed that the mires are not aligned, the proper procedure is to:**
    a) adjust the joystick to realign
    b) adjust the pressure reading accordingly
    c) adjust the pressure reading using the appropriate chart
    d) back off the eye, adjust the joystick, then reapplanate

31. **Between measuring the two eyes, it is helpful to ask the patient to:**
    a) look left then right to help him or her relax
    b) blink to redistribute the fluorescein
    c) blot his or her eyes with a tissue
    d) look straight ahead without blinking

32. **Each mark on the applanation tonometer drum stands for:**
    a) 10 mm Hg
    b) 2 mm Hg
    c) 1 mm Hg
    d) 2 g/mm^2

33. **The reading on the applanation tonometer drum is 2. The patient's IOP is:**
    a) 20 mm Hg
    b) 4 mm Hg
    c) 2 mm Hg
    d) 4 g/mm^2

34. **In properly aligned applanation tonometry:**
    a) there are no factors that affect the IOP
    b) the mires will pulsate slightly with the heartbeat
    c) the mires will pulsate slightly when the patient breathes
    d) accuracy is ensured if the patient does not blink

35. **When the applanation tonometer mires pulsate, the IOP:**
    a) is the lowest of the readings
    b) is the highest of the readings
    c) is the difference between the 2 readings
    d) is at the midpoint between the 2 readings

36. **One must make an adjustment to the applanation tonoprism if the patient's corneal astigmatism is:**
    a) greater than 1 D
    b) greater than 2 D
    c) greater than 3 D
    d) greater than 4 D

37. **If compensation for high corneal astigmatism is not made to the applanation tonometer, the IOP measurement could be in error by:**
    a) 1 mm Hg
    b) 2 to 3 mm Hg
    c) 4 to 5 mm Hg
    d) 8 to 10 mm Hg

38. **In order to compensate for high astigmatism with the applanation tonometer, the biprism should be aligned as follows:**
    a) the steepest axis aligned with the red line on the holder
    b) the plus axis aligned with the red line on the holder
    c) 45 degrees from the minus cylinder should be placed in the 90-degree position
    d) the minus axis aligned with the red line on the holder

39. **A scarred, irregular cornea is difficult to measure with the applanation tonometer because:**
    a) there is decreased scleral rigidity
    b) one cannot instill topical anesthetic because of tissue melt
    c) one cannot use fluorescein because it will infiltrate the tissue
    d) the mires are irregular, making it difficult to judge the endpoint

Complications

40. **The most common complication of contact tonometry is:**
    a) fainting
    b) allergy to anesthetic drops
    c) cardiac arrest
    d) conjunctivitis

41. **Corneal abrasions from tonometry can best be reduced by:**
    a) use of anesthetic
    b) proper fixation
    c) proper lighting
    d) holding the lids securely

42. **Measuring IOP is contraindicated in any patient:**
    a) who is nervous about the procedure
    b) who has possible optic nerve disease
    c) who has vision below 20/200
    d) who might have a penetrating injury

43. **Any type of contact tonometry must be avoided, if possible, in which patient?**
    a) patient with acquired immune deficiency syndrome (AIDS)
    b) patient with a corneal graft
    c) patient with epidemic keratoconjunctivitis
    d) children younger than 8 years of age

44. **If the patient has known human immunodeficiency virus (HIV), the assistant should:**
    a) refuse to take a pressure on the patient
    b) use only the noncontact tonometer
    c) wear gloves during contact tonometry
    d) place a tissue on the tonometer prism

45. **A patient who reports an allergy to topical anesthetics:**
    a) should have his or her IOP checked with a noncontact tonometer
    b) should be irrigated after contact tonometry if topical anesthetic is used
    c) cannot have a pressure check of any kind
    d) should tough out contact tonometry without drops

46. **All of the following can result in a falsely high IOP reading *except*:**
    a) breath holding
    b) moving the eye during the measurement
    c) straining to lean into the slit lamp
    d) squeezing the eyelids

Other Tonometry Methods[4]

47. **Schiøtz tonometry measures IOP by:**
    a) measuring the force it takes to equalize the eye's internal pressure
    b) measuring the force exerted on the instrument by the eye
    c) measuring the force it takes to flatten an area of the cornea
    d) measuring the force it takes to indent the cornea

[4]My JCAHPO® VOW has indicated that COA® candidates would be expected to know about alternate forms of tonometry.

48. **The Schiøtz tonometer readings:**
    a) are read from the instrument in millimeters of mercury
    b) are read from the instrument in gram weights
    c) must be converted to millimeters of fluorescein by use of a calculator
    d) must be converted to millimeters of mercury by use of a chart

49. **The Schiøtz tonometer should be disinfected:**
    a) at the beginning of each day
    b) at the end of each day
    c) between each patient
    d) when it appears dirty

50. **Patient position for Schiøtz tonometry is:**
    a) sitting up to the slit lamp
    b) sitting up in the exam chair
    c) lying back in the exam chair
    d) sitting at a 45 degree angle

51. **The patient is apprehensive about having that "air puff" test. She is most likely referring to:**
    a) the TonoPen
    b) the corneal sensitivity test
    c) a corneal biopsy
    d) noncontact tonometry

52. **The noncontact, or "air puff," tonometer measures:**
    a) the IOP directly
    b) either the time or force required to indent the cornea
    c) either the time or force required to flatten the cornea
    d) either the time or force required to photograph the cornea

53. **The noncontact tonometer is most useful for:**
    a) monitoring patients with glaucoma
    b) differentiating between ocular hypertension and glaucoma
    c) finding patients with low-tension glaucoma
    d) screening situations

Intraocular Pressure Dynamics[5]

54. **The aqueous humor is produced by the:**
    a) ciliary muscle
    b) ciliary body
    c) trabecular meshwork
    d) iris

[5]Although not listed as a specific criteria, my JCAHPO® VOW says that "the basic dynamics of IOP are referred to under tonometry."

55. **The composition of the aqueous is most like:**
    a) blood plasma
    b) tears
    c) saliva
    d) mucus

56. **The flow of aqueous in the eye follows this pattern:**
    a) angle, posterior chamber, pupil, anterior chamber
    b) angle, anterior chamber, pupil, posterior chamber
    c) pupil, posterior chamber, anterior chamber, angle
    d) posterior chamber, pupil, anterior chamber, angle

57. **As it exits the eye, aqueous humor flows in this pattern:**
    a) canal of Schlemm, trabecular meshwork, episcleral arteries
    b) trabecular meshwork, canal of Schlemm, episcleral veins
    c) trabecular meshwork, nasolacrimal duct, episcleral arteries
    d) canal of Schlemm, episcleral veins, trabecular meshwork

58. **IOP is determined by:**
    a) systolic and diastolic blood pressure
    b) rate of aqueous production and resistance to outflow
    c) pressure in the ophthalmic artery and vein
    d) cranial pressure transferred to the eye through the optic nerve

59. **Reduction and control of elevated IOP is based on:**
    a) lowering the diastolic and systolic blood pressure
    b) lowering cranial pressure
    c) increasing aqueous production and/or decreasing outflow
    d) decreasing aqueous production and/or increasing outflow

60. **Which of the following regarding aqueous and IOP is *not* true?**
    a) IOP is generally higher in the morning than in the evening.
    b) IOP is slightly higher in the posterior chamber than in the anterior chamber.
    c) Aqueous has no effect on the optical system of the eye.
    d) Aqueous provides nutrition and waste removal for internal ocular structures.

61. **Regarding the normal diurnal variation of IOP:**
    a) IOP is higher early in the morning
    b) IOP is lower early in the morning
    c) IOP reaches a peak around noon
    d) IOP is lowest around noon

62. **The diurnal curve of IOP in a glaucoma patient:**
    a) may vary by 4 mm Hg
    b) may vary up to 10 mm Hg
    c) is less than in an eye without glaucoma
    d) shows no variation in morning versus evening

63. **Elevated IOP as seen in chronic open-angle glaucoma is believed to be the result of:**
    a) decreased function of cells in the trabecular meshwork
    b) obstruction of the trabecular meshwork by particles
    c) overproduction of aqueous
    d) optic nerve damage

64. **Patients who experience an increase in IOP while using corticosteroids are called:**
    a) ocular hypertensives
    b) glaucoma suspects
    c) steroid regulators
    d) steroid responders

65. **If the cornea is extremely thick or scarred:**
    a) the IOP measurements will always be underestimated
    b) the IOP measurements will always be overestimated
    c) the IOP measurements can be accepted with reservations
    d) no tonometric measurement will be accurate enough to satisfy clinical needs

66. **You are about to do applanation tonometry on a patient, and she asks, "Will this tell you if I have glaucoma?" You answer:**
    a) "Yes, but Dr. Jackson will give you the results."
    b) "Only if the reading is abnormal."
    c) "No, this is just a screening."
    d) "Eye pressure is just one part of diagnosing glaucoma."

Explanatory Answers

1. b) The moveable arm that holds the biprism can be bent if care is not taken.
2. c) This recommendation comes from the manufacturer.[6] It is never a good idea to spray cleaner directly onto an instrument.
3. d) Technically, cleaning removes soil and debris and some germs. Disinfecting is the removal of all or most germs except bacterial spores (which are killed by sterilization). External debris is removed first (or at the same time) in order to allow all instrument surfaces to come into contact with the disinfectant.
4. d) Because the tonometer tip contacts the cornea and tear film, it must be disinfected (or a fresh, disinfected tip inserted) between each patient.
5. c) A 10-minute soak of bleach (1:10 dilution) or hydrogen peroxide is the best disinfection method. A moist tissue will not disinfect, nor will a quick "swipe" with alcohol (although some references suggest a 10-second wipe as acceptable). The autoclave will melt the tonometer tip.
6. b) Repeated exposure to alcohol can cause the numbers and lines on the side of the tonometer tip to fade and disappear.
7. a) Alcohol and hydrogen peroxide can cause marked discomfort, so the tip should be rinsed well and dried before using.
8. c) A calibration bar is placed in a special attachable holder when calibrating an applanation tonometer. If the calibration is not accurate, the instrument must be returned to the manufacturer.

[6]Available at: www.haag-streit-usa.com/pdf/disinfect.pdf

9. a) Movement of the tonometer arm should occur within 0.50 of the drum setting of 2. If you must turn the drum *more* than 0.50 before the arm will move, this indicates that the instrument is not accurate. Thus, when you are calibrating at 2, the arm should "rock" between the 1.95 and 2.05 reading on the drum.[7,8]

10. b) The calibration bar is marked to check the 0, 20, and 60 mm Hg readings on the tonometer. Especially pay attention to the calibration at 20 mm Hg, as this is often the crucial point in patients with glaucoma.

11. b) Remember, the drum readings are multiplied by 10, so the 20 mm Hg reading would translate to "2" on the drum.

12. d) Answers a through c might sound good, but the only way to recalibrate the tonometer is to return it to the manufacturer for servicing.

13. d) The applanation tonometer flattens the cornea and measures the amount of pressure required to do so. (By contrast, indentation tonometry measures the amount of pressure required to indent the cornea.)

14. a) Applanation tension is measured in millimeters of mercury (mm Hg).

15. c) The inner edges of the mires should touch when the reading is taken.

16. c) Wide mires (too much fluid) result in falsely high readings.

17. b) Thin mires (not enough fluid) result in falsely low readings.

18. b) The tonometer should not contact the eyelid at all.

19. a) Astigmatism over 3 D must be compensated for (see answers 36-38). There is no way to set the tonometer to compensate for a pterygium, scar, or graft—all of which can cause an inaccurate reading.

20. a) The applanation tonometer does not displace a significant enough amount of aqueous to cause even a more pliable eye to distend.

21. a) With the biprism, you have visual proof (the mires) of correct alignment.

22. a) The mires appear in only one ocular, making it monocular, not binocular. The other statements are true.

23. d) You do not need a conversion chart with applanation tonometry. The measurement is read directly off the drum.

24. Matching

proper position for measurement	c)
reading is too low	a)
reading is too high	h)
vertical position is off	e)
too close	d)
too far back	g)
too much fluorescein	f)
not enough fluorescein	b)

25. b) If you remove the lens and rinse it right away, you may be able to get the dye out before the lens is too stained.

26. a) To perform applanation tonometry, the light source should be at a 60 degree angle with the cobalt blue filter and full illumination.

[7]In the Cassin text, the range of movement for the tonometer arm at drum setting 2 is given as 1.8 and 2.2. I could not corroborate this with any other reference. All others say 1.95 and 2.05.

[8]When calibrating at the 6 drum setting, the movement should be no more than 5.9 and 6.1. Manufacturer details for calibration of the Haag-Streit tonometer is available at: www.haag-streit-usa.com/pdf/procedures-for-checking-tonometer-calibration.pdf.

27.   c) Applanation tensions are easier if the patient will open both eyes. The patient must look straight ahead for proper alignment. The patient should not hold his or her breath, as this can cause a falsely elevated IOP reading.

28.   b) The reading will be most accurate if the patient is relaxed.

29.   c) Have him loosen his tie and collar and try again. (The physician would be the one to order answers a or b.) The Schiøtz is less accurate than the applanation tonometer.

30.   d) Pull the tonometer off the cornea just slightly before adjusting position. Do not slide the tip around on the cornea.

31.   b) We ask the patient not to blink during the test, so the second eye may tend to be a little dry. A quick blink will spread the dye across the cornea.

32.   b) Each mark on the tonometer drum represents 2 mm Hg.

33.   a) If the number 2 on the drum is on the marker line, the IOP is 20. Each mark is 2 mm Hg, but each number is 10 mm Hg.

34.   b) The mires may pulsate slightly with the heartbeat (not with breathing). Even with accurate alignment, however, there are other factors that can induce error.

35.   d) Take the reading at midpoint between the readings during the pulsations.[9]

36.   c) The "magic number" is 3 D when it comes to resetting the tonoprism for astigmatism. Failure to do so may result in an erroneous measurement (see answers 37 and 38 for more information).

37.   b) If the biprism is not adjusted properly for the astigmatic cornea (more than 3 D), the IOP measurement could be 2 to 3 mm Hg off.

38.   d) Turn the biprism so that the axis (in minus cylinder) is in line with the red mark on the tonometer holder. It is best to get the cylinder reading from the keratometer rather than the patient's glasses prescription, because the glasses may also correct for lenticular astigmatism. (*Note:* Some sources say to turn the biprism 45 degrees from the flattest axis, which *is* the point indicated by the red line on the holder.)

39.   d) If the cornea is irregular, the mires will also be irregular. This makes it tough to tell when the inner edges are meeting.

40.   d) Spreading conjunctivitis from one patient to the next is the most common complication of contact tonometry.

41.   b) If the patient will fixate properly, holding the eye still, the risk of corneal abrasion is minimized. (Holding the lids securely would help, but b is the best answer.)

42.   d) A patient with a penetrating injury has an opening for bacteria to be introduced into the eye via fingers, eye drops, tonometer tip, etc. In addition, aqueous could be forced out of the eye during applanation.

43.   c) Epidemic keratoconjunctivitis is extremely contagious! There is no contraindication in any of the other cases.

44.   c) HIV has been isolated from human tears, so gloving is a wise precaution. (However, to my knowledge, there have been no reports of the virus being spread through contact with tears.)

45.   a) Use the noncontact tonometer on the patient who is sensitive to topical anesthetic, and you cannot go wrong. Answer b could be done if your doctor orders it. (The words "cannot...of any kind" should have clued you in that answer c was wrong.) I have done an occasional applanation tension using tear drops only, but it is not ideal.

[9]This is the standard "textbook" answer; some physicians may want the highest pressure indicated by the pulsations as a matter of individual preference.

46. b) Moving the eye during measurement changes alignment but does not falsely elevate the reading.
47. d) Schiøtz tonometry measures IOP by indentation.
48. d) The Schiøtz reading must be converted to mm Hg by use of a graph or chart.
49. c) Because the Schiøtz comes in direct contact with the cornea and tear film, it must be disinfected between each patient.
50. c) The patient must lie flat on his or her back for the reading.
51. d) Noncontact tonometry is often called the "air puff" test.
52. c) The noncontact tonometer may measure either time or force required to flatten the cornea.
53. d) The noncontact tonometer is adequate for screening, but will miss some elevated pressures. Thus, it is not sensitive enough for monitoring or diagnosing glaucoma.
54. b) The ciliary body, at the base of the iris (but not the iris itself), is responsible for aqueous production.
55. a) Blood plasma is most like aqueous in composition, with some difference in trace elements.
56. d) The aqueous flows out of the posterior chamber, through the pupil, into the anterior chamber, and then through the angle.
57. b) The flow of aqueous humor exiting the angle goes through the trabecular meshwork, into the canal of Schlemm, and from there into the episcleral veins. (Remember that veins carry blood to the *heart*. Arteries bring blood to an *organ*.)
58. b) IOP results from the combination of the amount of aqueous produced over time and its ability to drain out of the eye.
59. d) In order to lower the IOP (theoretically, at least), decrease the amount of aqueous being produced and/or increase the draining of it.
60. c) While slight, the aqueous does exert a refractive influence on light entering the eye. The IOP is slightly higher in the posterior chamber because the aqueous meets some resistance as it encounters the margin of the pupil. The circulating aqueous also acts to bring nutrients to and remove wastes from the eye's internal structures. Regarding answer a, see answer 61.
61. a) IOP varies during the day ("diurnal"). It is usually higher early in the morning and lower during the afternoon. (In monitoring glaucoma, many physicians will vary the time of day that a patient comes in for IOP checks, to get a clearer idea of how treatment is affecting the pressure.)
62. b) The diurnal curve of the IOP in a patient with glaucoma may vary up to 10 mm Hg, being higher in the morning. The average (nonglaucomatous) eye varies only by about 4 mm Hg. Thus, this larger fluctuation is a factor in both diagnosis and treatment of glaucoma.
63. a) The degeneration of the trabecular meshwork (in function and/or cell density) as seen in open-angle glaucoma is *not* a product of the normal aging process. It seems to be disease-specific. Obstruction by particulate matter would be a secondary glaucoma. While over-production of aqueous does exist, it is not the primary entity in open-angle glaucoma.
64. d) Steroids do not cause a rise in IOP in every patient, but those patients who do experience an IOP increase while on steroids are known as *steroid responders*.
65. d) This opinion comes from Brubaker in his excellent article entitled *Tonometry*.[10] Other sources agree.
66. d) Although often called "the glaucoma test," tonometry by itself is not adequate to diagnose glaucoma.

[10]Brubaker RF. Tonometry. Available at: www.oculist.net/downaton502/prof/ebook/duanes/pages/v3/v3c047.html.

Chapter 18

Visual
Assessment

Ledford JK.
*Certified Ophthalmic Assistant: Exam
Review Manual, Third Edition* (pp. 285-300).
© 2012 Taylor & Francis Group.

Visual Acuity

1. **Which of the following is the standard test done on virtually every patient at every visit?**
   a) pupil evaluation
   b) slit-lamp exam
   c) visual acuity
   d) tonometry

2. **The standard testing distance of 20 feet is used to test visual acuity because:**
   a) this is the distance at which the letters subtend 5 minutes of arc
   b) this is the length of most eye exam rooms
   c) this relaxes accommodation
   d) this stimulates accommodation

3. **The figures on an eye chart or acuity card—whether letters, numbers, symbols, or pictures—are known as:**
   a) Snellens
   b) optotypes
   c) points
   d) Allens

4. **The top number (numerator) of the notation "20/20" means:**
   a) the size of the optotypes
   b) the vision of a "normal" eye
   c) the test distance
   d) the patient's acuity

5. **The bottom number (denominator) of the notation "20/20" means:**
   a) the normal eye can recognize optotypes of this size from 2 feet away
   b) the normal eye can recognize optotypes of this size from 20 feet away
   c) an acuity quotient of 1%
   d) the testing distance is 1 foot

6. **A visual acuity of 20/20 or better (corrected or uncorrected) indicates all of the following *except*:**
   a) the media are clear
   b) the optic nerve is functioning properly
   c) the fovea is being used for fixation
   d) the rod cells are functioning normally

7. **A person with 20/80 vision:**
   a) sees at 80 feet what the normal eye can see at 20 feet
   b) sees at 20 feet what the normal eye can see at 80 feet
   c) can see better than 20/20
   d) has a refractive error

8. **The patient's acuity is noted to be 10/40. This indicates:**
   a) a test distance that is one-fourth of normal
   b) a test distance of 40 feet
   c) a test distance of 20 feet
   d) a test distance of 10 feet

9. **A visual acuity of 20/15 means that:**
   a) the patient was 15 feet away from the chart
   b) the patient missed five of the optotypes
   c) the patient could not see 20/20 optotypes
   d) the patient's vision is better than 20/20

10. **A vision of 15/20 is tested how far from the target?**
    a) 0.5 feet
    b) 10 feet
    c) 15 feet
    d) 20 feet

11. **The patient's acuity is noted to be 5/200. Convert this to a standard "20/X" acuity notation.**
    a) 20/40
    b) 20/400
    c) 20/800
    d) 20/1000

12. **The illumination in the examination room during the distant acuity test:**
    a) should be no less than half of the chart's illumination
    b) should be no less than one-fifth of the chart's illumination
    c) should be increased
    d) should be turned off

13. **Which of the following is an inadequate occluder?**
    a) near vision card
    b) 3 × 5 index card
    c) eye patch
    d) patient's hand

14. **A patient should be told not to squint during the acuity test because:**
    a) squinting will give a falsely low acuity
    b) squinting will give a falsely high acuity
    c) squinting will make the pupil enlarge
    d) squinting will make the pupil smaller

15. **Which of the following acuity tests is appropriate for an illiterate patient?**
    a) Snellen letters, numbers, and pictures
    b) Snellen letters, Sheridan Gardner test, and numbers
    c) Snellen letters, E game, and numbers
    d) E game, Landolt C, and sometimes numbers

16. **All of the following could cause falsely low distance acuity readings *except*:**
    a) a fingerprint on the projector bulb
    b) smudges on the chart, mirrors, or slides
    c) an old projector bulb
    d) a laminated acuity chart closer than 20 feet

17. **The standard acuity chart or projector can produce a falsely high sense of the patient's usable vision because:**
    a) it is low contrast
    b) it is high contrast
    c) it does not have any contrast
    d) it is more accurate than a potential acuity meter reading

18. **The standard Snellen chart may not be adequate for evaluating how a patient really sees because:**
    a) it is not as accurate as a visual field test
    b) it does not measure macular function
    c) the "real world" is a mixture of shadows and contrast
    d) it is easy to memorize

    For Questions 19 and 20, use the following eye chart:
    EGNUS 20/50
    FPEDZ 20/40
    OFLTZ 20/30
    APEOF 20/25
    EVOTZ 20/20

19. **The patient reads "EGNUS" then "PPFOS." Vision is recorded as:**
    a) 20/50 + 1
    b) 20/40 – 4
    c) 20/50
    d) 20/40 + 1

20. **The patient reads "FPEDZ, OPLFZ, ADPSP." Vision is recorded as:**
    a) 20/40 + 3 + 1
    b) 20/25 – 4 – 1
    c) 20/30 – 2 + 1
    d) 20/30 – 2

21. **If the patient cannot read the Snellen 20/400 line until he is 10 feet from it, vision is recorded as:**
    a) 20/10
    b) 10/400
    c) 2/40
    d) 10/200

22. **A new patient's records have the following: VA cc 20/40 OD, 20/20 OS. Which of the following is *true*?**
    a) The patient's vision was checked without glasses.
    b) The patient's vision was checked with glasses.
    c) The patient's vision was checked with both eyes together.
    d) The patient's vision was checked with a pinhole.

23. **In the same patient as above, which of the following is *true*?**
    a) The vision in the patient's right eye is 20/20.
    b) The vision in the patient's left eye is 20/40.
    c) The vision in the patient's left eye is 20/20.
    d) The patient's cumulative vision is 20/60.

24. **If the patient is unable to read the Snellen 20/400 line:**
    a) vision does not need to be evaluated further
    b) a refractometric measurement should be done
    c) vision can only be checked with a Snellen chart
    d) decrease testing distance until he or she can recognize the 20/400 figure

25. **If a patient is unable to read the largest letters on the chart, another option is to:**
    a) have him or her count fingers at increasing distances
    b) switch to an illiterate chart
    c) refrain from further vision testing
    d) have him or her move further back from the chart

26. **If a patient is unable to count fingers at 6 inches, the next option is to:**
    a) record "blind" on the patient's record
    b) do a glare test
    c) do a contrast sensitivity test
    d) see if he or she can detect hand movement

27. **The hand motion test:**
    a) should be done by increasing the testing distance after each accurate response
    b) should be done by moving the hand 3 inches in front of the patient's face
    c) can be done at any distance from the patient because the distance is irrelevant
    d) should be done with both eyes opened

28. **Under what circumstances would you use a penlight (or muscle light) to evaluate a patient's vision?**
    a) When he or she has failed to read the Snellen chart.
    b) When he or she has failed to count fingers.
    c) When he or she has failed to see hand motion.
    d) When he or she has failed the glare test.

29. **The difference between light perception and light projection is:**
    a) light perception is the ability to locate the light; light projection is the ability to see the light
    b) light perception vision is better than light projection
    c) light perception is the ability to see light; light projection is the ability to locate the light
    d) light perception can be done with children; light projection is done in adults

30. **If the patient is unable to see *or* locate the light, his or her vision is recorded as:**
    a) no light perception (NLP)
    b) legally blind
    c) malingering
    d) subnormal

31. **When checking a patient's near vision, it is important to:**
    a) have the patient wear his or her usual reading glasses
    b) have the patient use a pinhole instead of any usual reading glasses
    c) remove contact lenses, if worn
    d) check both eyes together rather than one at a time

32. **The patient should be told to hold the near card:**
    a) at whatever distance gives the best vision
    b) at 14 to 16 inches
    c) at 1 meter
    d) in his or her lap

33. **Each of the following represents normal near vision *except*:**
    a) 14/14
    b) J2
    c) N5
    d) L1

34. **Vision with both eyes together:**
    a) is never checked
    b) is usually slightly better than each eye tested alone
    c) is usually slightly worse than each eye tested alone
    d) should be checked without correction

35. **If the patient consistently misses the letters on the right side of the chart:**
    a) this is unimportant
    b) he or she should be pressure patched immediately
    c) a visual field defect may be present
    d) he or she is obviously malingering

36. **Your patient informs you that, because you checked her vision at last week's appointment, she does not need it checked today. You should:**
    a) honor her wishes and skip the test
    b) explain why vision needs to be checked at every visit
    c) write "patient is uncooperative" in the chart
    d) tell your physician

37. **Visual acuity in a patient with posterior subcapsular cataracts will usually worsen when tested:**
    a) in bright light
    b) in dim light
    c) at near as opposed to distance
    d) after being dilated, in dim light

38. **It is appropriate to include notes with the visual acuity measurement to indicate:**
a) the patient's attention during the test
b) accuracy of occlusion
c) illumination of the chart
d) illumination of the room

39. **It is appropriate to include notes with the visual acuity measurement to indicate:**
a) the use of contact lenses or low-vision aids
b) how wide open the patient's eyes were during the test
c) the pupil width during the test indicating accommodation
d) eye redness that might affect the vision

40. **In an ocular emergency, visual acuity should be checked:**
a) only after instilling numbing drops
b) only if the patient complains of vision loss
c) in every case
d) on a case-by-case basis

41. **A malingerer is:**
a) a patient who cannot read
b) a patient who cannot verbalize
c) a patient who intentionally and falsely claims to have poor vision
d) a patient who has poor vision due to hysteria

42. **The "crowding phenomenon" affects the visual acuity of patients with:**
a) astigmatism
b) strabismus
c) amblyopia
d) ametropia

43. **Because of the "crowding phenomenon," it is best to check visual acuity:**
a) in a room with no other people present
b) with both eyes open
c) using isolated figures
d) using a row of figures

44. **In checking visual acuity of children, the most important information is:**
a) whether or not the vision is 20/40 or better
b) the patient's vision with both eyes opened
c) any difference between the acuity of the two eyes
d) whether or not the vision in each eye is 20/20

45. **The presence of vision in an infant may be tested by:**
a) noting the child's reaction to his or her mother
b) noting the child's reaction if his or her mother leaves the room
c) seeing if the child's eyes follow a moving light
d) seeing if the child's eyes follow a squeaking toy

46. **Which of the following notations means that a 6-month-old infant's vision is probably normal?**
    a) Allen card vision of 10/10
    b) fixates on a bright light in dark room
    c) searching movements, OU
    d) central, steady, and maintained

47. **All of the following are true regarding the preferential looking test (using Teller or similar visual acuity cards) *except*:**
    a) it may be used for any nonverbal patient, infant or otherwise
    b) the patient will automatically look at the card with the stripes
    c) there is a tendency to underestimate vision with this test
    d) the stripes are graded for finer and finer acuity

48. **A 3-month-old may be tested for amblyopia by which of the following methods?**
    a) Worth 4 dot testing
    b) rating central, steady, and maintained
    c) preferential looking technique
    d) stereo testing

49. **A 6-month-old baby continues to look at you happily if you cover her right eye. If you cover her left eye, she becomes distracted and tries to move away from the cover. This may indicate:**
    a) vision is equal in both eyes
    b) vision is better in the right eye
    c) vision is weaker in the right eye
    d) vision is weaker in the left eye

50. **In the patient above, an appropriate notation of her vision would be:**
    a) prefers OD
    b) prefers OS
    c) covers OS easier
    d) vision steady and maintained

51. **When checking vision in young children, it is important to:**
    a) move quickly, because they get bored and tired
    b) move slowly, because they take longer to understand
    c) move slowly, so they are not tempted to malinger
    d) stop if the child seems tired

52. **Which of the following are the earliest and easiest letters recognized by children?**
    a) HTOV
    b) ABC
    c) XYZ
    d) EGK

53. **When teaching a child the E game for the first time, it is best to:**
    a) send an E card home and let the parents practice with the child
    b) practice with the child for 20 minutes prior to the real test
    c) disregard the first acuity taken
    d) tell the child how important it is that he or she do well

54. Clinically, amblyopia is diagnosed when the:
a) best-corrected vision of each eye differs by two or more acuity lines
b) best-corrected vision of each eye differs by four or more acuity lines
c) uncorrected vision of each eye differs by four or more acuity lines
d) patient cannot appreciate binocular/stereoscopic vision

55. Which of the following is appropriate when testing a preschooler for amblyopia?
a) single Allen cards
b) isolated projected figures
c) a full line of figures
d) single Es

56. It is best to check an amblyopic eye first, because:
a) the child will object to having the strong eye covered
b) the child will object to having the amblyopic eye covered
c) the child might memorize the chart if the strong eye is tested first
d) it is important to learn if the stronger eye has been occluded

57. A disadvantage to the Allen cards is:
a) most children do not recognize the pictures
b) the testing distance must be standardized
c) it is difficult to record
d) it presents single pictures instead of a row of figures

58. When testing the vision of a child with the Allen cards, a difference in the testing distance of how many feet between the eyes is considered significant?
a) 1 foot
b) 2 feet
c) 3.5 feet
d) 5 feet

59. A child should be told what regarding the visual acuity test?
a) "This test will show me how smart you are."
b) "If you fail the test, you will get to wear glasses."
c) "The letters will get too small to read, but do the best you can."
d) "You will have to spend the day here at the office until you cooperate."

60. If a child struggles with identifying the letters, you should:
a) have the child count your fingers
b) try numbers, rings, pictures, or Es
c) skip the vision test
d) encourage the child to try harder

61. When checking visual acuity on a preschool child, it is important to:
a) be sure he or she can consistently identify the pictures
b) be sure he or she can have both eyes uncovered
c) use your hand as an occluder
d) check vision at 10 feet instead of 20

62. **When a small child becomes uncooperative during the exam, it is best to:**
    a) have the parent leave the room
    b) have the parent scold the child
    c) push on with the exam to get it done quickly
    d) change gears by chatting for a moment

63. **When a child responds incorrectly to a test item, the assistant should:**
    a) tell the child he or she is doing a good job
    b) tell the child he or she is not trying hard enough
    c) scold the child
    d) have the parent scold the child

Potential Acuity Meter Measurement

64. **The potential acuity meter (PAM) is commonly used to evaluate macular function in the presence of:**
    a) glaucoma
    b) retinal disorders
    c) optic nerve disease
    d) media opacities

65. **Before performing a PAM test, it is important to:**
    a) set the eye piece
    b) enter the patient's refractive error
    c) calibrate the unit
    d) have the patient wear his or her best correction

66. **Your patient has cataracts. The surgeon may want a PAM measurement on him or her if the patient also has:**
    a) macular degeneration
    b) glaucoma
    c) dry eye
    d) high astigmatism

67. **Which of the following might warrant a PAM test?**
    a) preoperative posterior capsulotomy
    b) preoperative refractive surgery
    c) preoperative laser trabeculectomy
    d) preoperative laser iridotomy

68. **All of the following are true regarding a PAM test *except*:**
    a) the patient should be dilated
    b) ask the patient, "Do you see anything?"
    c) do not check the pupils just prior to testing
    d) position the patient firmly in the chinrest

69.   The target in a PAM is a(n):
a) Amsler chart
b) eye chart
c) set of mires
d) grid pattern

Pinhole Acuity

70.   Your patient sees 20/200 without correction in the right eye. You have performed refractometry and have improved this to 20/40. Which of the following tests could help you know whether or not this is the best acuity possible?
a) duochrome
b) pinhole
c) PAM
d) contrast sensitivity

71.   Which of the following is *not* true regarding the pinhole?
a) If vision improves with the pinhole, a refractive error is present.
b) It compensates for media opacities.
c) It can be used if a patient has forgotten his or her glasses.
d) It increases contrast.

72.   An intelligent, literate patient sees 20/400 without correction, 20/200 with the pinhole, and 20/200 with correction. The most reasonable assumption is:
a) he or she needs a change of glasses
b) he or she is malingering
c) he or she is uncooperative
d) he or she has some type of ocular pathology

73.   A patient is found to have 20/80 without correction, then to have 20/25 with a pinhole. This would be written as:
a) VA cc 20/80, PH 20/25
b) VA sc 20/80, PH 20/25
c) VA sc 20/25, PH 20/80
d) VA sc 20/80, PH 20/80

Explanatory Answers

1.   c) Visual acuity evaluation is the most basic of tests in any eye care office.
2.   c) Accommodation is stimulated, in part, by diverging light rays (ie, light rays leave an object and spread outward as they travel; the closer an object is, the more sharply the light diverges before reaching the eye and accommodation is stimulated). We do not wish the patient to accommodate during distance testing. Light rays are nearly parallel at 20 feet, so this was selected as a practical testing distance.
3.   b) Visual acuity testing figures are called optotypes.
4.   c) The upper number (numerator) of the standard "20/20" fraction stands for the test distance.

5. b) The test distance is the standard 20 feet (the numerator). The denominator (bottom number) is the distance at which someone with normal vision can correctly recognize optotypes of this size. Thus, 20/20 denotes an eye that can see "normally," or what the normal eye should see from 20 feet away.

6. d) Visual acuity tests the cone cells, not the rods.

7. b) The person with 20/80 vision sees at 20 feet (the test distance, numerator) what a person with normal vision can see from 80 feet away (the denominator). Thus, the patient with 20/80 vision has to be 60 feet *closer* to the optotype than someone with normal vision, before he or she can correctly identify it. The patient may have a refractive error, but subnormal vision can have many causes.

8. d) The numerator (top number) always refers to test distance; thus, 10/40 indicates a test distance of 10 feet.

9. d) A visual acuity of 20/15 means that the patient sees at 20 feet what the normal eye sees at 15. Thus, the *normal/average* eye has to get 5 feet *closer* before it can correctly identify the optotypes. Having vision better than 20/20 is sometimes called "super vision."

10. c) The numerator indicates the test distance; thus, the patient was 15 feet from the target or chart.

11. c) Remember how to change a fraction: If you multiply (or divide) both the numerator and denominator by the same number, you keep the correct ratio, and the fractions are equal. The conversion looks like this: 5/200 = 20/X
    You can see that if you multiply the first numerator (5) by 4, you will get the desired 20 numerator. Thus, you must also multiply the denominator (200) by 4. This means that X equals 800 and the answer is 20/800.

12. b) The illumination in the room should be no less than one-fifth of the illumination on the chart.

13. d) The only adequate occluder is opaque with no openings for peeking. A patient using his or her hand might peek between fingers.

14. b) Squinting acts like a pinhole and, thus, may improve the vision. In visual acuity testing, we want the measurement to reflect the patient's usual vision, so no squinting allowed!

15. d) An illiterate patient might be tested with the E game or Landolt C. Many illiterate patients can recognize numbers. (Of course, pictures might be used, too, but did not appear in a proper answer combination. Be sure to read all items in an answer.) The "functionally literate" can usually recognize letters, but this situation was not identified in the question.

16. d) If the testing distance is closer than 20 feet, the letters seem larger, and the patient's acuity would be falsely high. (A laminated chart was specified because projector-and-mirror systems can be calibrated to account for different testing distances.)

17. b) Because the standard acuity chart has high contrast (absolute black on stark white), the measured acuity might be falsely higher than the patient's actual visual ability.

18. c) The standard Snellen chart employs black letters on a bright white background. In other words, it has high contrast. How much of our world is of such high contrast? Most of what we see are shades and shadows. Therefore, the Snellen chart may give an exaggerated sense of the patient's acuity. Low-contrast situations—which are difficult even for a person with *normal* contrast sensitivity—may be virtually debilitating to a person with low-contrast sensitivity. Cataracts are notable among ocular disorders that can cause this problem.

19. a) The patient read the entire 20/50 line correctly, but got only one letter correct on the 20/40 line: 20/50 + 1.

20. c) The patient read the 20/40 line correctly, missed two on the 20/30, and got one right on the 20/25 line: 20/30 – 2 + 1.

21. b) If the patient recognizes the letter from 10 feet away, the numerator should be 10, hence 10/400.

22. b) The notation "cc" means with correction.

23. c) The abbreviation OD refers to the right eye, and OS refers to the left eye. Thus, the patient sees 20/40 in the right eye and 20/20 in the left.

24. d) If the patient cannot recognize the 20/400 figure, one option (and the only option offered here as an answer) is to have him or her walk up to the letter until it is recognized. Remember, however, this necessitates changing the numerator to reflect the true test distance.

25. a) Instead of having the patient walk closer to the chart, you could do a count fingers test, moving further away each time until the patient can no longer count fingers accurately.

26. d) A patient who cannot count fingers at 6 inches is not necessarily blind, nor can he or she see well enough to do a glare or contrast. Find out if he or she can detect hand motion.

27. a) If the patient can detect hand motion, move further away until he or she can no longer detect motion. This distance is recorded (eg, hand motion 3.5 feet OD). Each eye is tested separately.

28. c) If the patient cannot detect hand motion, the next step is to see if he or she can detect the presence of light.

29. c) Light perception means the patient can perceive the presence of light. In light projection, the patient can detect from which direction the light projects, which is considered a higher level of vision than light perception alone.

30. a) Absence of the ability to detect the presence of light is recorded as NLP.

31. a) A patient should wear his or her habitual reading correction for the near vision test. (Your physician might want a corrected and uncorrected near vision measurement, but that is not offered as an answer here. You have to work with the answers listed.)

32. b) The near card is designed to be held at 14 to 16 inches. (*Note:* During refractometry, the near card can be placed at the patient's preferred distance.)

33. d) Answers a through c are all normal near-vision acuities. There is no such designation as "L1."

34. b) Vision with both eyes is usually better than with either eye alone. (Of course, there are exceptions. The word "usually" is your clue here.)

35. c) A visual field defect might cause the patient to be unable to see a portion of the chart. The patient's consistency is the clue in this case. While he or she might be malingering, the assumption is that there is a problem until proven otherwise.

36. b) Taking visual acuity in the ophthalmic/optometric office is like checking blood pressure in the general practitioner's office. It is done every time, providing a long-term record of the patient's visual function. Explain this to the patient, and she will most likely cooperate.

37. a) A posterior subcapsular cataract can cause visual acuity to plummet in bright light because the constricted pupil forces the patient to try to look directly through the opacity.

38. a) It is proper to make noteworthy records of your observations of the patient during testing. This could include the patient's apparent motivation, attention, or mental capacity. Occlusion must always be accurate, and illumination should be standard with every patient.

39. a) It is important to make thorough, accurate notes regarding any correction the patient uses during the visual acuity test.

40. d) While checking vision is the general rule, there might be some cases where the injury is so severe that visual acuity is temporarily not so important.

41. c) A malingerer falsifies his or her responses, generally for some type of gain.

42. c) A person with amblyopia may have better acuity if optotypes are presented singly. Thus, a row of optotypes ("crowded") gives a more accurate acuity.

43. d) See answer 42.

44. c) It is most crucial to find amblyopia at as early an age as possible, while it is still correctable. So, finding a difference between the two eyes is more important than the actual vision. (An exception might be the child with low vision, but that was not offered as a response.)

45. c) If an infant's eyes locate and follow an object, vision is considered present and noted as "fix and follow." A squeaking toy will not work because it makes noise. A blind infant will still respond both to the mother and her absence.

46. d) An infant with normal vision will move his or her eye (assuming one is occluded for the test) to look at an object pretty much straight-on. This is the central component, in that the child is using central vision, and not looking to the side of the object. The infant should also look at the object steadily, without searching movements. Fixation should be maintained even when the other eye is suddenly unoccluded. These components, when present, are abbreviated as CSM. (*Note:* The Allen cards are inappropriate for a nonverbal infant. In addition, visual tests on infants are usually done in normal lighting.)

47. c) The cards used in the preferential looking test are divided in half; one half is a gray square, and the other is black with stripes. The cards vary in stripe frequency (ie, the stripes get closer and closer together). The test can be used on any nonverbal patient, checking each eye alone and both eyes together. The card is presented to the patient as the examiner observes through a hole in the card's center. The patient will automatically look at the striped side of the card, if acuity is intact. The finer the stripes that the patient responds to, the better the acuity. However, overestimation of acuity (not underestimation) can occur, especially where amblyopia is present.

48. c) Of the tests listed, only the preferential looking technique can be used to diagnose amblyopia in an infant. While the preferential looking technique does not give an actual acuity level, it can identify a difference in acuity between the two eyes, which strongly indicates amblyopia. Rating an infant's vision as central, steady, and maintained is not useful in this case; even an eye with poor vision can maintain steady, central looking.

49. c) The child will not want her only good eye covered, and she loses concentration when you cover the left eye. She will not care if you cover the weak right eye.

50. b) The child prefers to use her good, left eye.

51. a) Speed is the name of the game when working with kids, who tire and bore easily.

52. a) Children most often learn and recognize the letters HTOV first.

53. a) Let the parents work on the E game at home. A 20-minute practice session will wear the child out before the test is ever done! Answer d puts pressure on the child. Disregarding the first acuity will not work—how do you know when the acuity is accurate?

54. a) If the eyes are best-corrected and there is a difference of two or more acuity lines in the vision of the eyes, the diagnosis is amblyopia. An amblyopic patient will do more poorly on or fail the stereo test, but so will other patients with other eye problems.

55. c) An amblyopic eye can identify figures more easily if they are isolated than if they are presented in a group. This is called the crowding phenomenon. An accurate assessment of vision on an amblyopic eye can be obtained only by using a row of age-appropriate optotypes.

56. c) While we usually check the right eye first, a patient with amblyopia in the left eye should be checked left eye first. If you check vision in the stronger eye first, the child might memorize the optotypes and try to fake you out. Then everyone loses, especially if you have been using patching therapy. He or she may certainly object to having the strong eye covered, but this is no reason to check it first.

57. d) Single pictures, as with the Allen cards, may give a falsely high acuity if the patient has amblyopia (see answer 55).

58. d) In Allen card testing, a difference between the two eyes of 5 feet or more is considered a positive finding for amblyopia.

59. c) Answers a, b, and d are intimidating. Untutored, most kids assume you are trying to find out how smart they are. Let them know ahead of time that *nobody* sees all the letters. This takes some of the pressure off.

60. b) A child may "know" the alphabet (as in be able to sing the "ABC" song), but not be able to identify letters. Try Es, rings, pictures, or numbers.

61. a) If the child does not know what the pictures are, how can you test vision? It does not matter if the child calls the horse "doggie," as long as he or she does it every time. Each eye is tested separately at 20 feet using an opaque occluder.

62. d) If a small child's patience wears thin during the exam, give him or her a short break. You might distract him or her with a toy or ask fun questions. (What is your favorite food? Do you have a cat at home?) Having the parent leave will probably make the child more anxious. Scolding is not indicated unless the child is being downright naughty.

63. a) Scolding and shaming are not good ideas. While you would not tell the child that his or her answer is correct, you can still praise him or her for answering at all.

64. d) The PAM transmits a tiny, bright eye chart to the back of the eye, bypassing media opacities. Its most common use is in evaluating macular function in the presence of cataracts (especially very dense ones where the physician has a hard time viewing the macula directly).

65. b) There is a knob on the side of the unit where you must dial in the spherical equivalent[1] of the patient's refractive error.

66. a) The PAM will help the surgeon know whether the patient's postoperative vision will be improved enough to make the surgery worthwhile.

67. a) The posterior capsulotomy is treatment for a cloudy lens capsule following cataract surgery. It is a media opacity and thus might warrant a PAM reading prior to the procedure.

68. d) The chinrest is actually moved out of the way so the patient can talk without disrupting fixation.

69. b) The target in a PAM is an eye chart that is projected directly onto the retina, bypassing moderate opacities in the ocular media.

70. b) The pinhole will compensate only for refractive error, not pathology. The refractometric measurement should correct the patient to at least the pinhole vision.

71. b) The pinhole does not improve poor vision caused by opacities in the ocular media.

72. d) The patient sees no better with correction than with the pinhole, so changing the glasses will not help. The residual poor acuity would be due to pathology.

73. b) The notation "sc" means without correction; PH means the pinhole was used.

---

[1]For information on spherical equivalent, see Chapter 3, answers 56 and 58.

Chapter 19

Visual Fields

Ledford JK.
Certified Ophthalmic Assistant: Exam
Review Manual, Third Edition (pp. 301-318).
© 2012 Taylor & Francis Group.

Visual Field Basics[1]

1.   **The extent of vision beyond the central fixation point is known as the:**
      a) binocular field
      b) visual field
      c) neurological field
      d) pathway of light

2.   **The peripheral vision of a normal person is:**
      a) 60 degrees temporal, 60 degrees inferior, 75 degrees nasal, and 95 degrees superior
      b) 75 degrees temporal, 60 degrees inferior, 95 degrees nasal, and 60 degrees superior
      c) 95 degrees temporal, 60 degrees inferior, 75 degrees nasal, and 60 degrees superior
      d) 95 degrees temporal, 75 degrees inferior, 60 degrees nasal, and 60 degrees superior

3.   **The configuration of the normal visual field is delimited by:**
      a) the ear and nasal bridge
      b) the brow and nose
      c) the location of the fovea
      d) the size of the optic nerve

4.   **The key to performing any type of peripheral vision exam is to have the patient:**
      a) maintain fixation
      b) look at the moving target
      c) gaze into all four quadrants
      d) use both eyes

5.   **An object on the patient's right will be perceived by the patient's:**
      a) temporal retina OU
      b) nasal retina OU
      c) temporal retina OS and nasal retina OD
      d) foveae OU

6.   **The anatomic pattern of the nerve fibers produces visual field defects:**
      a) that are total blind spots
      b) that correspond to the location of the rods and cones
      c) that correspond to the location of the nerve fibers
      d) that respond well to treatment

7.   **The "blind spot" as plotted on a visual field test corresponds to:**
      a) the macula
      b) the fovea
      c) the optic disc
      d) the angle

[1]While not listed as a JCAHPO® criteria item, it is prudent to have a basic understanding of the visual field.

8. **On the visual field, the average blind spot is located:**
   a) 25 degrees temporal to fixation
   b) 5 degrees nasal to fixation
   c) 15 degrees nasal to fixation
   d) 15 degrees temporal to fixation

9. **Visual nerve fibers terminate at the:**
   a) brain stem
   b) occipital cortex
   c) thalamus
   d) pituitary

10. **Conversion of the visual field map into a three-dimensional representation results in:**
    a) isopters
    b) the island of vision profile
    c) a comparative analysis
    d) threshold gray-tone analysis

11. **The peak of the island of vision profile corresponds to the:**
    a) optic nerve
    b) center of the crystalline lens
    c) nerve fiber layer
    d) fovea

12. **The blind spot would be represented on the island of vision profile as:**
    a) a bottomless hole
    b) a peak
    c) a shallow dip
    d) a deep pit

13. **In the island of vision analogy, vision exists in:**
    a) a sea of blindness
    b) a sea of vision
    c) an expanse of vision
    d) a time-space continuum

14. **The validity of all visual field testing depends on:**
    a) the technical skill of the operator
    b) the patient's ability to maintain fixation
    c) the complexity of the screening program
    d) the illumination capabilities of the technique used

Amsler Grid

15. **The Amsler grid is used to document visual field defects:**
    a) within the central 30 degrees
    b) within the central 20 degrees
    c) within the central 10 degrees
    d) from 30 degrees outward

16. **All of the following warrant an Amsler grid exam *except*:**
    a) the patient with macular degeneration
    b) the patient complaining of a central blot in the vision
    c) the patient complaining that letters are distorted when reading
    d) the patient with a pituitary tumor

17. **When checking a patient with the Amsler grid, it is important to do all of the following *except*:**
    a) cover one eye at a time
    b) use good reading light
    c) have the patient use his or her regular reading glasses
    d) hold the chart 1 meter away

18. **When checking a patient with the Amsler grid, he or she is told to:**
    a) look at the upper left corner
    b) look at the lower right corner
    c) look at the center dot
    d) look at the bottom center

19. **When checking a patient with the Amsler grid, it is helpful to tell the patient:**
    a) not to touch the grid because oils from the skin will mar it
    b) to outline any missing or distorted areas with a pencil
    c) that the test is not conclusive
    d) that the test is not very accurate

20. **Each of the following is an advantage of the Amsler grid *except*:**
    a) it is useful for bedridden patient exams
    b) most people easily understand it
    c) it is handy for home use by the patient
    d) it is useful in monitoring field loss in glaucoma

21. **Each of the following is a standard question to ask when performing an Amsler grid check *except*:**
    a) "Are you aware of the page beyond the grid?"
    b) "Are all the lines straight and square?"
    c) "Are you aware of all four corners of the grid?"
    d) "Is any part of the grid missing?"

Confrontation Fields

22. **You are assisting the physician during screening eye exams at a nursing home with minimal equipment. To check a patient's peripheral vision, you will most likely perform a(n):**
    a) tangent screen
    b) confrontation visual field
    c) Goldmann visual field
    d) automated visual field

23. **What is the given assumption in confrontation field testing?**
    a) The patient has 20/20 vision.
    b) The fields are tested in the central area.
    c) The examiner's field is normal.
    d) The procedure is fully qualitative.

24. **The confrontation field:**
    a) requires the use of elaborate equipment
    b) will not pick up gross visual field defects
    c) can be performed on a patient in any position
    d) cannot be performed on children

25. **Which of the following is *not* true regarding the confrontation visual field test?**
    a) It is a subjective test.
    b) Only the examiner's fingers should be used as a target.
    c) The eye not being tested is occluded.
    d) A defect can be either described in words or drawn out in the chart.

26. **In the standard version of confrontation field testing, one tests the patient's peripheral vision:**
    a) in the standard positions of gaze
    b) in the center of fixation
    c) in the four quadrants
    d) superiorly and inferiorly

Automated Perimetry

27. **Matching. Match the term to the correct definition:**

Terms	Definitions
constricted	a) the central point at which the patient looks during testing
fixation	b) diameter lines designated in degrees
infrathreshold	c) point where a stimulus is seen 50% of the time
meridians	d) a stimulus that is too small or too dim to be seen
scotoma	e) a stimulus that exceeds threshold and is seen more than 50% of the time
step	
suprathreshold	f) internal area where threshold is not seen
threshold	g) field is moved inward from expected normal
	h) constriction, sometimes very sharp, along the 180-degree meridian

28. **Maintenance measures for automated perimeters include all of the following *except*:**
    a) a surge protector for the electrical outlet
    b) initializing (formatting) the hard drive once a week
    c) replacing ink and paper when indicated
    d) covering the instrument when not in use

29. **Abrasions or marks on the perimeter bowl surface may be treated by:**
    a) touching up with correction liquid
    b) covering with white nylon tape
    c) touching up with white enamel paint
    d) a new manufacturer-applied coating

30. **At the beginning of each day before using an automated perimeter:**
    a) the background reflectance must be calibrated
    b) the stimulus illumination must be calibrated
    c) the technician should run a diagnostic test
    d) check the amount of printer paper in the machine

31. **Regarding data entry on an automated perimeter:**
    a) one may use all the data from a previous test
    b) the computer automatically makes changes from one test to another
    c) the computer automatically saves displayed data, even if the machine is shut off
    d) it must be entered in the prescribed manner or the computer will not find it later

32. **All of the following are true regarding the floppy disks used in an automated perimeter *except*:**
    a) they are sensitive to magnetic fields
    b) they should be left in the computer at all times
    c) an extra copy should be stored apart from the testing site
    d) a log book should be kept to cross-reference files

33. **Before starting automated fields, it is a good idea to perform a confrontation field on the patient. In addition to providing the examiner general information about possible gross defects, this also serves to:**
    a) locate the blind spot
    b) educate the patient about fixation and response
    c) quantitate possible defects
    d) evaluate the patient's visual acuity

34. **The best type of lens to use for the near add during automated perimetry is:**
    a) the patient's own glasses
    b) a lens from any trial lens set
    c) sphere only
    d) a lens with a thin rim

35. **Calculation of the add for automated perimetry includes the factors of:**
    a) full distance correction and age-related add
    b) full distance correction and habitual add
    c) full distance correction, age-related add, and bowl depth
    d) full distance correction and a 30-cm bowl depth

36. **The trial lens(es) should be placed:**
    a) with the sphere closest to the eye and as close to the eye as possible
    b) with the cylinder closest to the eye and as close to the eye as possible
    c) with the sphere closest to the eye at the patient's habitual vertex distance
    d) with the cylinder closest to the eye at the patient's habitual vertex distance

37. **The trial lens is used when testing:**
     a) the entire visual field
     b) the central 30 degrees
     c) the central 40 degrees
     d) the peripheral field

38. **The smallest size pupil diameter for adequate mapping of the periphery is:**
     a) 0.5 to 1.5 mm
     b) 2.5 to 3.0 mm
     c) 3.5 to 5.0 mm
     d) 6.0 to 7.0 mm

39. **Occlusion of the eye not being tested for visual fields is best done by:**
     a) having the patient close his or her eye
     b) the patient's hand
     c) a piece of tape running from upper to lower lid
     d) a "pirate patch" that can be disinfected

40. **The visual field patient should be told all of the following *except*:**
     a) you will not see every light
     b) some of the lights will be dimmer or smaller than others
     c) be sure to look at the light once you see it
     d) press the button as soon as you are aware of the light

41. **The visual field patient should be positioned so that he or she:**
     a) is not leaning forward at all
     b) is on an eye level with the fixation target
     c) has his or her chin jutted forward as far as possible
     d) has his or her forehead tilted forward as far as possible

42. **What is the best way for a visual field patient who is physically unable to push the buzzer button with the thumb to indicate his or her response?**
     a) The test cannot be done.
     b) Have him or her push the upside-down buzzer against the tabletop.
     c) Have him or her give a verbal response.
     d) Have him or her nod when the stimulus is seen.

43. **If the visual field patient's head is tucked into a chin-down position:**
     a) the brow may obstruct the upper field
     b) the cheek bone may obstruct the lower field
     c) the eye cannot be aligned properly
     d) fixation will be impossible

44. **If a male visual field patient has a beard:**
     a) tape the facial hair back out of the way
     b) request that he shave before the test
     c) position him so there is as little hair as possible in the chinrest
     d) no special modifications are necessary

45. **Which of the following is the most comfortable position during the visual field exam?**
    a) The feet should not touch the floor.
    b) The back should be curved gently.
    c) The patient should not have to lean forward at all.
    d) The back should be straight, with feet flat on floor.

46. **Adaptations that might allow a wheelchair-bound patient to be positioned at the perimeter include all of the following *except*:**
    a) placing a sturdy board across the wheelchair armrests and having the patient sit on the board
    b) raising the table so the chair will fit under it, and using pillows to help prop the patient
    c) removing the wheelchair armrests so that the chair will slide under the table
    d) removing the footrests so the chair will fit closer to the table

47. **In general, the longer the test time:**
    a) the less reliable the patient becomes
    b) the more reproducible the test
    c) the more accurate the test because more data are provided
    d) the more reliable the patient becomes

48. **To provide for patient comfort and rest during an automated visual field, the patient should be:**
    a) told to hold down the button to pause the test after every couple of stimuli
    b) told to close his or her eye whenever needed
    c) encouraged periodically to continue, then allowed to rest between testing eyes
    d) allowed to take a break every 5 minutes

49. **Which of the following is *true* regarding visual field screening techniques?**
    a) they are difficult for patients because of the time required
    b) they are not practical for evaluating large groups
    c) the main purpose is to rule out pathology
    d) they cannot be used to confirm changes in prior fields

50. **When testing a return patient for an annual automated field exam, it is important to:**
    a) use the same test parameters as the previous test
    b) use the same correcting lens as before
    c) not fatigue the patient with test instructions
    d) save the results on the same floppy disk

51. **You are halfway through the field when your patient begins to complain that her eye is stinging and watering. This might indicate that you forgot to instruct the patient to:**
    a) maintain fixation
    b) use artificial tears before the test
    c) blink often during the test
    d) take her allergy medication before the test

52. **Once the automated visual field test has begun, the technician should:**
    a) encourage the patient frequently
    b) be totally quiet
    c) leave the room
    d) speak only if the patient repeatedly loses fixation

53. **Fixation losses may be minimized by:**
    a) telling the patient where the next kinetic stimulus is going to appear
    b) telling the patient that you can see his or her eye during testing
    c) using the correct near add
    d) enlarging the fixation point for every patient

54. **Match the automated field terms with the definitions. Each will be used more than once:**

    Terms
    fixation loss
    false-positive
    false-negative
    fluctuation

    Definitions
    a) evaluates the patient's understanding of the test
    b) the patient does not respond to the brightest target available in an area where he or she previously responded to a dimmer light
    c) the patient responds to a target that appears within the previously designated blind spot
    d) the patient responds to the sound of the perimeter when no stimulus was presented
    e) a measure of the patient's consistency
    f) evaluates the patient's alertness
    g) some perimeters will retest the points that were evaluated just before this occurred
    h) this factor can be affected by certain eye diseases
    i) a higher number indicates that the patient is giving varying responses to the same point
    j) may be detected continually by a photoelectric sensor

55. **During automated visual fields, if the patient repeatedly responds to the blind spot check, yet seems to be maintaining fixation:**
    a) encourage the patient to continue to fixate
    b) relocate the blind spot
    c) pause the test and allow the patient to rest
    d) turn off the fixation monitor

56. **All of the following could cause the perimeter to be unable to find the blind spot except:**
    a) the other eye is not adequately occluded
    b) the patient is not fixating
    c) you have selected the wrong eye to be tested
    d) the presence of a scotoma

57. **Target exposure time on an automated perimeter is usually:**
    a) 0.1 to 0.4 seconds
    b) 0.5 to 0.7 seconds
    c) 0.9 to 1.0 seconds
    d) 1.5 to 2.0 seconds

58. **Your patient seems to have a slow response time. In order to get the most accurate results possible, you should:**
    a) change the stimulus presentation interval
    b) let the patient rest frequently
    c) use a different testing strategy
    d) turn off the gaze monitor

59. **"At threshold" means that the patient responds to a given stimulus at the same location:**
    a) 25% of the time
    b) 50% of the time
    c) 75% of the time
    d) 100% of the time

60. **In automated perimetry, threshold is dependent on all of the following *except*:**
    a) background and stimulus intensity
    b) patients' age
    c) patients' level of stereopsis
    d) distance of stimulus from the fovea

61. **A patient might not respond to a suprathreshold stimuli:**
    a) by chance
    b) because it is too dim
    c) because it is too small
    d) because it is too large

62. **The main challenge in testing the visual fields of low-vision patients is:**
    a) patients' inability to understand the test
    b) patients' inability to see the fixation area
    c) finding the appropriate threshold
    d) finding the appropriate correcting lens

63. **If the patient has poor vision and cannot see the fixation target in the center of the automated perimeter:**
    a) activate an alternate/eccentric fixation pattern
    b) turn off the fixation monitor
    c) increase the size of the stimulus
    d) use a +3.00 correcting lens to provide more magnification

64. **A "normal" screening test means that:**
    a) the patient has no visual field defect
    b) the patient has no field defect detectable by this test
    c) confrontation visual fields are adequate for future testing
    d) the patient does not have glaucoma

65. **Which of the following is *not* true regarding test results found with an automated perimeter?**
    a) The data can be rearranged into a variety of printouts.
    b) It is valid only if the same person performs the test each time.
    c) The data can be compared with the patient's previous test(s).
    d) The data can be compared to normal age-related values.

66. **On the numeric printout of an automated field, the number zero indicates that:**
   a) the stimulus was seen 100% of the time
   b) the stimulus was below threshold
   c) the dimmest stimulus was used
   d) the brightest stimulus was not seen

67. **A point that is not seen is represented on a gray-scale printout by:**
   a) a white area
   b) a dot
   c) a black area
   d) an X

68. **The comparison printout on an automated perimeter is designed to:**
   a) compare the patient's results to normal
   b) compare the patient's test with and without a correcting lens
   c) compare the patient's current results to a previous test
   d) compare the patient's responses to one stimulus with another

69. **Which of the following ocular disorders is frequently followed by visual field testing on a regular basis (every 6 to 12 months)?**
   a) cataracts
   b) macular degeneration
   c) glaucoma
   d) retinal detachment

70. **The physician has requested an automated visual field to be performed "taped and untaped." Most likely, this patient is being evaluated for:**
   a) blepharoplasty
   b) cataract surgery
   c) driver's license renewal
   d) glaucoma

71. **The visual field in a high hyperope will be:**
   a) compressed, with a blind spot closer to fixation than normal
   b) expanded, with a blind spot farther from fixation than normal
   c) compressed, with a smaller blind spot than normal
   d) expanded, with a larger blind spot than usual

72. **A high myope will have a field that is:**
   a) compressed, with a blind spot closer to fixation than normal
   b) expanded, with a blind spot further from fixation than normal
   c) compressed, with a smaller blind spot than normal
   d) expanded, with a larger blind spot than usual

Explanatory Answers

1. b) Vision beyond fixation is the visual field. Binocular field is the visual field with both eyes. A neurological field is a particular method of testing. The pathway of light refers to the ocular structures through which light must pass to reach the retina.

2. d) The normal visual field is approximately 95 degrees temporal, 75 degrees inferior, 60 degrees nasal, and 60 degrees superior. You could pick this out even if the numbers were slightly different, if you remember that the temporal field is the widest and the nasal and superior fields are the narrowest.

3. b) The superior and nasal fields are limited by the anatomical boundaries of the brow and nose. (The superior field also is limited by the lids, which are not mentioned in this question.)

4. a) Without proper fixation, any test of peripheral vision is invalidated. Generally, the eyes are checked separately.

5. c) An object on the patient's right will stimulate the temporal retina of the left eye and the nasal retina of the right eye. The foveae (plural of fovea) are used during central fixation, not for peripheral vision.

6. c) Because the nerve fibers fan out in a specific anatomic pattern, visual field defects occurring in the nerve fibers also follow the same pattern. This makes diagnosis easier because the patterns are identifiable.

7. c) The optic disc has no rods or cones to receive light impulses. It is, therefore, an area of blindness commonly called the "blind spot." The macula and fovea are at the center of the visual field and are normally the areas of highest sensitivity. The angle refers to the internal point where the cornea and iris meet.

8. d) The average blind spot is located 15 degrees temporal to fixation. (The optic disc is anatomically located in the nasal part of the retina, which picks up the temporal field.)

9. b) The visual nerve fibers terminate into the occipital cortex of the brain. (The eye-related fibers that terminate in the brain stem, only 10% of all the fibers, are concerned with pupillary action and are not visual.)

10. b) The island of vision profile is a three-dimensional representation of the visual field. An isopter is a boundary. Comparative analysis and threshold gray-tone analysis are automated perimetry programs.

11. d) The peak of the island represents the area of highest visual sensitivity, the fovea.

12. a) The blind spot is devoid of light receptor cells and would be represented by a bottomless hole. A peak is the point of highest sensitivity. A dip and a pit have a bottom, indicating that a stimulus *could* be found to which that area would respond.

13. a) The island of vision is afloat in a sea of blindness, because anything that is not seen is in a blind area. (The time-space continuum is a term I borrowed from *Star Trek*.)

14. b) The validity of any type of field testing depends on the patient's ability and willingness to maintain fixation. Automated perimetry requires minimal technical skill as compared to the manual Goldmann. Other factors involved (but not listed as responses) are the patient's response time, vision, and mental capabilities.

15. b) The Amsler grid is used in the central 20 degrees of field.

16. d) The patient with a suspected or known pituitary tumor will have formal fields versus an Amsler grid.

17. d) The Amsler grid should be held at normal reading distance, 14 to 16 inches. (A meter is a little over 3 feet.)

18. c) The patient is to fixate on the central dot on the grid.

19. b) If the patient notices any distorted or blank areas, he or she should outline it on the grid. This gives the physician an idea of what part of the retina might be affected, as well as providing a permanent record of the defect.

20. d) The Amsler grid is not generally used to monitor glaucoma field defects, which occur outside the inner 20 degree field until very advanced.

21. a) Answer a moves the testing area off the grid, which is beyond the central 20 degrees of the patient's field. The other answers are standard Amsler grid questions.

22. b) The confrontation visual field requires no equipment and can be done even on a patient who is lying down.

23. c) In confrontation visual field testing, the assumption is that the examiner's visual field is normal. The patient need not have 20/20 vision. The peripheral area, rather than the central area, is tested. The test is not qualitative.

24. c) One advantage of the confrontation field is that it can be performed on a patient in any position (ie, sitting or lying down). Properly done, the test will pick up gross defects. Most school-aged children can cooperate for a confrontation field test.

25. b) In some cases, a small test object (frequently, the red cap of an eye drop bottle) is used instead of the more common use of the examiner's fingers. Confrontation field testing is a subjective test, requiring a response from the patient. The field is checked one eye at a time, and any defect can be described or drawn.

26. c) In the standard confrontation field test, the patient is asked to identify the number of fingers that the examiner holds up in the periphery of each quadrant. If a defect is detected in this manner, then more meridians may be examined. Other versions of the test involve:
   - moving a target (finger or object) from the periphery inward until the patient first reports seeing it
   - asking the patient to identify hand motion in each quadrant
   - presenting fingers in two quadrants simultaneously and asking the patient the total
   - presenting a colored target (eg, a red bottle cap) in each quadrant and asking if there is any difference in color intensity

27. Matching:

constricted	g)
fixation	a)
infrathreshold	d)
meridians	b)
scotoma	f)
step	h)
suprathreshold	e)
threshold	c)

28. b) Initializing or formatting a disk erases all of the information on it. You never will initialize the hard drive. This not only would erase data files but program files as well.

29. d) Only the manufacturer can "treat" the perimeter bowl finish. Answers a through c are blatantly wrong.

30. d) Check the printer paper supply each day before beginning. Automated perimeters are self-calibrating and run their own internal diagnostic without any prompting, so tasks in answers a through c are not necessary.

31. d) Data must be entered the same way every time. If you enter Charles Aaron for one test and Aaron Charles for the next, the computer will not know they are the same patient. Data from a previous test needs to be updated. For example, the lens prescription might have changed. The computer only knows what you tell it. Data are lost if the instrument is turned off before the information is saved.

32. b) Floppy disks should be removed from the instrument before the computer is turned off.

33. b) Performing a confrontation field on the patient prior to formal perimetry serves to reinforce the idea that "you will not be looking directly at the target" and "you need to look straight ahead during the entire test." Confrontation fields will not quantitate defects or give visual acuity.

34. d) A lens with a thin rim is the best type of trial lens to use. The patient's glasses, or a trial lens with a thick rim, will most likely cause artifactual field losses because the edge of the frame or the lens rim will block off part of the patient's side vision. Cylinder correction for astigmatism may sometimes be required, so "sphere only" is not a correct answer.

35. c) In automated perimetry, the near add calculation must include the patient's full distance correction, an age-related add, and the bowl depth. Bowl depth can range from 30 cm (equal to a Goldmann perimeter) to 50 cm. Most computerized perimeters calculate the add for you once you input the distance prescription and the patient's age.

36. a) The near add should be placed with the sphere closest to the patient's eye (if cylinder is also required) and as close to the patient's eye as possible. Vertex distance is not usually considered when going from glasses to trial lens.

37. b) The trial lens is used to compensate for the patient's need for a near add and is thus used for the central 30 degrees. Most automated perimeters will prompt you when to insert/remove a trial lens if the test chosen evaluates the field beyond 30 degrees.

38. b) If the pupil is smaller than 2.5 to 3.0 mm, consider dilating the patient before proceeding with the test.

39. d) A patch that can be disinfected (such as a plastic "pirate" patch) should be used. It is not advisable to use a patch and place a tissue under it because this may cause a corneal abrasion. Some clinics use a flesh-toned stick-on occlusion patch. This is a good option because there is no strap to potentially interfere with testing on the other eye, and a fresh one would be used for each patient. (***Note:*** In the past, a white patch was recommended. However, when researching for this edition, I was unable to find any printed reference to this. Several of my colleagues had heard of the white patch rule, but none of us had the same logic for using one. I had been taught that it would keep the eye from dark-adapting, which would be a problem when that eye was uncovered and tested. Another technician had heard it was to avoid affecting reflectivity from the bowl. Yet another thought it was an issue of cleanliness.)

40. c) Patients should be told *not* to look at the stimulus. Telling patients up front that they will not see every light reduces a lot of stress, because normally they think, "I must be doing terribly because I do not see anything." Tell them that they may go for a while without seeing anything. They also should know that they are to respond regardless of the size or brightness of the stimulus. Patients should respond as soon as they are aware of the light and not wait for it to get crystal clear.

41. b) The eye should be level with the fixation area. It is okay if the patient has to lean forward a little as long as the back is straight and not hyperextended or hunched over. The plane of the face should be parallel to the plane of the back of the bowl or screen. If the chin is jutted forward, this will minimize the lower field. If the forehead is jutted out, the size of the superior field is reduced.

42. b) Patients who cannot press the buzzer may turn the buzzer upside down and press the button into his or her knee, leg, armrest, or tabletop. Giving a verbal response or a nod will interfere with fixation and positioning and, of course, will not register on an automated perimeter.

43. a) A patient with the chin tucked down has a reduction of the superior field because of interference by the brow. You must visually check the head position, because it still is possible to align the eye and for the patient to fixate even if the head is malpositioned.

44. c) If a man has a full beard, have him put his chin beyond the chinrest, then slide back into the chin cup. Then, the hair can be parted to either side of the chin cup so as not to interfere with the lower field. A beard can cushion the chin in the cup, making it difficult to maintain alignment.

45. d) The patient's back should be straight, not hyperextended, even if he or she has to lean forward a little. Feet should be flat on the floor, thighs parallel to the floor.

46. a) Perching the wheelchair-bound (or any) patient on a board for the test would be uncomfortable and probably dangerous. Remove parts of the wheelchair, if possible, in order to accommodate. If you remove the armrests, be sure the patient is not going to fall out of the chair. Propping with pillows may help with comfort and positioning.

47. a) The longer the test continues, the greater the patient's fatigue, boredom, and "hypnosis." These all lower reliability. The test may stretch on because the program does not find that the data are reliable.

48. c) Give patients verbal encouragement. This helps them stay alert and motivated. For example, tell patients they are doing well, or that they are halfway through. Answer a might be considered correct by some. My opinion is that if you tell patients to hold down the button and pause whenever they want to, it will lengthen the test and add to the stress, instead of helping the patient. It is better to let pauses remain in the control of the technician. A patient should not be allowed to sit at the machine with his or her eyes closed during the test. Resting every 5 minutes might be allowed in extreme cases, but not as a general rule.

49. c) The main purpose of screening techniques is to give a yes/no answer to the question: Is this patient's peripheral vision grossly normal? In general, screening techniques are quicker and practical for evaluating large groups of people. (Not all at once, of course!) They also are useful in comparing a patient's screening results from one test to the next.

50. a) In order for tests to be comparable, they must be run with the same parameters. Otherwise, you are trying to compare apples and stones. The correcting lens used for one test may not be appropriate for the next, however. The patient always should be instructed, even if he or she has done numerous field tests. There is no need to back up files on the same floppy disk.

51. c) Burning, watery eyes are symptoms of dryness. In the case of a visual field exam, dryness is usually caused by staring. Before starting the test and sometime during the test, remind the patient to blink. You can stop the test and instill artificial tear drops, if necessary.

52. a) Communication during an automated field is almost constant. The droning of the machine and rhythm of responses can be tiring for even the most alert patients. Automated fields are taxing; therefore, reinforce the patient often. Leaving the room is not a good idea. Even the best patient can slip out of alignment.

53. b) Just knowing that you are watching makes the patient more motivated to hold fixation. A few Goldmann perimeter advocates tell the patient where the next kinetic stimulus is coming from, but most technicians do not feel this is a good idea. Using the near add may clear the fixation target, but cannot be used to plot the outer isopter. The fixation point needs be enlarged only for low-vision patients. Fixation in a visually and mentally capable patient is a matter of willpower.

54. Matching:

fixation loss	c), g), j)
false-positive	a), d)
false-negative	b), f)
fluctuation	e), h), i)

55. b) If the patient seems to be fixating, yet the instrument is registering fixation losses, have the program relocate the blind spot or reduce the fixation stimulus. If the blind spot is not placed accurately, the patient will respond when the light is flashed in that area. Reducing the intensity of the stimulus may help, as well.

56. d) The presence of a scotoma anywhere in the field would not affect the instrument's ability to find the blind spot. The other three situations would. Even technicians experienced in doing fields occasionally forget to patch the untested eye. If the patch is on and the instrument cannot locate the blind spot, you should double-check the patch placement: it could have slipped enough to let the patient "peek." If the patient is looking around and not fixating, he or she may respond to every stimulus, and the machine will be unable to find the blind spot. Alternately, if you accidentally tell the perimeter to check the right eye and then patch the right as if testing the left, the blind spot will be on the opposite side from what the instrument expects, and the perimeter will be unable to find it.

57. a) Most automated perimeters present the target for somewhere between 0.1 and 0.4 seconds.

58. a) Some perimeters will automatically change the presentation rate to accommodate a "slower" patient. Alternately, the time interval can be increased by manually changing the testing speed.

59. b) Threshold refers to a response to a given stimulus, at a given location, 50% of the time.

60. c) Stereopsis is a binocular phenomenon. Visual field testing is monocular. The intensity of the background and stimulus affects threshold, in that a dimmer background increases contrast and a brighter stimulus is easier to see. Threshold decreases with age and with distance from the fovea.

61. a) A suprathreshold stimulus is not seen 100% of the time, but rather is considered to be seen only 95% of the time. It is extrapolated that suprathreshold could be missed 5% of the time, in part by chance alone.

62. b) Because of poor vision, many low-vision patients have difficulty seeing the fixation area and maintaining fixation on it. Many automated perimeters have an alternate fixation area made up of several lights instead of just one that may be used in low-vision testing situations.

63. a) Most automated perimeters have an alternate fixation pattern that can be used for low-vision patients. This pattern is offset from normal fixation, so you may hear it called an eccentric fixation pattern. If the eccentric fixation pattern is activated, the instrument automatically adjusts the blind spot and other points to coincide. Turning off the fixation monitor will not help the patient see the fixation point any better, nor will using a larger target. The correcting lens must be calculated for each patient; a +3.00 lens used across the board is unacceptable.

64.   b) Normal for a screening test does not necessarily mean that there is no field loss. It means that there is no field loss detected at this time by this particular instrument and this particular testing strategy. Screening programs can miss shallow defects that indicate the early stages of disease. The need for future formal visual field tests depends on the patient's diagnosis and complaints. Screening tests are not adequate in glaucoma evaluation. Diagnosis of glaucoma requires elevated pressures, nerve damage, and consideration of central corneal thickness, in addition to field loss.

65.   b) One of the beauties of automated perimetry is that it is largely independent of operator bias and expertise.

66.   d) The numbers represent retinal sensitivity. A zero means that the brightest stimulus on the unit was shown and not seen. Lower numbers indicate that the target had to be made brighter before it was seen and are more commonly elicited in the periphery. The higher numbers around the fovea represent dimmer lights and greater retinal sensitivity.

67.   c) A point that is not seen would appear as a black area on the gray-scale printout.

68.   c) The comparison printout is designed to compare a patient's previous test to the present test.

69.   c) Routine visual field testing is standard of care for the patient with glaucoma. Many clinicians will alternate visual field testing and retinal scanning every 6 months. While the other disorders will exhibit visual field changes, they are not monitored on a routine basis like glaucoma.

70.   a) Before agreeing to pay for a blepharoplasty, most insurance companies will want a visual field test. This is performed twice: once with the lids in their relaxed, drooped position (possibly showing a loss of the upper visual field) and another with the upper lids taped up, out of the way (simulating how much upper field would be restored if the surgery was done). Correction of a field loss moves the surgery from cosmetic to functional.

71.   a) A high hyperope will exhibit a compressed field with a blind spot displaced closer to fixation than normal. This happens because the prismatic effect of a plus-diopter lens changes the image location.

72.   b) By contrast, a high myope will have an expanded field with a blind spot further away from fixation than normal. This happens because the prismatic effect of a minus-diopter lens changes the image location (in an opposite manner to the plus-diopter lens, as in answer 71).

Appendix A

Study and Test-Taking Strategies

Ledford, JK.
*Certified Ophthalmic Assistant: Exam
Review Manual, Third Edition* (pp. 319-328).
© 2012 Taylor & Francis Group.

It seems that humankind is always looking for purpose in everything we do. We like having goals. Having a goal for your studying will give you purpose and motivation to keep going and to improve. Your short-term goal may be to complete the reading for a given study session or to review specific material. Your long-term goal is to pass that test! This section is designed to help you study, review, and manage stress.

Hitting the Books

Reading Savvy

It may be your tendency to zip through everything you read. In and of itself, fast reading is not necessarily poor reading. The key in study-reading is to comprehend what you read, regardless of your reading speed. Here are several suggestions to help you increase your reading speed and comprehension:

1. Before you start, know *why* you are reading. In our case, we are seeking to learn and understand new material. We are looking for information.
2. Glance over the headings and subheadings to get a quick grasp of the main ideas before you start to read (more on this later).
3. When reading the material for the first time, take it slow and easy.
4. Look up any words you do not know. Increasing your vocabulary will increase your cumulative reading speed.

There are several bad habits that will slow down your reading. You will need to eliminate them. Here are the biggest offenders and what to do about them:

1. Using your finger or a pencil to track along as you read. If you have trouble keeping your place, use a ruler or a straightedge under the line you are reading.
2. Moving your whole head as you read across the page. Instead, you should move your eyes across the page, keeping your head still.
3. Moving your lips as you read. (To find out if you do this, hold a pencil between your lips while reading. Do not bite or grip it with your teeth, just hold it gently between your lips. If the pencil waggles and falls out as you read, you are afflicted!) The remedy is to put the pencil between your lips every time you read for a week or so. Concentrate on holding the pencil still. You should eventually be able to retrain yourself and kick the habit.
4. Reading each and every word independently. Train yourself to read groups of words instead.

Good reading habits can be learned. With practice (and you will be getting plenty of that!), your reading skills will gradually improve. If you have a serious reading deficit, you should consider professional counseling.

Study Strategy

Like reading, good study habits can be learned and developed over time. If you have an interest in the topic, it is easier to study. Your study will be focused and purposeful. In the exam/certification game, your study habits can make or break you.

With a little bit of preplanning, your study time will become second nature. To avoid hit-and-miss studying, you need to plan your work and then work your plan, as the saying goes.

First, choose a place where you will study. I know you have heard this before, but here it is again: Study in the same place every session. The ideal study conditions include the following:

1.   Ample desk room—a good writing surface with enough space to spread out. If you can create a place for yourself that is off-limits to anyone else, that would be best. Then, you can leave your materials there and will not have to regather everything each session.
2.   Good lighting.
3.   Comfortable temperature. It will be hard to study huddled over a space heater in the basement!
4.   A sturdy, comfortable chair. (But not too comfortable.)
5.   No distractions, or at least minimal distractions. We usually think of distractions as noise. But there may be visual distractions as well. It is even been suggested that you remove your family's picture from your desk! Certainly, studying in front of a window would be distracting. We will talk about minimizing family interruptions later.

There is one other type of distraction, and it is the toughest one to eliminate: drifting brain syndrome. These are internal distractions—thoughts that pop into your head unbidden as you try to study. You may be worried about paying the rent or your daughter's football game (she is the quarterback!). The dog may have fleas, and the 2-year-old may have temper tantrums. But try to put these things aside as much as possible when you come to your study time. All of your problems will still be there when you have finished your assignment.

Once you have carved out your study niche, the next item on the agenda is *when* you are going to study. You need to be a good time manager because you are probably adding studying to an already crowded schedule of obligations. Trying to fit your studying between or after other activities can lead to problems.

To help decide what time is best for you, consider what part of the day you are at your best. Try to schedule at least some of your studying during that time. For "morning people," that means studying early in the morning, before the day really starts. If mornings make you queasy, study at night after the kids are in bed. Either the early morning or late night time slot will eliminate, or at least minimize, those family distractions we were looking at earlier.

So, set a definite time you will study, and commit yourself to it. Set your highest priorities, and put them on your calendar. For now, studying for your exam will have to be one of those high priorities. Add other less important things around your study schedule as you are able. To help carve out your study time, try to become more efficient in your other tasks. Check out books that will teach you how to save time doing things. Your family will not cave in if you do not squeeze your own orange juice or fix your own car. This need to study is temporary, anyway. Teach the kids how to make peanut butter and pickle sandwiches (and, ask them to make you one, too, while they are at it!)

How long should you study each day? That depends in part on how much time you have before the date of your exam. But you should understand that the shorter the study time, the sooner you will forget what you have learned. In fact, you may not learn much at all, having stored the information in your short-term memory. Most of it will pop back out after the test. As you plan your study time, remember that, to be efficient and avoid fatigue, you should give yourself a 10-minute break after every 45 minutes or so of intense study. This break time must be included as a vital part of your study schedule.

Organizing a Study Schedule

Having a schedule for study has several advantages:

1. It puts you in control. You are never biting your pencil wondering what to do next.
2. It decreases anxiety. You are not overwhelmed by all those areas on the criteria list because you know that each item is going to be covered.
3. You will work efficiently. You will know you have a certain number of pages to cover. You will not spend time flipping through your book trying to decide what to read next.

Creating a study schedule for yourself is a matter of listing what you need to accomplish, then fitting that into the amount of time you have. Giving yourself 6 months to get ready for the exam should be plenty of time to proceed at a relaxed but steady pace. Of course, everyone is different, and each person's situation is unique. Here is a sample 6-month plan. You will need to accomplish the work listed regardless of the time you have available, so this should be helpful whether you have 6 months or (heaven forbid!) 6 weeks. The test can be taken at any time (although you must register beforehand), but to make things easy, suppose you plan to take the test in July.

- January—Obtain the criteria booklet and an application. Review the requirements, and obtain the necessary paperwork (proof of home study course, etc). Assemble study texts, and use indices and tables of content to find information appropriate to content areas. Make a list of the topics and corresponding books and page numbers. (Do not waste time with material that is not on the test!) Decide when you will study (days and times), and divide the material accordingly. Allow several weeks before the test for review.
- February to March—Begin your study schedule.
- April—Continue your study plan. Submit your application to JCAHPO® (this usually takes approximately 4 to 6 weeks to process.)
- May—Finish study plan. JCAHPO® will have sent an eligibility notice within 4 to 6 weeks of receiving your application, so you should hear from them this month. If accepted, you now have 90 days to take the exam. Go ahead and schedule your exam appointment with the test center. (JCAHPO® does *not* do this for you!) Make arrangements for travel and accommodations, if necessary.
- June—Review. Incorporate a diet and rest plan.
- July—Final days of review.

Square *What?*

Okay. So you have chosen a time and a place. You formulated a study schedule, which gives you a goal for each study period. Your textbook is on your desk, and you are ready to get to work. What is next?

Next is a nifty little method of study-reading called the SQ3R[1] method. The letters and number are a mnemonic for the five general steps for good study-reading. SQ3R stands for survey, question, read, recite, and review. Here is how you use it:

1. Survey. Before reading, leaf through the pages you will be covering that study period. Skim the headings and subheadings, pictures, and captions for an overview. As you glance over the material, you will probably recognize some of it. This scanning process will give direction to your reading and aid in your concentration.

[1]Carmen RA, Adams WR. *Study Skills: A Student's Guide for Survival.* New York, NY: John Wiley & Sons; 1972.

2. Question. From your survey, formulate some mental questions about what you are going to read. What do you expect to learn? Turn the headings into questions. For example, suppose you notice the subheading "Control Centers for Eye Movements." You could ask yourself: "What are these control centers? How do they affect eye movement? What types of eye movements are there?" Also ask yourself, "What do I already know about this topic?" These questions will help you concentrate as you look for the answers. If you have trouble doing this, you may want to actually write down your questions for several sessions just to get the hang of it. After that, you can just keep them in your head.

3. The 3 Rs.

    a. The first R refers to the actual reading. As you read, you will be checking for three items. First, you will be looking for the answers to the questions you have just formulated during the questions stage. Second, you will be paying attention to those "little extras"—captions, graphs, illustrations, and so forth. Third, you will be alert to words and phrases that are boldface, italicized, or underlined. Look up any words you do not know. Do not panic if you did not seem to catch on after reading the material for the first time. Do not freeze up! Relax. Read it again. Try to lay your problems aside. Focus on your reading.

    b. The second R stands for recite. After you have read a short portion of your assignment, stop and summarize it. Condense the material into key words and phrases that will jog your brain to remember what you just read. There are several ways to do this. First, recite orally. This gives you extra stimulation by involving your hearing, not just your vision. A second method of recitation is to go back over the material quickly and underline or mark important parts of the text. Underline only key words or phrases, not entire sections. Later, when you glance over the material and see the words you highlighted, you will remember what you read about. A third way to recite is to make notes after you read, jotting down key words and main ideas. Summarize the material in your own words. You could even make these notes on index cards, creating valuable flash cards for later study.

    c. The last R of SQ3R stands for review. After you have read the entire assignment, stopping several times to recite, you should go back over all the material one more time. Look over the headings again, thinking over what each section was about. Let the marked words and phrases jog your memory.

Each day when you sit down to study, it is important to crank up and get going; do not dawdle or daydream. Take a break after 45 minutes or so of straight reading. Reward your brain and body with a nice long stretch. Your eyes need a break, too. But instead of closing them, gaze at something far off in the distance for a minute or so. This will relax the ciliary muscle and help prevent accommodative spasms.

Be sure to reward yourself in some way when you have finished. Watch TV or take a bubble bath. (But, be cautious about rewarding yourself with food! If you do that, you will probably find that you have gained a bit of weight by exam time. Then, the self-discipline you have been using to study will have to be applied to dieting. Yuck!) So if you want to reward yourself with a snack, stick to fruit and carrot sticks. You will be doing yourself a favor!

How to Prepare for the Test

Managing Pretest Stress[2]

Things might have been pretty relaxed when all you had to do was read. Now that test time is close, the heat is on, and you may be feeling the pressure. Actually, a moderate amount of stress is good for you. Not enough stress, and you may be too carefree. Too much stress, and you may freeze. So, let us take an honest look at the situation.

What is at stake? This is not a do-or-die risk we are talking about. You can retake the test if you need to. Regardless of the results, you will come out alive.

Uncontrolled stress is not productive. Focused stress can help you think more clearly and sharpen your perception. Later, we will talk about what to do if you panic during the test. But for now, you need to relax so you can review productively. There are several ways you can prepare yourself for the exam and control your stress.

1. Academic preparation. Study! The other three are useless without this one. We will talk about reviewing in a minute. If you have taken the test before, take extra time to strengthen weak areas.

2. Psychological preparation. Think positive! Build yourself up. Remind yourself of the benefits of passing. I was studying for my COMT® exam during the Summer Olympics. I got a lot of encouragement from watching the competition. I knew I would never compete in an Olympics, but I had my own important job to do. I was reaching for my own gold. The athletes did not give up, no matter what; I would not either. By the same token, do not compare yourself with others. Look at the test as an opportunity rather than an adversary.

   a. Avoid self-pity by planning to reward yourself in some way when the test is over.

   b. It might seem odd to mention this as part of your psychological readiness, but avoid smoking or chewing gum when you study. You will not be allowed to do either during the exam, and that might throw you off.

   c. Get some information about the test itself. Knowing what to expect reduces stress. How many questions are there? What topics are covered? What type of questions might be asked? How long do you have to take the test? Do you need to take pencils and paper? All these are answered for you in the criteria booklet. Also, talk to friends who have taken the test.

   d. Visit JCAHPO®'s website (www.jcahpo.org) for a practice test.

   e. If possible, visit the test site ahead of time. Then the place will be familiar.

   f. If you have a history of panic during tests, consider getting counseling ahead of time. Also, there are some things you can do to handle panic—we will cover them later.

3. Physical preparation. Proper food and rest is important all the time, not just the night before the test. In the weeks before the exam, reduce sugars and increase protein and vitamins.

4. Logistical preparation. Make early plans on how to get to the test site, and have a backup plan ready. Be sure to take your admission card and ID. Do not forget your watch and any materials you may require.

[2]Elifson JM, Gordon B. *Strategies for Passing the Georgia Regents' Exam.* Raleigh, NC: Contemporary Publishing Co. of Raleigh; 1982.

Review Techniques

Study Material

Now that your reading is completed, you are armed with some formidable study aids. From the "question" part of SQ3R, you have study questions. From the "recite" portion of SQ3R, you have a highlighted text, written notes, and flash cards. Dig out your old home study course test. (Make sure the answers are correct!) Some books have questions at the end of the chapter. Of course, you will plan on spending time daily with this book. Ask questions at work about anything you do not understand. Talk to others who have taken the test and pick their brains for what they remember. You might want to make a new schedule to allot specific review times for specific material.

The test includes diagrams (you match the letter on the picture to the correct answer) and single best answer questions (a statement or questions followed by four possible answers, one of which is best, ie, multiple choice). Both of these types of questions call for recognition more than recall. If your study methods include asking yourself the tougher type of fill-in-the-blank and short answer questions, you will be even better prepared for the actual exam.

Another study aid you might consider is a formal COA® review class. These are offered by various individuals and groups across the country, often over a weekend. There are many advantages to such a course. First, you get the benefit of being taught by someone who has already taken and passed the exam. Second, you have a chance to rub shoulders with others who, like you, are determined to pass. Finally, you will come home with handouts and other valuable material to study. The class should also help you identify your areas of strength and weakness.

Instead of a review course, you might attend a seminar or similar meeting that allows you to choose the courses you want. Select classes that fall into the content areas. Contact JCAHPO® for a list of review classes and seminars near you.

The Review Session

Successful review starts long before a mere 4 weeks prior to your exam. It is a fact of life: You have to study the material before you can review it! But since you made and followed a reading schedule months ago, you are ready to review. Way to go!

When reviewing, start with the material you feel least confident about, then move to the easier topics. Do not worry yourself over what they "might" ask. Concentrate on what they are most likely to ask.

Go back through your reading material, skimming what you marked. The next time you go through it, skip over what you know. Then grab a friend and recite, going over the material verbally. If you did not make flash cards when you originally read the material, do so now. This will help you with memorization (covered in the next section).

How to Memorize[3]

Memorization is a key factor in exam preparation. Here are some suggestions:

1. Repetition—practice! This is another reason why flash cards are so great. You can pull them out of your pocket while you are in line at the grocery store and get in 5 minutes of study. Going over the material again and again really gets it into your conscious and subconscious brain.

2. Association—associate new information with something you already know. Mnemonics are merely intended to assist the memory. Do you remember Roy G. Biv? That silly name is the mnemonic used to memorize the colors in the spectrum. Each letter of the name stands for one of the hues. (Cannot remember them? Go look it up!) You can make up mnemonics for yourself. Here is one of my favorites: The edges of a minus lens bow inward, giving the lens the appearance of being caved in. That is how I remember that it is a concave lens.

3. Stimulation—of as many senses as possible. Making your own note and flash cards serves several purposes. Your sight is stimulated by reading, touch by writing, and hearing when you recite aloud.

Fifteen to 20 minutes at a time of intense memorization is enough. Committing material to memory is more intense than reading, so give yourself more frequent breaks.

Study Groups

Study groups can be a great way to review the material for your exam. Besides having someone to study with, group study can help you manage stress simply by knowing that you are not alone. There are others who are going through the rigors of test preparation! Ideally, find someone who has already taken and passed the exam to function as group leader. If there is no one available to be your guide, you could take turns at being the facilitator. One person might be especially good at a particular task or subject and could conduct that review.

Use the same strategies in a group that you have for your own private study. Set a specific time and place, and be sure to schedule breaks. This is a review, so everyone should have a good understanding of the material already. Try to stay on target, but do not forget that laughter is a great stress-reliever. Listen and learn from each other. Someone else may have a fresh perspective that will "turn the lights on" for some topic you may have been struggling with. Or, they may have a mnemonic or some other way of remembering that will help you. Be sure to share your discoveries, too. Use the same review materials in the group as you would alone. Another idea is to ask each group member to write several multiple choice questions to share. Perhaps each person could do a different content area.

Remember SQ3R? Use R#2 (recite) as a study aid. Have a partner scan your reading material and ask you to do the following:

1. Explain the chapter title, headings, and subheadings.
2. Define bold or italicized words and phrases.
3. Answer questions based on the pictures and tables.
4. Answer questions from the end of the chapter, this book, or old home-study tests.

[3]Lass A, Wilson E. *The College Student's Handbook.* New York, NY: David White; 1965.

There are several cautions about study groups, however. If anyone in the group tends to panic or be anxious, they can affect the whole group. If encouragement doesn't help, you might have to ask them to refrain from making negative comments. If you are beginning to get upset yourself, it might be better to study alone.

Close Encounters of the Examination Kind

Test Day

Actually, let us look at Test Day minus one. The day before your exam needs to be as laid-back as possible. Eat well, and get plenty of rest. Plan what you will wear tomorrow (something comfortable!) so you will not be scrambling around in the morning. If you must travel to the test site and spend the night before, allow plenty of time to get there. If possible, drive by the test center so you know where it is. Ideally, go in, and look at the room itself. This will help you psychologically. Review your notes for about an hour before going to bed. Refuse to upset yourself by thinking about all that you do not know.

Now, the alarm rings, and it is test day. Get up early enough so you are not rushed. Eat a good breakfast that includes protein, but avoid eating anything too heavy in the 2 hours just prior to test time. Remember your admission card, ID, and wristwatch. Scratch paper and a pencil will be provided for you. Arrive early. Choose a distraction-free seat. It is probably best not to talk to others about the test beforehand. Try to relax. Focus on being calm and self-confident.

How To Take a Test

Listen to the proctor. Read instructions carefully. Be sure to enter your name and number correctly. Ask for any computer help that you need; the staff will be glad to help you.

In the COA® exam, you have 3 hours to answer about 200 questions (an additional 30 minutes is *added* to look over the exam tutorial). That is about 1 minute per question. Use this information to pace yourself. When your time is half over, if you haven't worked to the halfway point, go there anyway.

Read the entire question before looking at the answers. Think of an answer before you read the choices. Read each choice before selecting an answer.

A multiple choice question is actually a group of true/false questions. Try out each answer. Does it make the statement true or false? One answer will be "truer" than all the rest. Answer the easy questions, then go back to those you are not sure of or have to figure out. You might jot a note or two regarding a tougher question to help you when you come back. When you have been through the test once and are going back to answer the harder questions, continue to pace yourself. If you feel the need to spend more time on a question, move on again and come back later. Your subconscious will be looking through your brain's files for the answer while you continue on. When you come back to a question, it may have "soaked" long enough, and the answer will come right to you. Multiple choice questions often contain one answer that is obviously wrong, one or two answers that appear reasonable, and one or two correct answers. (If there are two, one is more correct than the other.) If the answer to a question is not obvious to you, eliminate any answers that you are sure are wrong. Then, try to pick the best answer from those that are left.

If the question involves math, read the problem carefully. What do they want to know (lens power, cylinder axis, minus cylinder)? Estimate the answer before you start the actual calculations.

Every now and then, one question will contain the answer or hints to another. Lucky you! But do not waste too much time looking back through trying to find something.

Do your best to concentrate on one question at a time.

Beware of the following words: none, most, never, always, must, only, all, some, usually, sometimes, every, many, few, often, seldom, more, equal, less, best, good, bad, worst, exactly, and may. If used in the question, be sure to read very carefully.

If you finish before time is up, go back over the test to those questions you were not sure about.

Managing Panic

If you panic, stop (before you freeze). Take a brief break. Close your eyes. Talk to yourself. Remember all you did to prepare for the exam. Then breathe! Inhale for 3 seconds, hold it for 12, then exhale for 6 seconds. This helps even out your blood gas level and puts you in control. Remind yourself that you know what to do—you have a plan. Refocus on the task at hand. Concentrate on one question at a time, not on the whole test. Imagine yourself in a familiar setting, at work on a task that you know you can perform. Hold that thought, then get back to work.

A Final Word

All of the certification exams are now computerized, but do not let that stop you. Access and move around on the JCAHPO® Web site. Most important, take the practice test on the site, and relax a little. The computer allows you to mark a question and come back to it later, as well as change an answer. No more worrying whether or not you filled in the circle completely, or got off on your numbering. Hooray! Plus, you get an immediate pass/fail notice, although it is not official until you hear from JCAHPO® 2 to 4 weeks later. But you have prepared well. Go out there and shine!

Appendix B

Suggested Reading and Resources

Ledford, JK.
*Certified Ophthalmic Assistant: Exam
Review Manual, Third Edition* (pp. 329-332).
© 2012 Taylor & Francis Group.

American Academy of Ophthalmology. Ophthalmic Medical Assisting: An Independent Study Course.

Association of Technical Personnel in Ophthalmology (ATPO). COA® Certification Review Flashcards. Joint Commission on Allied Health Personnel in Ophthalmology, 2025 Woodlane Dr., St. Paul, MN 55125.

Bittinger M. *General Medical Knowledge for Eyecare Paraprofessionals*. Thorofare, NJ: SLACK Incorporated.

Boess-Lott R, Stecik S. *The Ophthalmic Surgical Assistant*. Thorofare, NJ: SLACK Incorporated.

Burlew-Quartey JA. *Disinfection of equipment in the ophthalmology clinic*. Available at: http://webeye.ophth.uiowa.edu/asorn/AM2008/Handouts/105.pdf. (Good slide show on disinfection of various pieces of ophthalmic equipment from trial frames to probe tips.)

Cassin B, ed. *Fundamentals for ophthalmic technical personnel*. Philadelphia, PA: Saunders; 1995.

Cassin B, Rubin ML. *Dictionary of Eye Terminology*. 5th ed. Triad Communications, 2006.

Choplin N, Edwards R. *Field Testing With the Humphrey Field Analyzer*. Thorofare, NJ: SLACK Incorporated.

Choplin N, Edwards R. *Visual Fields*. Thorofare, NJ: SLACK Incorporated.

Cunningham D. *Clinical Ocular Photography*. Thorofare, NJ: SLACK Incorporated.

DuBois L. *Clinical Skills for the Ophthalmic Examination: Basic Procedures*. 2nd ed. Thorofare, NJ: SLACK Incorporated.

Duvall B, Kershner RM. *Ophthalmic Medications and Pharmacology*. 2nd ed. Thorofare, NJ: SLACK Incorporated.

Gayton JL, Kershner RM. *Refractive Surgery for Eyecare Paraprofessionals*. Thorofare, NJ: SLACK Incorporated.

Gayton JL, Ledford JR. *The Crystal Clear Guide to Sight for Life*. Lancaster, PA: Starburst; 1996.

Gwin N. *Overview of Ocular Disorders*. Thorofare, NJ: SLACK Incorporated.

Hands-Only CPR. www.handsonlycpr.org/.

Hansen VC. *A Systematic Approach to Strabismus*. 2nd ed. Thorofare, NJ: SLACK Incorporated.

Hargis-Greenshields L, Sims L. *Emergencies in Eyecare*. Thorofare, NJ: SLACK Incorporated.

Herrin M. *Instrumentation for Eyecare Paraprofessionals*. Thorofare, NJ: SLACK Incorporated.

Identify the ocular side effects of systemic medications. Review of Optometry Online. Available at: http://cms.revoptom.com/index.asp?ArticleType=SiteSpec&page=osc/105682/lesson.htm. Excellent (though slightly dated) article on ocular side effects of systemic drugs.

Infection Prevention Online Courses. Available at: www.engenderhealth.org/ip/index.html. Offers various courses regarding hand hygiene, aseptic technique, sterile technique, etc. Really good!

IOLMaster video. (Free registration required.) Available at: www.meditec.zeiss.com/C1256CAB00599F5D?Open

Joint Commission on Allied Health Personnel in Ophthalmology. Learning Systems Interactive Software Courses 1-6 (Keratometry, Lensometry, Tonometry, Ocular Motility, Retinoscopy/Refinement & Visual Fields). JCAHPO®: 2025 Woodlane Dr., St. Paul, MN 55125.

Joint Commission on Allied Health Personnel in Ophthalmology. Preparing for the certified ophthalmic assistant exam: A study guide. JCAHPO®: 2025 Woodlane Dr., St. Paul, MN 55125.

Kershner R, Duvall B. *Ophthalmic Medications and Pharmacology*, 2nd ed. Thorofare, NJ: SLACK Incorporated.

LASIK vs LASEK Comparison Chart. Available at www.the-lasik-directory.com/lasik_lasek_chart.html.

Ledford JK, Hoffman J. *Quick Reference Dictionary of Eyecare Terminology*. 5th Edition. Thorofare, NJ: SLACK Incorporated.

Ledford JK, Sanders V. *The Slit Lamp Primer*. 2nd ed. Thorofare, NJ: SLACK Incorporated.

Ledford JK. *Handbook of Clinical Ophthalmology for Eyecare Professionals*. Thorofare, NJ: SLACK Incorporated.

Ledford JK. *The Complete Guide to Ocular History Taking*. Thorofare, NJ: SLACK Incorporated.

Ledford JK. *The Little Eye Book: A Pupil's Guide to Understanding Ophthalmology*. 2nd ed. Thorofare, NJ: SLACK Incorporated.

Lens A. *Optics, retinoscopy, and refractometry*. 2nd ed. Thorofare, NJ: SLACK Incorporated.

Lens A, Nemeth SC, Ledford JK. *Ocular Anatomy and Physiology*. 2nd ed. Thorofare, NJ: SLACK Incorporated.

Lens A, Werner E, Duvall B. *Cataract and Glaucoma for Eyecare Paraprofessionals*. Thorofare, NJ: SLACK Incorporated.

Medical Terminology. Available at: www.globalrph.com/medterm.html.

Ophthalmic Equipment Terminology chart. Available at: http://bsmconnectionasc.com/Resources/Glossary/GlossaryOfTermsOphthalmicEquipmentTerminology.pdf.

Pickett K. *Overview of Ocular Surgery and Surgical Counseling*. Thorofare, NJ: SLACK Incorporated.

Riordan-Eva P, Cunningham E, eds. *Vaughn & Asbury's General Ophthalmology*. 18th ed. New York, NY: Lange Medical Books/McGraw-Hill; 2011.

Schuman JS, Puliafito CA, Fujimoto JG, eds. *Everyday OCT: A Handbook for Clinicians and Technicians*. Thorofare, NJ: SLACK Incorporated.

Schwartz GS. *The Eye Exam: A Complete Guide*. Thorofare, NJ: SLACK, Incorporated.

Stein HA, Stein RM, Freeman MI. *The Ophthalmic Assistant: A Text for Allied and Associated Ophthalmic Personnel*. 8th ed. Philadelphia, PA: Elsevier Mosby; 2006.

Bibliography

Ledford, JK.
*Certified Ophthalmic Assistant: Exam
Review Manual, Third Edition* (pp. 333-336).
© 2012 Taylor & Francis Group.

About Scribes. Available at: www.scribemd.com/PDF/ScribeMD_outline.pdf. Accessed 3/9/11.

AllAlliedHealthSchools. Surgical Assistant vs. Surgical Tech. Available at: www.allalliedhealthschools. com/faqs/surgical-assistant.php. Accessed 3/9/11.

Ambrosio R Jr, Wilson S. LASIK vs LASEK vs PRK: Advantages and indications. Available at: www.ncbi. nlm.nih.gov/pubmed/12759854. Accessed 11/24/10.

American Academy of Professional Coders. Medical Coding. Available at: www.aapc.com/medicalcoding-glossary/MEDICAL_CODING.aspx. Accessed 3/4/11.

American Health Information Management Association. Medical Coding. Available at: www.ahima.org/coding. Accessed 11/25/10.

American Health Information Management Association. Coding Classification Systems. Available at: www. ahima.org/coding/standards.aspx. Accessed 11/25/10.

American Heart Association. Hands-only CPR. Available at: www.handsonlycpr.org. Accessed 6/14/11.

American Heart Association. New CPR guidelines from the American Heart Association. Available at: www. americanmedical-id.com/blogs/new-cpr-guidelines-from-the-american-heart-association. Accessed 6/14/11.

American Optometric Association. Intraoperative floppy iris syndrome (IFIS) associated with systemic alpha-1 blockers. Available at: www.aoa.org/x10462.xml. Accessed 1/9/11.

Aseptic Technique. Available at: www.surgeryencyclopedia.com/A-Ce/Aseptic-Technique.html. Accessed 11/25/10.

Backer LA. Strategies for better patient flow and cycle time. Available at: www.aafp.org/fpm/2002/0600/p45.html. Accessed 10/16/10.

Barnabas Health Behavioral Health Network. The extra mile: quality assurance & outcome measurements. Available at: www.barnabashealth.org/hospitals/psychiatric/outpatient/index.htm. Accessed 7/18/11.

Berry M. Help is on the way for: tests. Chicago, IL: Childrens' Press; 1985.

Brouhard R. How to do CPR on a child. Available at: http://firstaid.about.com/od/cpr/ht/08_Child_CPR. htm. Accessed 6/14/11.

Brouhard R. How to do infant CPR. Available at: http://firstaid.about.com/od/cpr/ht/08_Infant_CPR.htm. Accessed 6/14/11.

Brouhard R. How to perform adult CPR. Available at: http://firstaid.about.com/od/cpr/ht/06_cpr.htm. Accessed 6/14/11.

Compliance Assistance Quick Start: Health Care Industry. Available at: www.osha.gov/dcsp/compliance_assistance/quickstarts/health_care/index_hc.html. Accessed 10/13/10.

Doctor's Initial Report State of New York—Workers' Compensation Board. Available at: www.wcb.state. ny.us/content/main/forms/c4.pdf. Accessed 10/13/10.

DuBois L. *Clinical Skills for the Ophthalmic Examination: Basic Procedures.* 2nd ed. Thorofare, NJ: SLACK Incorporated; 2005.

Duvall B, Kershner R. *Ophthalmic Medications and Pharmacology.* 2nd ed. Thorofare, NJ: SLACK Incorporated; 2006.

Federal Trade Commission. 16 CFR Part 456 [RIN 3084–AA80] Ophthalmic Practice Rules. Available at: www.ftc.gov/os/2004/01/040130ophthalmicpracticesfrn.pdf. Accessed 7/26/11.

Flynn HW, Scott IU. Intravitreal injections: controversies, guidelines. Available at: www.revophth.com/index.asp?page=1_654.htm. Accessed 11/24/10.

Frazier L, Whitaker N. Ischemic optic neuropathy and amiodarone: a case report and review. *Clinical & Refractive Optometry.* 2006;17:7, 258-261. Available at: www.ce4optometry.com/mediconcept/17.7Whitaker.pdf. Accessed 1/9/11.

GDx VCC brochure. Available at: www.zeiss.com/88256DE3007B916B/0/827FB176E93010BE882576AA 006D2F63/$file/gdxvcc_brochure_gdx_294.pdf. Accessed 7/11/10.

Glaucoma Research Foundation. Five common glaucoma tests. Available at: www.glaucoma.org/learn/diagnostic_test.php. Accessed 12/7/10.

Hauswirth K, Sherk SD. Aseptic technique. Available at: www.surgeryencyclopedia.com/A-Ce/Aseptic-Technique.html. Accessed 3/18/11.

Hayden BC, Kelley L, Singh AD. Ophthalmic ultrasonography: theoretic and practical considerations. Available at: www.arauto.uminho.pt/pessoas/smcn/MAIO/ultra-som/ultra%20sound%20review%20Hayden%202008.pdf. Accessed 2/5/11.

Heidelberg Engineering GmbH. Quantitative three-dimensional imaging of the posterior segment with the Heidelberg Retina Tomograph. Available at: www.agingeye.net/glaucoma/heidelberg.pdf. Accessed 7/11/10.

Woodcliff Lake Ophthalmology, LLP. HIPAA Compliance. Available at: www.bergeneye.com/hipaa_privacy.htm. Accessed 7/26/11.

Krumpaszky HG, Dannheim R, Klauss V, Selbmann HK. Quality management, possibilities and chances in ophthalmology. Available at: www.ncbi.nlm.nih.gov/pubmed/7655192. Accessed 1/11/11.

LASIK vs LASEK comparison chart. Available at: www.the-lasik-directory.com/lasik_lasek_chart.html. Accessed 11/27/10.

Lenz E, Shaevitz MH. *So you want to go back to school.* New York, NY: McGraw-Hill; 1977.

Leung CK, Chan W, Chong KK, et al. Comparative study of retinal nerve fiber layer measurement by Stratus OCT and GDx VCC, I: correlation analysis in glaucoma. Available at: www.ncbi.nlm.nih.gov/pubmed/16123421. Accessed 7/11/10.

McQuaid KI. The technician's role in intravitreal triamcinolone acetonide injections. Available at: www.atpo.org/TechniciansRoleinIVTA.pdf. Accessed 1/11/11.

Medical Coding: education, career, and resources. Available at: http://medical-coding911.blogspot.com/2010/01/modifiers-usage-cpt-coding.html. Accessed 3/4/11.

Medmont International Pty Ltd. Medmont E333 Corneal Topographer User Manual. Available at: www.medmont.com.au/files/E300.pdf. Accessed 2/5/11.

The MSDS FAQ: Introduction. Available at: www.ilpi.com/msds/faq/parta.html. Accessed 10/13/10.

Northeast Wisconsin Retina Associates. Intraocular injection of medication. Available at: http://newretinamd.com/surgical_procedures/intraocular_injections.php. Accessed 4/9/11.

Ocular diseases could be in your genes. Available at: www.revoptom.com/content/d/web_exclusives/p/16744/c/16751/. Accessed 1/9/11.

Ophthalmic photography. Ophthalmic Photographers' Society. Available at: www.opsweb.org/?page=Ophthalmicphoto. Accessed on 2/5/11.

Premier Emergency Medical Specialists Scribe Program. www.pemsscribes.com/Program_Details.html. Accessed 8/1/10.

Quality Assurance. Available at: http://medical-dictionary.thefreedictionary.com/quality+assurance. Accessed 7/18/11.

Rumpakis JMB. Coding eye exams. *Optom Manag.* Available at: www.optometric.com/article.aspx?article=71233. Accessed 11/6/10.

Schachat AP, Lee PP, Wu W. A quality assurance program for an inpatient department of ophthalmology. Available at: http://archopht.ama-assn.org/cgi/content/summary/107/9/1293?maxtoshow=&hits=10&RESULTFORMAT=&fulltext=quality+assurance&searchid=1&FIRSTINDEX=0&resourcetype=HWCIT. Accessed 1/11/11.

Scott IU. Intravitreal injections: safety guidelines. Available at: http://cms.revophth.com/index.asp?page=1_858.htm. Accessed 1/11/11.

Sliney DH, Mainster MA. Ophthalmic laser safety: tissue interactions, hazards, and protection. *Ophthalmology Clinics of North America.* 1998;11(2):157-164. Available at: www.ophthalmology.theclinics.com/article/PIIS0896154905700419/fulltext. Accessed 07/05/2010.

Srinivasan V, Thulasira RD. Ophthalmic instruments and equipment: a handbook on care and maintenance. 2nd ed. Available at: http://laico.org/v2020resource/files/instruments_book.pdf. Accessed 1/8/11.

Svensson L, Bohm K, Castren M, et al. Compression-only CPR or standard CPR in out-of-hospital cardiac arrest. Available at: www.nejm.org/doi/pdf/10.1056/NEJMoa0908991. Accessed 6/25/11.

Understanding corneal topography. Available at: http://cms.revoptom.com/handbook/oct02_sec3_6.htm. Accessed 1/10/11.

Veterans Health Administration. Documentation Tips for Nurses. VA Training Module. Accessed 7/30/10.

What is medical coding? Available at: www.medicalcodingcertification.com/what-is-medical-coding.html. Accessed 11/6/10.

What is a medical coding specialist? Available at: http://degreedirectory.org/articles/What_is_a_Medical_Coding_Specialist.html. Accessed 11/6/10.

Whitman GJ, Niziak E, Newton SL, Palumbo DS, Sweeney DP, Saini S. Socioeconomics of imaging: quality assurance in outpatient CT. Available at: www.appliedradiology.com/Issues/1997/10/Articles/Socioeconomics-of-Imaging--Quality-assurance-in-outpatient-CT.aspx. Accessed 7/18/11.

Why use scribe services? Available at: www.emscribesystems.com/why-scribe-services. Accessed 8/1/10.

Zangwill LM, Bowd C, Berry CC, et al. Discriminating between normal and glaucomatous eyes using the Heidelberg Retina Tomograph, GDx Nerve Fiber Analyzer, and Optical Coherence Tomograph. Available at: www.ncbi.nlm.nih.gov/pubmed/16123421. Accessed 7/11/10.

Printed in the United States
by Baker & Taylor Publisher Services